COGNITIVE THERAPY
WITH CHILDREN AND ADOLESCENTS

Also from Philip C. Kendall

Child and Adolescent Therapy, Fourth Edition:
Cognitive-Behavioral Procedures
Philip C. Kendall, Editor

Cognitive-Behavioral Therapy
for Impulsive Children, Second Edition
Philip C. Kendall and Lauren Braswell

Cognitive Therapy with Children and Adolescents

A Casebook for Clinical Practice

THIRD EDITION

Edited by

PHILIP C. KENDALL

THE GUILFORD PRESS

New York   London

Copyright © 2018 The Guilford Press
A Division of Guilford Publications, Inc.
370 Seventh Avenue, Suite 1200, New York, NY 10001
www.guilford.com

Printed in the United States of America

This book is printed on acid-free paper.

Last digit is print number: 9 8 7 6 5 4 3 2 1

The authors have checked with sources believed to be reliable in their efforts to provide
information that is complete and generally in accord with the standards of practice that
are accepted at the time of publication. However, in view of the possibility of human error
or changes in behavioral, mental health, or medical sciences, neither the authors, nor
the editor and publisher, nor any other party who has been involved in the preparation
or publication of this work warrants that the information contained herein is in every
respect accurate or complete, and they are not responsible for any errors or omissions or
the results obtained from the use of such information. Readers are encouraged to confirm
the information contained in this book with other sources.

Library of Congress Cataloging-in-Publication Data

Names: Kendall, Philip C., editor.
Title: Cognitive therapy with children and adolescents : a casebook for
   clinical practice / edited by Philip C. Kendall.
Description: Third edition. | New York : The Guilford Press, [2018] |
   Includes bibliographical references and index.
Identifiers: LCCN 2017028508 | ISBN 9781462528233 (paperback) |
   ISBN 9781462532162 (hardcover)
Subjects: LCSH: Cognitive therapy for children. | Cognitive therapy for
   teenagers. | Cognitive therapy for children—Case studies. | Cognitive
   therapy for teenagers—Case studies. | BISAC: PSYCHOLOGY / Psychotherapy /
   Child & Adolescent. | MEDICAL / Psychiatry / Child & Adolescent. | SOCIAL
   SCIENCE / Social Work.
Classification: LCC RJ505.C63 C65 2018 | DDC 618.92/891425—dc23
LC record available at https://lccn.loc.gov/2017028508

About the Editor

Philip C. Kendall, PhD, ABPP, is Distinguished University Professor and Carnell Professor of Psychology at Temple University, where he is also Director of the Child and Adolescent Anxiety Disorders Clinic. Dr. Kendall has been a researcher, scholar, and clinician since the 1970s. He has made seminal contributions to the treatment of anxiety disorders in youth; cognitive-behavioral theory, assessment, and treatment; research methodology; and the conceptualization and understanding of the psychopathology and treatment of children and adolescents. With more than 650 research publications and books, Dr. Kendall has been a Fellow at the Center for Advanced Study in the Behavioral Sciences and has received numerous awards, including the Aaron T. Beck Award for Significant and Enduring Contributions to Cognitive Therapy from the Academy of Cognitive Therapy, the Distinguished Scientist Award from the Society for a Science of Clinical Psychology, Distinguished Career Research Awards from the Society of Clinical Child and Adolescent Psychology (Division 53) and the Society of Clinical Psychology (Division 12) of the American Psychological Association, and the inaugural Research Recognition Award from the Anxiety and Depression Association of America.

Contributors

Anne Marie Albano, PhD, ABPP, is Professor of Medical Psychology in Psychiatry, Director of the Clinic for Anxiety and Related Disorders, and Clinical Director of the Youth Anxiety Center at Columbia University Medical Center/New York Presbyterian Hospital. She is engaged in clinical care and research in the area of internalizing conditions of youth, and in the training of emerging professional psychologists and mental health workers.

Arthur D. Anastopoulos, PhD, is Professor of Human Development and Family Studies at the University of North Carolina at Greensboro, where he also directs a specialty attention-deficit/hyperactivity disorder (ADHD) clinic. Throughout his career, he has maintained clinical and research interests in the assessment and treatment of ADHD across the life span, with a current focus on emerging adults with ADHD who attend college.

Kristen Anderson, LCSW, is cofounder of the Chicago Center for Evidence Based Treatment and former Clinical Director of the University of Chicago Eating Disorders Program. Her primary research interest is the treatment of eating disorders across the developmental life span and the use of telemedicine in delivering psychotherapy.

Wayne A. Bowers, PhD, ABPP, is Clinical Professor of Psychiatry at the University of Iowa College of Medicine. He is a Fellow in the Academy of Cognitive Therapy and the Academy for Eating Disorders. His areas of interest include using cognitive therapy to treat eating disorders, treatment of severe and enduring eating disorders, and ethical aspects in the care and treatment of eating disorders.

Allison C. Bray, PhD, is a licensed psychologist in the behavioral medicine division at LeBauer Healthcare/Cone Health System in Greensboro, North Carolina. Her clinical and research interests include the assessment and treatment of ADHD and comorbid depression and anxiety in youth and adults.

Rachel Brookland, MS, is a doctoral student at the Philadelphia College of Osteopathic Medicine. She received her master's degree in mental health counseling from the Philadelphia College of Osteopathic Medicine and is interested in children with generalized anxiety disorder and chronic illnesses.

Simone Budzyn, BA, is a research assistant working with Martin E. Franklin in the Child and Adolescent OCD, Tic, Trich and Anxiety Group (The COTTAGe) at the Perelman School of Medicine at the University of Pennsylvania. Her research and clinical interests are focused on the treatment of anxiety and related issues in sexual- and gender-minority youth.

Matthew K. Burns, PhD, is Associate Dean for Research at the College of Education and Professor of School Psychology at the University of Missouri. He has published over 175 articles and book chapters in national publications, and has coauthored or coedited 12 books. Dr. Burns is a past editor of *School Psychology Review* and *Assessment for Effective Intervention* and is one of the leading researchers in the use of assessment data to determine individual or small-group interventions. He has published extensively on response to intervention, academic interventions, and facilitating problem-solving teams.

Melissa Coolong-Chaffin, PhD, NCSP, is Associate Professor of School Psychology at the University of Wisconsin–Eau Claire, where she is also a reading specialist in the Human Development Center and Codirector of the Academic Intervention Clinic. Her research and teaching interests include developing academic and social–behavioral interventions for struggling students, and training preservice educators in assessment approaches to developing and monitoring interventions.

Kristen M. Culbert, PhD, is Assistant Professor of Psychology at the University of Nevada, Las Vegas. She completed postdoctoral research fellowships in eating disorders at The University of Chicago and Michigan State University. Her research and clinical interests focus on the etiology and treatment of eating disorder symptoms across the life span.

John F. Curry, PhD, ABPP, is Professor of Psychiatry and Behavioral Sciences, and Psychology and Neuroscience at Duke University. He is a Fellow of the American Psychological Association and the Academy of Cognitive Therapy. His research and clinical interests focus on the treatment of adolescent disorders, particularly depression and substance abuse.

Norman B. Epstein, PhD, is Professor of Family Science and Director of the Couple and Family Therapy program in the School of Public Health at the University of Maryland, College Park. He is a pioneer in the development of cognitive-behavioral therapy (CBT) with couples and families. His research, writing, teaching, and training of clinicians have focused on cognitive processes in relationship adjustment and dysfunction, couple and family coping with stress, cross-cultural studies of couple and family relationships, and treatment of aggression in couple relationships.

Hannah E. Frank, MA, is a graduate student at Temple University working with Philip C. Kendall. Her research interests are in the dissemination and implementation of evidence-based treatments for youth with anxiety disorders.

Martin E. Franklin, PhD, is Associate Professor of Clinical Psychology in Psychiatry and Director of the Child and Adolescent OCD, Tic, Trich and Anxiety Group (The COTTAGe) at the Perelman School of Medicine at the University of Pennsylvania. He has developed and maintained clinical research on the psychopathology and treatment response of individuals with anxiety and related conditions across the developmental spectrum. His work has included multisite randomized controlled trials designed to examine the relative and combined efficacy of CBT and pharmacotherapy, augmentation of selective serotonin reuptake inhibitor pharmacotherapy with CBT, and response to CBT in very young children. Dr. Franklin is an expert in clinical trials methodology, development of CBT protocols for efficacy and effectiveness trials, and CBT in the clinical trials context.

Elizabeth A. Gosch, PhD, ABPP, is Professor of Psychology at the Philadelphia College of Osteopathic Medicine and Chief Clinical Supervisor at the Temple University Child and Adolescent Anxiety Clinic. Dr. Gosch is also president-elect of the Clinical Child and Adolescent Board of the American Board of Professional Psychology. Her research focuses on anxiety and emotional regulation in youth.

Lauren Hoffman, PsyD, is a postdoctoral fellow in the Department of Psychiatry, Division of Child and Adolescent Psychiatry, at Columbia University Medical Center. Dr. Hoffman specializes in using CBT to treat anxiety and mood disorders in children, adolescents, and young adults. Her research interests include the interrelated nature of internalizing disorders and bullying, as well as the use of technology in psychological treatments.

Rebecca Kanive, PhD, is an educational consultant and a school psychologist in the Wayzata Public Schools in Hennepin County, Minnesota. Her work focuses on developing and implementing an evidence-based mathematics intervention program in elementary and middle school settings.

Philip C. Kendall, PhD, ABPP. See "About the Editor."

Connor M. Kerns, PhD, is Assistant Research Professor of Psychology and Community Health and Prevention at the A. J. Drexel Autism Institute at Drexel University. Dr. Kerns has received grant funding from the Autism Science Foundation and the National Institutes of Health to research mental health conditions in children with autism spectrum disorder (ASD). She has published extensively on the overlap, assessment, and treatment of anxiety disorders in ASD.

HaeDong Kim, MS, MDiv, is a research assistant and doctoral student in family science at the University of Maryland, College Park. He received his master's degree in couple and family therapy from the University of Maryland and his Master of Divinity from Presbyterian College and Theological Seminary in Seoul, South Korea. His clinical and research interests are focused on racial minority/multicultural families and the long-term influences of racial socialization practices in these families.

Hillary E. Kratz, PhD, is a staff psychologist at the University of Pennsylvania. Her research and clinical interests are in the treatment of pediatric anxiety, obsessive–compulsive disorder, trichotillomania, and tic disorders, and on the assessment and treatment of anxiety among children with autism.

Daniel Le Grange, PhD, is the Benioff UCSF Professor of Children's Health, and Eating Disorders Director in the Department of Psychiatry and UCSF Weill Institute for Neuroscience at the University of California, San Francisco. He has devoted his career to the development and evaluation of psychosocial treatments for adolescents with eating disorders.

Howard A. Liddle, EdD, ABPP, is Professor of Public Health Sciences and Psychology at the University of Miami. The developer of multidimensional family therapy (MDFT), Dr. Liddle has led a treatment research program focusing on youth substance abuse and delinquency for 30 years.

John E. Lochman, PhD, ABPP, is Professor and Doddridge Saxon Chairholder in Clinical Psychology at the University of Alabama, where he also directs the Center for Prevention of Youth Behavior Programs. He also is Adjunct Professor in the Department of Psychiatry and Behavioral Sciences at the Duke University Medical Center. Dr. Lochman has received Lifetime Achievement Awards from the Society of Clinical

Child and Adolescent Psychology (Division 53 of the American Psychological Association) and the American Board of Professional Psychology. His research focuses on risk factors, social cognition, and intervention and prevention in children with aggressive behavior problems.

Rogelio J. Mercado, MA, is a doctoral candidate in clinical psychology at Temple University working with Philip C. Kendall. His research focuses on cognitive factors that underlie the overlap between autism and anxiety. His clinical work has focused on treating anxiety in anxious youth with and without ASD.

Allison E. Meyer, BA, MA, is a graduate student in clinical psychology at Duke University. Her research interests are in the areas of anxiety and mood disorders of youth, with particular focus on the stress-generating effects of internalizing disorders.

Qshequilla P. Mitchell, PhD, MPH, is a research scientist at the Center for the Prevention of Youth Behavior Problems at the University of Alabama. She provides the child and parent components of Coping Power to small groups of early adolescents who display moderate to high levels of aggressive behaviors. Her research focuses on the racial and ethnic mental health disparities among rural youth.

Sarah H. Morris, MA, is a doctoral student in the Department of Psychology at the University of Pennsylvania. She has worked with her advisor, Martin E. Franklin, on a number of scientific articles and chapters in the area of pediatric obsessive–compulsive spectrum disorders. She is currently completing her predoctoral clinical internship at the Warren Alpert Medical School of Brown University.

Sarah R. O'Rourke, PhD, is a medical instructor in the Department of Psychiatry and Behavioral Sciences at Duke University School of Medicine. Her clinical and research interests include evidence-based assessment and treatment of youth with ADHD, anxiety disorders, and chronic health conditions.

Dustin A. Pardini, PhD, is a child clinical psychologist whose research and clinical work has focused on examining the development and prevention of severe delinquency and substance abuse among youth. Dr. Pardini is currently Associate Professor of Criminology and Criminal Justice at Arizona State University. His program of research has resulted in over 100 peer-reviewed publications and book chapters.

Cynthia L. Rowe, PhD, is Research Associate Professor of Public Health Sciences at the University of Miami Miller School of Medicine. Her research focuses on refining, testing, and disseminating family-based interventions for adolescents with substance abuse and related problems. She works with her colleagues to promote the translation of research findings into practice and to train providers to implement MDFT.

Stephen E. Schlesinger, PhD, is a psychologist in private practice in Chicago and Oak Park, Illinois. His publications have focused on cognitive-behavioral treatment of couple and family problems, as well as substance abuse.

Megan Wolensky, MS, is a doctoral candidate in clinical psychology at the Philadelphia College of Osteopathic Medicine, where she is currently completing her internship. She has been a professional speaker on childhood disorders, including ADHD and anxiety.

Preface

Since the publication of the second edition of *Cognitive Therapy with Children and Adolescents: A Casebook for Clinical Practice* in 2003, the field of mental health treatment for youth has seen many significant advances in treatment. New developments from the results of empirically based clinical research have given rise to better interventions, improved programs, and clinically sensitive procedures supported by the empirical research.

One compelling finding has been the identification of the key elements of effective treatments common across target disorders. Interventions that are now woven into many effective programs include problem solving, affective education, changing self-talk, role playing, rewards, and enactive behavioral experiments. We focus in this edition on how these transdiagnostic treatment strategies vary by specific disorders and how they are applied to address a known difficulty associated with each disorder. For example, behavioral experiments may test the "anticipated catastrophe" of a child experiencing anxiety (exposure) or may be implemented to test whether an event produces the desired outcome for teens who need to incorporate pleasurable activities to lift their depressed moods.

The current edition covers the main mental health conditions facing children and adolescents. The authors, each an expert in his or her field, teach readers how to implement effective treatment procedures. Each chapter provides the theoretical foundations for the intervention strategies, a brief review of the relevant research literature, and descriptions of the measures used to assess the problem and evaluate the outcome. The bulk of each chapter is devoted to detailed descriptions of the treatment strategies and the materials used in treatment. The role of parents, developmental differences, and multicultural issues are each considered. To further the direct application of the treatment strategies, case examples are provided.

The accumulating body of evidence demonstrates that numerous mental health conditions in youth can be treated effectively. I am delighted to present this new edition, detailing these exciting findings and clinical strategies for effective treatment of youth in need of mental health services.

Contents

CHAPTER ONE

Working with Youth

Philip C. Kendall

Précis: A Casebook with
Empirically Supported Treatments?

Psychology has long striven to provide optimal care to those in need. A seminal meta-analysis (Smith & Glass, 1977) of the effects of psychological therapy summarized the findings to that date, and the findings allowed the authors to state that the results provided convincing evidence of the efficacy of psychological treatments. In retrospect, their work opened the door to an expanded focus on empirical support for psychological treatments and subsequently the degree to which psychological treatments are effective for children and adolescents (Weisz et al., 2017). Much has transpired over these 40 years.

Within a historical context, a great deal of research has been designed to answer the question, Does psychotherapy for children and adolescents work? As Kazdin (2000) noted, there were more than 1,500 published empirical studies of psychotherapy for youth as of his review in 2000, and we now know that psychological therapy for youth can be effective. Despite support for the efficacy of psychological therapy for children and adolescents, we are not yet at a point where we can definitively answer the question posed by Kiesler (1966) and reasked by Paul (1967): "What treatment, by whom, is most effective for this individual with that specific problem, under which set of circumstances?" Research has, however, identified

1

specific treatment strategies that are effective for identifiable child and adolescent mental health problems. Indeed, this very volume offers a casebook with empirically supported treatments.

Is there an incompatibility in the phrase "casebook with empirically supported treatments"? A "casebook" connotes a series of theoretical details with illustrative and descriptive cases, whereas "empirically supported treatments" connotes a restricted list of science-evaluated therapies. Do these notions blend or stay separate? Are they compatible (or compatibull)? In fact, these seemingly incompatible concepts are very compatible. Indeed, in the chapters of this book you will find clinically rich theoretical material and descriptions of specific cases that have been treated with approaches that have evidence to support their use.

What are empirically supported treatments? An extended discussion of this important theme is beyond the scope of this volume, but a few important points merit consideration. Although one must acknowledge the somewhat arbitrary nature of determining the sufficiency of evidence required for the label "empirically supported treatment," the label is a meaningful indicator that scientific evaluations support the application of the treatment (Hollon & Beck, 2013).

The following labels are typically used (after Chambless & Hollon, 1998).

1. A *well-established treatment* has been supported either by (a) two or more quality group-design studies conducted by different investigators that have demonstrated efficacy by being superior to a pill placebo, psychological placebo, or another treatment and/ or by being found to produce equivalent outcomes to a previously established treatment using studies with sufficient statistical power; or (b) a large series of single-case design studies that have demonstrated efficacy while using good experimental designs and by comparing the intervention to another treatment. In both, the studies must have specified the characteristics of the client samples and used treatment that was guided by manuals.
2. A *probably efficacious treatment* has been identified by (a) the presence of at least two studies demonstrating that the treatment is more effective than a waiting-list control group; (b) at least two studies otherwise meeting the well-established treatment criteria but with both having been conducted by the same investigator, or only one good study demonstrating effectiveness by established criteria; (c) two or more quality studies that demonstrate effectiveness but are flawed by the heterogeneity of the client samples; or (d) a series of single-case-design studies otherwise meeting the well-established treatment criteria but that is not yet large enough to be deemed well established.

3. Last, an *experimental treatment* is one that does not yet have enough sound data to be deemed at least probably efficacious.

When seeking to implement an intervention with children and adolescents, those that have met the "empirically supported" label merit first consideration. Indeed, they have met rigorous, yet reasonable, criteria. A recent development in the evolving terminology is the emergence of "evidence-based practice in psychology" (EBPP). Evidence-based practice seeks to integrate science and practice in terms of psychological assessment, conceptualization, and intervention.

Within this context, cognitive-behavioral therapy (CBT) emerges as an evidence-based treatment that also typically qualifies as an empirically supported treatment. It is beyond the scope of this opening chapter to review the extensive research that provides impressive support for a variety of versions of CBT with youth, but there are other sources (e.g., Kendall, 2012a; Weisz & Kazdin, 2017; Weisz et al., 2017) that can be consulted. The contents of the present volume, authored by experts with clinical experience, provides case materials and clinical strategies for the implementation of these evidence-based *and* empirically supported treatments.

On the Need to Be Developmentally Informed

Psychological treatments for children and adolescents are optimally effective when implemented with consideration of developmental factors. Consider these key areas: (1) initiating treatment, (2) age-appropriate delivery, (3) differing levels of cognitive, emotional, and social understanding, (4) roles for parents, and (5) therapist style.

Initiating Treatment

Children and adolescents, unlike adults, rarely initiate psychological services for themselves. In contrast, parents, pediatricians, teachers, or other agents of society are typical referral sources for youth. This "treatment entry" distinction is crucial: Children and adolescents may not be eager or willing to discuss their problems or be "involved" in sessions. Therapists working with youth must create an experience that encourages youth to return. A maxim that we follow is this: "A goal for Session 1 is that the child/adolescent returns for Session 2." Rapport-building activities, depending on the age of the youth, may include get-to-know-you-games, taking a walk or tour of the area, doing some online surfing, and engaging in activities of the youth's choice. Even when parents bring their children and adolescents to a family therapy clinic, they commonly are focused on the child as the problem (see Epstein, Schlesinger, & Kim, Chapter 12, this volume), and the child may be reluctant to be there, not wanting to be criticized and blamed. A crucial initial task for the family therapist is to gain rapport with the child, demonstrating interest in his or her thoughts and feelings, minimizing the time that parents spend complaining about the child, and setting positive goals (including changes in the family that the child would desire).

Age-Appropriate Delivery

Fun activities can be an age-appropriate and effective way to facilitate the implementation of CBT for youth. Fun activities foster a collaborative relationship between client and therapist and can boost the learning of therapy content. Play activities can also be informative, allowing the therapist to observe the child's expectations and beliefs, as well as coping skills. Fun activities may include art projects, role plays, songs, board games, and computer time. For example, within the Coping Cat program for child anxiety (Kendall & Hedtke, 2006a, 2006b), therapists engage in a "body drawing" art activity that helps youth identify the locations where they feel their anxiety.

Computers are a contemporary delivery system for therapeutic content. Consider anxiety in youth, for example; for adolescents suffering with anxiety, there is the Cool Teens program (Cunningham et al., 2009), and for children ages 6–13 there is the Camp Cope-A-Lot (Kendall & Khanna, 2008) program that offers 12 modules with interactivities and challenges that foster coping and reduce anxiety (Khanna & Kendall, 2010).

Level of Cognitive, Emotional, and Social Understanding

Not all youth are comparably mature, so the implementation of any treatment, including CBT, requires knowledge about cognitive, emotional, and social development. A type of cognitive restructuring used with adults may not be understood by children; for example, a refutation of a personal belief might be taken as punitive rather than explorative. Children may not have the cognitive maturity or vocabulary to distinguish rational and irrational thoughts. By the same notion, they can label thoughts as "helpful or not helpful," or "sad or coping thoughts." The specific probabilities of anticipated outcomes may be difficult for youth, but children can understand that certain events have a "small" or "big" chance of happening, and they can be coached to gather evidence or "clues" about the possibility of an outcome occurring. Gosch, Brookland, and Wolensky (Chapter 4, this volume) illustrate the use of this process with a child experiencing fears of harm. Some parents use parenting techniques that are not appropriate for a child's developmental level (e.g., giving a young child complex rationales for desired behavior). The therapist needs to take development into account not only to guide his or her assessment and interventions but also to educate parents (see also Epstein, Schlesinger, & Kim, Chapter 12, this volume).

Therapists working with children and adolescents benefit greatly from an awareness of the ups and downs of typical normal development and the many and varied "temporary" issues that merit attention but perhaps not a diagnosis. Recognition of a developmental issue in social functioning, in cognitive ability, or in emotional understanding can trigger initial monitoring. Youth face social challenges at different points in their development; peer relationships and academic performance take on increased importance in adolescence. As needed, and when appropriate, developmental needs and social issues can become part of the goals of CBT. For example, see discussion of CBT for youth on the autism spectrum (Mercado, Kratz, Frank, Wolensky, & Kerns, Chapter 8, this volume) and eating disorders (Culbert, Anderson, Bowers, & Le Grange, Chapter 10, this volume).

Roles for Parents

For several reasons, including the fact that children and adolescents are not fully independent, it is critical to consider the role of parents when treating youth. Parents can serve as *consultants* (e.g., providing information about symptoms and impairment), *collaborators* (e.g., bringing their children to treatment, assisting with implementation of therapy techniques), or *co-clients* in the treatment itself (Kendall, 2012b; Epstein et al., Chapter 12, this volume; Rowe & Liddle, Chapter 7, this volume).

The nature and benefits of including parents in CBT for youth vary depending on the specific problem and the child's age (e.g., Culbert et al., Chapter 10, this volume). Younger children may benefit more when parents are involved from the beginning, whereas adolescents may accrue more gains when parents are not regularly included in treatment. Some treatments for disruptive behavior problems involve parent training as a core component of treatment and thus require parental involvement. On the other hand, CBT for child anxiety can be implemented in a child-focused format and, with adolescents, with less parental involvement. Despite the variations in the roles for parents in treatment, there remain the benefits that can be gained from parent education about child development, mental health, and coping strategies. For example, Child Anxiety Tales, an online parent-training program for parents with anxious children (see *www.CopingCatParents.com*), can be an early step in a stepped-care approach to addressing the problem.

Therapist Style

When working with children and adolescents, the CBT therapist fills multiple roles, including diagnostician, consultant, and educator. As diagnostician, the therapist uses multimethod, multi-informant assessment of the youth's symptomatology and functioning in multiple domains to create a case conceptualization. As a consultant, the therapist works with the youth and parents (and potentially others) to share perspectives and select treatment goals. As an educator, the therapist provides information about the disorder and the course of treatment. It can be helpful to view the therapist's role as that of a *coach* (Kendall, 2012b; Podell et al., 2013) for the youth (not the mean and screaming coach, but the coach who teaches and provides opportunities to learn and perform). The coaching analogy helps communicate that the therapist will provide information, provide opportunities to learn, teach coping skills, and provide opportunities to practice the use of coping skills in real situations. And the same is true in family approaches, in which the key parties are in the room together (see Epstein et al., Chapter 12, this volume).

Illustrative Components in Effective Psychological Treatments for Youth

As you will see in this casebook, many of the main components of effective treatments for children and adolescents reappear, with appropriate adjustments, in the procedures used for different social, behavioral, cognitive, and emotional problems (see also Ehrenreich-May & Chu, 2014; Nangle et al., 2016). Some of the core strategies are also similar to those used with adults, but visual aids, fun activities, and age-appropriate metaphors help make the concepts accessible for youth. Several illustrative treatment components (i.e., problem solving, affective education, cognitive change, modeling and role playing, behavioral contingencies, and relaxation) are described, but note that this list is not exhaustive and that the components are not isolated or applied solely on their own; they are interconnected and build upon one another.

Problem Solving

The problem-solving process generates potential solutions to a dilemma and systematically determines the most effective response (D'Zurilla & Goldfried, 1971). Core problem-solving strategies for children and adolescents (see Anastopoulos, O'Rourke, & Bray, Chapter 9, this volume; Culbert et al., Chapter 10, this volume) are generally consistent with those used with adults (Nezu, Nezu, Friedman, Faddis, & Houts, 1998) and in families (Epstein et al., Chapter 12, this volume). Youth are introduced to a series of steps that they refer to when they identify a problem. For children, the problem-solving steps may be made into an acronym to facilitate learning. For example, a treatment for youth with aggression called

Keeping Your Cool uses the acronym SPEAR (Nelson & Finch, 2008). The SPEAR sequence consists of S̲top: what's the problem? (understanding the situation); P̲lan: what can I do? (generating solutions); E̲valuate: what is the best solution? (choosing a plan of action); A̲ct: try it out; R̲eact: did it work? (self-evaluation). Other treatments use variations of the same fundamental problem-solving steps and tailor them to a specific disorder. Initially, the therapist helps the child generate solutions and process the outcome of selected strategies. As youth repeat the problem-solving process and apply it to a variety of situations, they learn to think ahead and better resolve future problems (Gosch, Flannery-Schroeder, Mauro, & Compton, 2006).

Problem solving has been incorporated into treatments targeting a variety of child and adolescent mental health problems. Youth with aggression tend to believe that their aggressive behavior is instrumental toward achieving a desired goal (Lochman & Dodge, 1994). An important part of engaging aggressive children in problem solving is helping them to recognize the advantages and disadvantages of each potential plan of action and to choose one with a reasonable outcome (see Lochman, Powell, Boxmeyer, & Jimenez-Camargo, 2011; Mitchell, Pardini, & Lochman, Chapter 6, this volume). Problem solving is a balanced approach that acknowledges the potential benefits of an unproductive or impractical solution, as well as the benefits of a more appropriate solution. In problem solving, the therapist validates the child's experience while also showing that problems can have several potential solutions (see the example for generalized anxiety disorder in Gosch et al., Chapter 4, this volume). It is also illustrative of the collaborative/coach style that is effective with youth. Treatments for aggressive children focus on developing nonaggressive strategies to express anger and alternative means to achieve a desired goal.

Problem solving has also been used with impulsive children (Kendall & Braswell, 1993). The components resemble those from other protocols with the addition of a step to maintain focused attention. For children with depression, problem solving (Stark, Streusand, Arora, & Patel, 2012) may require added attention to negative affect and thoughts that may be an obstacle preventing the youth with depression from taking action. Children are encouraged to do something pleasurable to improve mood and to facilitate problem solving. Therapists may need to pay special attention when youth with depression disqualify potential positive outcomes after a problem-solving strategy has been used effectively (Curry & Meyer, Chapter 5, this volume). Across target problems, considering unorthodox and even silly potential solutions is a welcomed part of brainstorming potential solutions with youth: They add fun to the process and constitute examples of solutions that can be eliminated. Deriving silly solutions to problems adds humor to the setting and highlights the sensibility of other solutions.

Learning about Feelings

Youth are not known for their grasp of the emotional side of their lives. Affective education helps the child recognize, differentiate, and express emotion. Affective education is implemented to be consistent with the youth's presenting problem and the stage of treatment. For example, for a teen who has reached a level of metacognitive development and thinking about his or her own thinking, sad experiences can become the grist for rumination. Therapists can help reduce this problem by, as appropriate, normalizing the youth's experience of sadness: A teen can be told that happiness and sadness are normal emotions experienced by everyone (including adults) but that, when they are too intense or too frequent, they need to be "adjusted."

Youth are taught to distinguish among emotional states. The therapist and young child client might cut out pictures of people from magazines and label their emotions. The labeling can be accomplished based on the situation in the picture and the facial expressions of the character. The labeling exercise can also include discussion about how the feeling might be different if the situation were different or if the child thought about the situation differently. Another option, perhaps for older youth, would be to play "feelings charades," in which the therapist and youth alternate acting out and guessing various emotions. It's not a teacher teaching emotions ("teachy" therapist style) but a collaborative interaction (Creed & Kendall, 2005; Podell et al., 2013) around the content of feelings. Indeed, in cases in which the youth takes off and runs with aspects of the affective education, the therapist can take a back seat.

Learning how to identify one's own physiological cues of emotional distress or arousal is part of affective education. Recognition of a trigger for anger or aggression or a bodily marker of emotional distress can then signal the child to stop and think and use problem solving. To raise physiological awareness, a youth may draw a picture of his or her body and highlight the parts that are active when emotionally charged (e.g., tightened face when angry; "butterflies" in the stomach or sweating palms when nervous). Youth and/or therapists can create a "feelings thermometer" to represent the range of a particular emotion, and the thermometer is then used as a visual aid to help children better comprehend the varying intensity of negative emotions (Lochman et al., 2011). For example, when children with depression reach a particular threshold on their "mood thermometer," they are encouraged to do something they enjoy (Stark et al., 2012). The thermometer can help reveal common triggers that elicit a particular negative emotion, and the mere construction of the thermometer can provide an opportunity for building rapport. Younger children often enjoy decorating and personalizing their feelings thermometer.

Changing Self-Talk (the Inner Dialogue)

Within the cognitive model, dysfunctional and distorted thoughts (self-talk) mediate the relationship between stressful life events and psychopathology (Beck, 1976). Within depression (see Curry & Meyer, Chapter 5, this volume), cognitive distortions refer to negative misperceptions about oneself, the world, or the future. Children with a variety of disorders display distorted thinking (Crick & Dodge, 1996; Kendall, 1993), and there are data to suggest that the content of the negative self-talk reflects the specific psychopathology. For example, a core cognitive feature in depression includes attribution of negative events to internal, stable, and global characteristics of the self and attribution of positive events to external, unstable, and specific causes. Externalizing disorders, on the other hand, are associated with distorted processing of ambiguous situations, such as angry youth seeing ambiguous situations as hostile and provocative (Lansford et al., 2006; Yaros, Lochman, Rosenbaum, & Jimenez-Camargo, 2014) and potentially requiring retaliation. Changing self-talk (also referred to as "cognitive restructuring") refers to the process of helping youth to see alternate ways to make sense of experiences. The process involves identifying distorted beliefs and/or negative self-talk, connecting thoughts to feelings and behaviors, challenging the validity of the thoughts and beliefs with evidence, and developing new and helpful patterns of thinking. This process plays a key role for traumatized youth, in which their cognitive distortions about the safety of the world can either be reaffirmed or shattered. The evidence comes from the youth's experiences in behavioral experiments and in exposure tasks both in and out of session. Given the importance of developmental level in matters that concern self-talk, this strategy is modified depending on the age and presenting problem of the child.

Children learn to recognize some of their unfounded negative thoughts early in cognitive restructuring. In one exercise, children are presented with various cartoons of people in ambiguous situations. Children fill in a blank thought bubble above the character's head to express the thoughts (Kendall & Hedtke, 2006a). After the child has identified the thoughts of others, the therapist can inquire about what is in the child's own thought bubble. For homework, children keep a journal, record their thoughts, and note the situation and their accompanying emotion. This self-monitoring exercise helps children become aware of the link between thoughts, feelings, and behaviors. The therapist can also take time to identify a situation from the child's life, write down thoughts, feelings, and behaviors, and review how the three components are interconnected. Integrating the mood thermometer into the discussion of thoughts (self-talk) is another way to show that emotions and thoughts influence one another.

After identifying maladaptive self-talk, children move on to challenging their thoughts and beliefs and eventually developing coping thoughts. Children can become "thought detectives" who objectively evaluate the validity of self-talk. The therapist and child examine maladaptive thoughts and ask, "What is the evidence for that?" or "What's another way of looking at it?" The latter question can be helpful for aggressive children who misinterpret ambiguous social cues as having hostile intent. In "decatastrophizing," the therapist asks, "If a feared or nonpreferred outcome happens or if your thought is true, so what?" By exploring the worst-case consequences of some thoughts, the child learns that he or she can very likely cope with the situation. A child learns to identify "thinking traps." Thinking traps, adapted from Beck's cognitive errors for adults (Beck, 2011), include mind reading (knowing what others are thinking), fortune telling (being certain about an ambiguous future event), and black-and-white thinking (dichotomizing things on a continuum), among others. Finally, therapists and children collaborate to develop coping thoughts. An aggressive child might try, "It may have been an accident; I won't get angry until I learn more"; or an anxious child might think, "I tried it a few times, and did OK, so I may do OK when I try it again."

Although not a formal component of cognitive restructuring, several treatments "externalize" the disorder. The idea is for the youth to realize that his or her symptoms do not define who he or she is but represent something to be managed or addressed. "Externalizing" reduces self-blame and distances the child from negative thoughts. A treatment for depression externalizes the collective symptoms into the "muck monster" (Stark et al., 2012). The child draws a picture of the monster and can direct his or her coping statements at it. In treating obsessive–compulsive disorder (OCD; see also Franklin, Morris, & Budzyn, Chapter 3, this volume), children name their symptoms (e.g., "stupid thing"), and a treatment goal is to reclaim control by "bossing back OCD" (March & Mulle, 1998).

Modeling and Role Playing

Modeling, a form of observational learning, allows a child or adolescent to acquire a new skill or improve on an existing one by viewing the behavior of others (despite receiving no explicit reinforcement). Modeling exemplifies social learning theory, in that individuals learn through observation in addition to direct experience (Bandura, 1977). Several types of modeling exist, including covert, filmed, live, and participant-guided modeling. Covert modeling strategies have the child imagine the therapist or another model dealing with a difficult situation. Children can visualize a model (a cartoon character, superhero, or celebrity), in addition to the therapist. In filmed modeling, children might watch a video, whereas in live modeling the therapist might demonstrate a behavior for a child. In some protocols, same-age peers proficient in a particular behavior serve as live models (e.g.,

Beidel, Turner, & Morris, 2000). In guided modeling, the therapist inter-acts with the child as they navigate the situation. Research has supported the benefits of participant-guided modeling.

Role-play activities provide a safe environment in which to practice new skills. In a role play, the therapist and child typically act out a scenario in which the child faces a challenge and uses problem-solving and coping skills. Role plays simulate real-life situations (see Rowe & Liddle, Chapter 7, this volume). They do not provide the real-life consequences, but they do provide the opportunity for therapist feedback. For example, the therapist could pretend to be the child's friend who is experiencing negative thoughts (Deblinger & Heflin, 1996). The child's task is to be a good friend and help his or her friend to challenge the negative thoughts. With practice and feedback, the child can internalize the skills and challenge his or her own thoughts. Similarly, children who have experienced trauma benefit from writing narratives about their traumatic experiences and, through repeti-tion, reducing the anxiety caused by the memory of the trauma.

Behavioral Contingencies

Behavioral contingencies include positive reinforcement, shaping, and extinction. Contingency management strategies promote targeted behav-ior and encourage treatment compliance. Research has found that reduc-tions in children's conduct problems following intervention occurs in part because of intervention-produced improvements in parents' abilities to be consistent in providing consequences (Lochman & Wells, 2002). Often, the initial reinforcers are tangible, whereas later in treatment they may be social or self-chosen rewards. It is important that rewards reflect the devel-opmental level of the child: Younger children may require concrete and frequent rewards (Crawley et al., 2010). However, rewards do not necessar-ily have to be large or material. Getting to be the person who chooses the meal for a family dinner, earning computer time, or spending time alone with a parent can all be effective rewards. In addition, therapists can print certificates of achievement to increase self-esteem and motivation after the child successfully completes a task. The certificate provides an opportunity for children to brag about their accomplishments to others, which in turn is reinforcing. Separate from the specific reinforcer, it is important that the reward be contingent and meaningful to the child.

In many of the empirically supported programs for youth, parents play a role and are taught how to use behavioral contingencies. Parents are taught to be consistent in their implementation and, depending on the age of the child, may be encouraged to set up a sticker chart or other system to track the child's progress. Effort and partial success are always rewarded (for family therapy, see Epstein et al., Chapter 12, this volume), particularly in children who have perfectionistic tendencies (Kendall & Suveg, 2006).

Relaxation

Relaxation training has been incorporated within some protocols to treat children. Youth can be taught to use relaxation as a means to reduce and/or cope with stress. Debate exists regarding the benefits of relaxation training, as well as the precise mechanism accounting for the effects of relaxation, with some researchers arguing that the process helps children regulate emotional and physiological responses to negative life events (Gosch et al., 2006), whereas others theorize that its effects are due to cognitive changes, such as increased self-efficacy and control (Conrad & Roth, 2007). There is also controversy regarding the necessity of relaxation training within some treatments for children. Some research on treatment of anxiety suggests that CBT may remain effective without relaxation training (Hudson & Rapee, 2000; Peris et al., 2015; Rapee, 2000). Although its centrality varies, relaxation is often a feature in programs targeting a variety of disorders in children.

Epilogue

As you enter this volume, you will find wise theoretical guidance, rich clinical descriptions, and lively case illustrations, all of which will add meaningful flesh to the initial bones described in this opening chapter. Consistent with optimizing practice, the cases and treatment procedures are both (1) organized by the nature of the primary presenting problem and (2) qualified as evidence-based and empirically supported. Enjoy.

References

Bandura, A. (1977). *Social learning theory.* Englewood Cliffs, NJ: Prentice Hall.
Beck, A. T. (1976). *Cognitive therapy and the emotional disorders.* New York: International Universities Press.
Beck, J. S. (2011). *Cognitive behavior therapy: Basics and beyond* (2nd ed.). New York: Guilford Press.
Beidel, D. C., Turner, S., & Morris, T. (2000). Behavioral treatment of childhood social phobia. *Journal of Consulting and Clinical Psychology, 68,* 1072–1080.
Chambless, D. L., & Hollon, S. D. (1998). Defining empirically supported therapies. *Journal of Consulting and Clinical Psychology, 66,* 7–18.
Conrad, A., & Roth, W. (2007). Muscle relaxation therapy for anxiety disorder: It works but how? *Journal of Anxiety Disorders, 21,* 243–264.
Crawley, S., Podell, J., Beidas, R., Braswell, L., & Kendall, P. C. (2010). Cognitive-behavioral therapy with youth. In K. S. Dobson (Ed.), *Handbook of cognitive-behavioral therapies* (3rd ed., pp. 375–410). New York: Guilford Press.
Creed, T., & Kendall, P. C. (2005). Empirically supported therapist relationship building behavior within a cognitive-behavioral treatment of anxiety in youth. *Journal of Consulting and Clinical Psychology, 73,* 498–505.

Crick, N. R., & Dodge, K. A. (1996). Social information-processing mechanisms on reactive and proactive aggression. *Child Development, 67,* 993–1002.

Cunningham, M., Wuthrich, V., Rapee, R., Lyneham, C., Schniering, J., & Hudson, J. (2009). The Cool Teens CD-ROM for anxiety disorders in adolescents. *European Child and Adolescent Psychiatry, 18,* 125–129.

Deblinger, E., & Heflin, A. (1996). *Treating sexually abused children and their nonoffending parents: A cognitive behavioral approach.* Thousand Oaks, CA: SAGE.

D'Zurilla, T., & Goldfried, M. (1971). Problem solving and behavior modification. *Journal of Abnormal Psychology, 78,* 107–126.

Ehrenreich-May, J., & Chu, B. (Eds.). (2014). *Transdiagnostic treatments for children and adolescents: Principles and practice.* New York: Guilford Press.

Gosch, E. A., Flannery-Schroeder, E., Mauro, C. F., & Compton, S. N. (2006). Principles of cognitive-behavioral therapy for anxiety disorders in children. *Journal of Cognitive Psychotherapy: An International Quarterly, 20,* 247–262.

Hollon, S. D., & Beck, A. T. (2013). Cognitive and cognitive behavioral therapies. In M. J. Lambert (Ed.), *Bergin and Garfield's handbook of psychotherapy and behavioral change* (6th ed., pp. 447–492). New York: Wiley.

Hudson, J., & Rapee, R. (2000). *Treating anxious children and adolescents: An evidence-based approach.* Oakland, CA: New Harbinger.

Kazdin, A. E. (2000). Developing a research agenda for child and adolescent psychotherapy. *Archives of General Psychiatry, 57,* 829–835.

Kendall, P. C. (1993). Cognitive-behavioral therapies with youth: Guiding theory, current status, and emerging developments. *Journal of Consulting and Clinical Psychology, 61,* 235–247.

Kendall, P. C. (Ed.). (2012a). *Child and adolescent therapy: Cognitive-behavioral procedures* (4th ed.). New York: Guilford Press.

Kendall, P. C. (2012b). Guiding theory for therapy with children and adolescents. In P. C. Kendall (Ed.), *Child and adolescent therapy: Cognitive-behavioral procedures* (4th ed., pp. 3–24). New York: Guilford Press.

Kendall, P. C., & Braswell, L. (1993). *Cognitive-behavioral therapy for impulsive children* (2nd ed.). New York: Guilford Press.

Kendall, P. C., & Hedtke, K. (2006a). *Coping Cat workbook* (2nd ed.). Ardmore, PA: Workbook.

Kendall, P. C., & Hedtke, K. (2006b). *Cognitive-behavioral therapy for anxious children: Therapist manual* (3rd ed.). Ardmore, PA: Workbook.

Kendall, P. C., & Khanna, M. (2008). *Camp Cope-A-Lot: The computer-assisted Coping Cat program.* Ardmore, PA: Workbook.

Kendall, P. C., & Suveg, C. (2006). Treating anxiety disorders in youth. In P. C. Kendall (Ed.), *Child and adolescent therapy: Cognitive-behavioral procedures* (3rd ed., pp. 243–294). New York: Guilford Press.

Khanna, M., & Kendall, P. C. (2010). Computer-assisted cognitive-behavioral therapy for child anxiety: Results of a randomized clinical trial. *Journal of Consulting and Clinical Psychology, 78,* 737–745.

Kiesler, D. J. (1966). Some myths of psychotherapy research and the search for a paradigm. *Psychological Bulletin, 65,* 110–136.

Lansford, J., Malone, P., Dodge, K., Crozier, J., Pettit, G., & Bates, J. (2006). A 12-year prospective study of patterns of social information processing problems and externalizing behaviors. *Journal of Abnormal Child Psychology, 34,* 715–724.

Lochman, J. E., & Dodge, K. A. (1994). Social-cognitive processes of severely violent, moderately aggressive, and nonaggressive boys. *Journal of Consulting and Clinical Psychology, 62,* 366–374.

Lochman, J. E., Powell, N., Boxmeyer, C., & Jimenez-Camargo, L. (2011). Cognitive-behavioral therapy for externalizing disorders in children and adolescents. *Child and Adolescent Psychiatric Clinics of North America, 20,* 305–318.

Lochman, J. E., & Wells, K. C. (2002). Contextual social-cognitive mediators and child outcome: A test of the theoretical model in the Coping Power Program. *Development and Psychopathology, 14,* 971–993.

March, J., & Mulle, K. (1998). *OCD in children and adolescents: A cognitive-behavioral treatment manual.* New York: Guilford Press.

Nangle, D. W., Hansen, D. J., Grover, R. L., Kingery, J. N., Suveg, C., & Contributors. (2016). *Treating internalizing disorders in children and adolescents: Core techniques and strategies.* New York: Guilford Press.

Nelson, M., & Finch, A. J. (2008). *Keeping your cool: The anger management workbook.* Ardmore, PA: Workbook.

Nezu, A., Nezu, C., Friedman, S., Faddi, S., & Houts, P. (1998). *Helping cancer patients cope: A problem-solving approach.* Washington, DC: American Psychological Association.

Paul, G. L. (1967). Strategy of outcome research in psychotherapy. *Journal of Consulting Psychology, 31,* 109–118.

Peris, T., Compton, S., Kendall, P. C., Birmaher, B., Sherill, J., March, J., et al. (2015). Trajectories of change in youth anxiety during cognitive-behavior therapy. *Journal of Consulting and Clinical Psychology, 83,* 239–252.

Podell, J., Kendall, P. C., Gosch, E., Compton, S., March, J., Albano, A. M., et al. (2013). Therapist factors and outcomes in CBT for anxiety in youth. *Professional Psychology: Research and Practice, 44,* 89–98.

Rapee, R. (2000). Group treatment of children with anxiety disorders: Outcome and predictors of treatment response. *Australian Journal of Psychology, 52,* 125–129.

Smith, M., & Glass, G. (1977). Meta-analysis of psychotherapy outcome studies. *American Psychologist, 32,* 752–760.

Stark, K., Streusand, W., Arora, P., & Patel, P. (2012). Childhood depression: The ACTION treatment program. In P. C. Kendall (Ed.), *Child and adolescent therapy: Cognitive-behavioral procedures* (4th ed., pp. 190–233). New York: Guilford Press.

Weisz, J. R., & Kazdin, A. E. (Eds.). (2017). *Evidence-based psychotherapies for children and adolescents* (3rd ed.). New York: Guilford Press.

Weisz, J. R., Kuppens, S., Ng, M., Eckshtain, D., Ugueto, A., Vaughn-Coaxum, R., et al. (2017). What five decades of research tells us about the effects of youth psychological therapy: A multilevel meta-analysis and implications for science and practice. *American Psychologist, 72,* 79–117.

Yaros, A., Lochman, J. E., Rosenbaum, J., & Jimenez-Camargo, L. A. (2014). Real-time hostile attribution measurement and aggression in children. *Aggressive Behavior, 40,* 409–420.

CHAPTER TWO

Treatment of Social Anxiety Disorder

Anne Marie Albano
Lauren Hoffman

The emotional and physical experience of social anxiety, that sense of unease and discomfort associated with being the focus of attention, especially during performance or evaluative situations, is well known to many and a common phenomenon throughout the life span. Blushing or shaking when giving an oral report in school or a talk to a large audience, "butterflies" or racing heart and thoughts of "What if this goes badly?" when asking someone out for a date or being called into the boss's office, and the hot, flushed feeling and thoughts of "Get me out of here" when dropping a full tray of food on the cafeteria floor or showing up empty handed to a potluck dinner—these reactions are considered normal expressions of social anxiety in response to specific events or situations. In contrast to these transient and prompted experiences of anxiety that occur and resolve relatively quickly, with the individual moving on with little to no disruption to his or her overall development and functioning, social anxiety disorder (SoD), otherwise known as social phobia, is the most frequently occurring anxiety disorder in youth and adults and the second most common of all mental health disorders (Kessler et al., 2005; Merikangas et al., 2010). SoD has its onset early in life, by early adolescence, and persists through adulthood (see Ranta, La Greca, García-Lopez, & Marttunen, 2016). This chapter focuses on the phenomenology and cognitive-behavioral treatment of SoD in youth. Descriptions of the symptoms and phenomenology of SoD are discussed in a developmental frame, to understand the distinction between expected, transient states of social anxiety and the disability and disturbance associated with the clinical disorder. The overall goal of the chapter is to provide mental health practitioners working with youth a developmental model for understanding and applying the cognitive behavioral approach to assessment and treatment of SoD.

Overview of SoD

The Parents

"He used to participate in sports and meet up with friends. But, in thinking back, I was the one arranging his activities. Once he got to middle school, he started to refuse to do things outside of our family events. As it is, we have to drag him to those."

"I kept hearing about my friends' kids, and was just so grateful that she wasn't going out to wild parties, online and texting all the time, or causing any trouble at school."

"She has always been very quiet, but I had no idea that she was in such pain and felt so alone."

The Youth

"I try to find the biggest kid in each class, and I sit right behind them. Most of the time I think that works and I'm not called on. But, I feel like vomiting while waiting for class to end."

"The other kids just seem to do things more easily than me, you know, like give talks and just talking together. I don't know what to say. I can't think of anything and know I'll be laughed at."

"I'm hoping college will be different than these last 12 years. Everyone will be friendly and I'll feel more confident meeting up with people once I'm out of this high school."

The experience of a modest degree of social fear in children from the earliest age is developmentally appropriate and not uncommon. Anxiety reactions may serve to protect a toddler from wandering away from parents or alerting caretakers to the presence of a stranger, for example. Between ages 3 and 8, the developing child is able to experience embarrassment, take others' perspectives, and understand the impact of negative evaluation on one's reputation or place in a group or setting. Social anxiety naturally increases in intensity and frequency as the youth's cognitive abilities are expanded and refined during later childhood and the adolescent years. Almost daily, middle school children and adolescents are subjected to heightened expectations for their performance in social and academic situations, managing their emotions and behavior with increasing independence from adults, and having to take responsibility for their actions and attitudes (Detweiler, Comer, Crum, & Albano, 2014; Velting & Albano, 2001). The repeated experience of various social and evaluative challenges results in a youth learning to manage each situation and control his or her anxiety, to accurately assess social risk and responding, and to problem-solve when things don't go as expected or outcomes are not as one would hope (see Albano & Pepper, 2013, Chap. 9). Hence, social anxiety is a normal, expected experience throughout childhood and adolescence that typically results in minor and transient upset and little disruption in functioning and that usually resolves with repeated experience and time.

Maladaptive and Interfering Symptoms and Associated Features

In contrast to transient social anxiety, the fifth edition of the *Diagnostic and Statistical Manual of Mental Disorders* (DSM-5; American Psychiatric Association, 2013) defines SoD as persistent fear of one or more situations wherein the individual is exposed to unfamiliar people or possible scrutiny (i.e., evaluation) by others and in which the individual fears embarrassment or humiliation. The feared situations are either avoided or endured with distress, and the fear persists 6 months or longer while interfering with the individual's usual routine and functioning. Although adults with heightened social anxiety or SoD may choose to avoid situations that prompt this anxiety, school-age youth are exposed to challenging social and evaluative situations with little choice about attendance, unless, contrary to what would be recommended by a clinician, the parents arrange for alternatives to the traditional school experience. Accounting for developmental differences between children and adults, DSM-5 requires that the fear be expressed when in contact with peers and not restricted to anxiety in relation to adults. Throughout the school year, youth are in constant contact with peers and expected to perform and manage social engagement and evaluation anxiety. Meeting other students at the start of school, engaging in group activities, giving oral reports, talking to peers on the school bus, eating together in the cafeteria, and being invited (or not) to a peer's birthday party are just some of the situations prompting anxiety in a typical school day. DSM-5 allows for the diagnosis of the generalized subtype of SoD, indicating fear and avoidance of a wide range of situations and activities, or the nongeneralized subtype, wherein the anxiety is more limited to specific situations, such as giving oral reports, speaking to unfamiliar persons, or situations requiring assertiveness. Table 2.1 is a partial list of situations and activities that prompt social anxiety reactions in youth and that are identified as highly feared and avoided by youth with SoD (see Beidel, Turner, & Morris, 1999; DiBartolo et al., 1998; Hofmann et al., 1999).

In response to the social anxiety trigger, DSM-5 further specifies that the anxiety reactions may be manifested in an age-appropriate manner, such as through crying, clinging to caretakers, or having tantrums as expressions of discomfort and distress. Children and adolescents will manifest panic attacks or symptoms of panic, such as increased heart rate, flushing, trembling, shaking, sweating, and depersonalization, and related physiological stress reactions (see Beidel et al., 1999; Mesa, Beidel, & Bunnell, 2014). Youth with SoD report higher levels of depressed mood, higher trait anxiety, and lower perceptions of cognitive competence than their nonanxious peers (Albano, Chorpita, & Barlow, 2003), as well as higher levels of loneliness and having fewer friends than their same-age peers (Beidel et al., 1999; La Greca & Lopez, 1998). The avoidance associated with social phobia may also extend to refusal to attend school in order to escape the negative affect associated with social and evaluative situations (Kearney & Albano, 2004). Further complicating the child's clinical presentation are family upset, potential academic decline, and an overall lag in meeting developmental expectations (Detweiler et al., 2014; Guerry, Hambrick, & Albano, 2015).

Prevalence, Age, Gender, Comorbidity, and Course

Although SoD can present at any time in childhood, the disorder is typically associated with later childhood and adolescence. Results from the National Comorbidity Survey Replication—Adolescent Supplement (NCS-A), indicate that 8.6% of adolescents (n = 10,123, ages 13–18 years) met criteria for SoD in their lifetimes (Burstein et al., 2011). Of these youth, 55.8% met criteria for the generalized subtype and 44.2% for the nongeneralized subtype. Burstein and colleagues found that the median age of onset was 9 years, 2 months in the NCS-A cohort. Regarding subtypes, generalized SoD had a younger age of onset (median = 8 years, 7 months vs. 9 years, 4 months) and was 1.7 times more likely to occur in older as compared with younger adolescents. The gender distribution of SoD is nearly equal with interesting trends: Males with generalized SoD demonstrated a significantly younger age of onset as compared with females with this subtype, although there is a trend toward more females experiencing the generalized subtype overall as compared with male adolescents.

Adolescents with SoD report moderate severity of their illness, upward of seven different social fears, and having a highly persistent condition (Burstein et al., 2011). In addition, youth affected with the generalized subtype endorsed higher levels of disability and longer duration of illness than

TABLE 2.1. Situations and Activities Prompting Social Anxiety in Youth

- Starting school (for the first time; a new school; a new school year)
- Finding someone to sit with on the school bus
- Meeting the teacher
- Joining other kids on a playground (at school or in a park)
- Conversations with peers (initiating, joining in)
- Asking a friend to get together
- Reading aloud in class or giving an oral report
- Being picked for a game or team
- Asking a question in class or being called on to answer
- Asking for help from the teacher
- Being wrong in front of others
- Being assigned to work with a group of kids
- Hanging out/walking through the hallway at school
- Entering class late
- Handing in homework
- Discussing a difference in opinion with others (teacher, peers)
- Having homework or classwork displayed for others to see
- Finding a place to sit in the cafeteria
- Going to a summer camp, day or overnight, and meeting new kids
- Performing (sports, dance, music) in front of others
- Going to a party alone (in younger children, going without a parent)
- Using social media or texting
- Asking someone for a date or being asked out on a date
- Interviewing for an internship, college, or a job
- Meeting someone for the first time
- Dealing with teasing
- Engaging with others at a party (playing games, talking, dancing)
- Refusing alcohol or drugs
- Eating or drinking while talking
- Sticking up for yourself or saying "No"

youth with the nongeneralized subtype in the NCS-A, and this subtype was also found to evidence greater severity of illness and higher use of services. SoD is highly comorbid with other anxiety disorders, oppositional defiant disorder, substance use disorders, and mood disorders (Burstein et al., 2011). Social phobia, similar to other anxiety disorders, runs a chronic and persistent course into adulthood and is associated with psychological and physical comorbidities, poor social and impaired role functioning, decreased educational attainment, and long-term dependence on family or social services (Comer et al., 2011; Mendlowicz & Stein, 2000).

Etiological Mechanisms and Cognitive–Behavioral Model

The cognitive-behavioral approach incorporates a diathesis–stress model of psychopathology in which learning history plays a meaningful role and interacts with neurobiological, familial, and sociocultural mechanisms (see Barlow, 2002; Rapee & Heimberg, 1997). This model suggests that biological factors such as genetics and temperament comprise a diathesis for problematic social anxiety (Asendorpf, 1994; Hayward, Killen, Kraemer, & Taylor, 1998; Lewis-Morrarty et al., 2012; Lewis-Morrarty et al., 2015). Further, the model recognizes that the realization of social anxiety symptoms is dependent on other risk and protective factors, including environmental variables such as parental rearing style (Chorpita & Barlow, 1998; Rubin, Hastings, & Asendorpf, 1999), negative or positive experience with peers (Cohen & Kendall, 2015), observational learning and selective attention to threat-related stimuli (Reeb-Sutherland et al., 2015).

Parents are often concerned and ask clinicians if they "caused" their child to be anxious, and they may compare the child to their own histories of anxiety or to their children without anxiety. They wonder if they transmitted the anxiety to their child, or if there could be a "chemical imbalance" causing the anxiety or possibly some known (e.g., bullying) or unknown traumatic event that may have occurred. As anxiety is multifactorial, transactional, and developmental, it is important to provide the parents and the youth with an understanding that anxiety is a normal, natural emotion inherent in all humans and in animals, and that social anxiety is unique to humans and possibly primates (see Albano & Pepper, 2013; Albano & Hayward, 2004). It is important to emphasize to families that normative levels of social anxiety occur throughout life, in addition to specific periods in which we expect to see increases in social anxiety, such as a transition to a new school level (middle to high school; high school to college) or initiation of a novel activity (e.g., initiating dating, starting an internship). For some individuals, social anxiety occurs at a continuously high level that is unnecessary or overly excessive for the situation, resulting in the distress and impairment that accompanies the disorder.

According to the cognitive-behavioral model, the development of the clinical condition of SoD for a particular child results from a possible biological vulnerability to more readily experiencing anxiety. Through a process of oversensitivity to anxiety-provoking cues (via biological risk factors such as temperament or genetics, environmental experiences, or cognitive style), the child develops heightened sensitivity to anxiety sensations and a cognitive bias to misinterpret threat, and he or she learns to react to and anticipate more negative outcomes in social situations than is realistic or necessary (see also Kendall, 2012). Understanding this model sets the stage to discuss with families openly and up front the problem of becoming drawn into the cycle of anxiety and inadvertently reinforcing escape from and avoidance of socially challenging situations. Certain parental child-rearing styles, specifically parental overprotectiveness and overcontrol, have been associated with the maintenance of anxiety disorders in youth (see Albano, 2013; Chorpita & Barlow, 1998). Studies of anxious children and their parents (Barrett, Rapee, Dadds, & Ryan, 1996; Chorpita, Albano, & Barlow, 1996), as well as adolescents with social phobia (Logsdon-Conradsen, 1998), demonstrate that parents selectively attend to ambiguous cues in the environment (e.g., the children are laughing on the playground as your child approaches and some are looking his way) and misinterpret these cues as threatening to the child. With the repeated experience of comforting and reassuring the anxious child, parents focus in on the ambiguous cue (laughing . . . some are looking his way) and give a verbal message to escape or avoid the situation, rather than to engage in constructive problem solving and approach behavior. When the parents themselves endorse higher trait anxiety, this overprotection is more evident (Logsdon-Conradsen, 1999). It is hypothesized that the child's anxiety has shaped the parents' natural tendency to protect and comfort, which in turn reinforces the child's anxiety, leading to more overprotection, and so on, contributing to the maintenance of anxious responding in the youth. Consequently, as the child ages through childhood to adolescence, repeated overprotection and overinvolvement by the parents in soothing and protecting the child results in fewer trial-and-error experiences by the child in managing various social and evaluative situations, self-soothing when anxious, gradual shaping and refinement of age-appropriate social problem-solving skills, and overall reinforcing of avoidance behavior.

The cognitive-behavioral model of social anxiety suggests that due to the complex diathesis, individuals with the disorder develop negative, stable beliefs about themselves, social situations, and other people, with the underlying belief that in situations in which one is the focus of attention or evaluation, something is likely to happen to cause embarrassment, humiliation and/or rejection. Moreover, the individual believes that he or she does not have the capabilities to manage the situation or outcomes, and, hence, he or she develops escape or avoidance behaviors that can generalize over time to similar situations. When confronted with a situation that is perceived as socially challenging (e.g., meeting someone new, taking a test, being called on), the individual's attention becomes focused internally on the physical sensations of anxiety, as well as on the negative self-talk (beliefs, images, ideas), resulting in real or perceived disruption in performance (see Rapee & Heimberg, 1997; Barlow, 2002). Cognitive-behavioral treatments for social anxiety include age-specific components geared toward educating the individual about the nature of anxiety, addressing negative and self-defeating self-talk, using skill-building modules to address specific issues, and exposing the individual to the feared situations and activities.

Efficacy of Cognitive–Behavioral Therapy

Cognitive-behavioral therapy (CBT) is efficacious in reducing the symptoms, disorder, and associated impairments of SoD in children and adolescents (see Higa-McMillan, Francis, Rith-Najarian, & Chorpita, 2016; Hollon & Beck, 2013). CBT involves teaching psychoeducation at an age-appropriate level, somatic management skills, cognitive restructuring techniques, and specific skills training applied in accordance with individual patient need (e.g., problem solving, social skills, communication training), along with gradual exposure to anxiety-producing situations. Many randomized clinical trials enrolled a heterogeneous sample of youth presenting with one or more of the "triad" of childhood anxiety disorders: SoD, separation anxiety disorder (SAD), and generalized anxiety disorder (GAD). These three conditions share the construct of anxiety, beginning in childhood or by early adolescence, running similar courses through adulthood, and responding similarly to pharmacotherapy and CBT (Albano & Kendall, 2002). Coping Cat (ages 7 to roughly 12 years; Kendall & Hedtke, 2006a, 2006b) and the C.A.T. Project (adolescent adaptation; Kendall, Choudhury, Hudson, & Webb, 2002a; Kendall, Choudhury, Hudson, & Webb, 2002b) are the gold-standard CBT, "Level 1" (best support/well established; see Higa-McMillan et al., 2016) treatment programs for the triad, with an "empirically supported" designation based on numerous individual, group, and family-based clinical trials (e.g., Kendall, 1994; Kendall et al., 1997; Kendall, Hudson, Gosch, Flannery-Schroeder, & Suveg, 2008), replication (e.g., Barrett, Dadds, & Rapee, 1996; Barrett, Duffy, Dadds, & Rapee, 2001), and evaluation in combination with and as compared with medication and pill placebo (Walkup et al., 2008). Of note, in examining outcomes for 842 youth ages 6–18 years treated with a family group CBT for broad-based anxiety disorders extending beyond the triad (SoD, SAD, GAD, specific phobia, and obsessive–compulsive disorder [OCD]), Hudson and colleagues (2015) found that the presence of SoD resulted in a slower rate of change and poorer diagnostic outcomes at posttreatment and follow-up than for children with other anxiety disorders. These results were not moderated by children's age or presence of comorbid depression.

Social anxiety is also targeted directly in disorder-specific CBT programs. These manual-guided treatments are focused on relieving symptoms and distress associated with social and evaluation anxiety and are often delivered in group format. Beidel, Turner, and Morris (2000) randomly assigned 67 children (ages 8–12) to 12 weeks of social effectiveness therapy for children (SET-C) or an active study-skills and test-anxiety comparison condition (Testbusters; Beidel, Turner, & Taylor-Ferreira, 1999). SET-C is a CBT approach with additional components of social skills training and peer pairing, whereby youth with social anxiety have weekly outings with peers without anxiety, arranged for ecological validity as exposure situations to test out anxiety management skills and foster habituation to feared situations. Independent evaluator ratings of clinical severity on the Anxiety Disorders Interview Schedule for Children (ADIS-C; Silverman & Albano, 1996) found that SET-C resulted in significantly greater remission rates compared with Testbusters (67% vs. 5%). In Australia, Spence, Donovan, and Brechman-Toussaint (2000) randomized 50 children (ages 7–14 years) diagnosed with SoD to 12 weeks of a child-focused CBT program, CBT plus parent involvement, or a wait-list condition. Both active treatment conditions resulted in higher rates of remission than the control condition at immediate posttreatment (58% vs. 87.5% vs. 7%). Treatment gains maintained and a nonsignificant trend was found at 1-year follow-up, suggesting a greater treatment effect for the CBT-plus-parent-involvement condition (53% vs. 81%).

In a study restricted to female adolescents, 35 girls who met criteria for SoD were randomized to receive 16 weeks of cognitive-behavioral group treatment for social anxiety in adolescents (CBGT-A; Albano, Marten, Holt, Heimberg, & Barlow, 1995; n = 12) or no treatment (n = 23; Hayward, et al., 2000). Youth receiving CBGT-A evidenced significantly greater remission rates compared with the no-treatment condition (45% vs. 4%). At 1-year follow-up, although no significant difference was found between the CBGT-A and no-treatment conditions (60% vs. 44%), trends emerged suggesting that CBGT-A prevented the development of subsequent depressive symptoms.

Assessment

Clinical evaluation of children and adolescents with SoD requires knowledge of normal development and the expected situations and issues that result in normative levels of social and evaluative anxiety reactions. It is essential that clinicians understand the variations in personality style, temperament, and introversion so as not to pathologize a naturally more quiet individual. Shy and introverted individuals will sometimes engage in CBT to learn specific strategies or address personal goals and issues, but a diagnosis of SoD is not automatically assumed. Most important for children and adolescents, parent involvement in the diagnostic and ongoing assessment process is essential to having a full understanding of the youth and to developing appropriate treatment plans and goals. This section reviews specific methods of assessment for social anxiety in youth.

Diagnostic Interviews

Structured or semistructured clinical interviews are the gold standard for diagnosing mental health disorders in clinical trials, and their utility in clinical practice is extended beyond reliable diagnosis to elucidating the triggers for symptoms and their severity and patterns of avoidance and escape and allowing the development of treatment targets and goals for CBT. Interviews provide the clinician with a guide for directly interviewing the child or adolescent separately from the parents, and, subsequently, allow him or her to combine the information using clinical judgment regarding the reliability of the report and knowledge of psychopathology and development. Interview methods, although high in utility and reliability when used by trained, competent clinicians, may be cumbersome in some practice settings in which time and cost constraints preclude their use (Albano & Hayward, 2004). However, diagnostic interviews provide a reliable tool for gathering both categorical and dimensional data, for making refined distinctions when comorbidity is present, and for gathering historical information regarding onset, course, and disability for clinical disorders (Albano & Hayward, 2004).

The *Anxiety Disorders Interview Schedule for Children—Child/Parent Versions* (ADIS-5; Albano & Silverman, in press), updated from the DSM-IV version (ADIS-IV), is the most often used semistructured interview to determine principal and comorbid diagnoses in clinical trials of anxiety disorders in youth (e.g., Walkup et al., 2008).The ADIS-IV demonstrated good interviewer reliability (e.g., interviewer kappa = .93; Silverman & Nelles, 1988), test–retest reliability (r = .76; Silverman & Eisen, 1992), and sensitivity to treatment effects (e.g., Kendall et al., 1997). Clinician Severity Ratings (CSRs) range from 0 ("no impairment") to 8 ("disabling impairment"); a rating of 4 represents clinical threshold warranting intervention.

Self- and Parent–Report Social Anxiety Measures

In contrast to clinician-administered diagnostic interviews, self-reports provide information on symptoms, avoidance, and distress in a relatively time- and cost-efficient manner and from varied informants (e.g., child, parent, teacher). Whereas diagnoses cannot be derived from these methods, dimensional ratings of various constructs of interest can be tracked throughout the course of treatment. Most measures take 10–15 minutes to complete, and many are available in or adaptable to tablet format or online with automated scoring. As noted in other chapters of this volume, self-report scales for assessing related constructs—such as other anxiety states, depression, broadband factors of internalizing and externalizing symptoms, parent levels of psychopathology, and family conflict—can add rich clinical information for the therapist in formulating the clinical picture and identifying areas for monitoring or intervention as direct targets of treatment. Following are three common scales used in assessing social anxiety in youth.

The *Social Phobia and Anxiety Inventory for Children* (SPAI-C; Beidel, Turner, & Fink, 1996) is a specialized self-report measure assessing symptoms of social anxiety in children ages 8–14 years. A separate parent version is also available (Higa, Fernandez, Nakamura, Chorpita, & Daleiden, 2006). The SPAI-C is composed of 26 items using a 4- point scale (0–3; "never" or "hardly ever" to "always") and contains five subscales: Assertiveness; General Conversation; Physical and Cognitive Symptoms; Avoidance; and Public Performance.

The *Social Anxiety Scale for Children—Revised* (La Greca, 1999; La Greca & Stone, 1993) also has an adolescent version and consists of 22 items assessing three factors: fear of negative evaluation, social avoidance and distress in new situations, and social avoidance and distress in general. Better reliability estimates are found with the 5-point as opposed to the 3-point rating formats (La Greca, 1998), and the overall scale has excellent psychometric properties.

The *Liebowitz Social Anxiety Scale for Children and Adolescents* (LSAS-CA; Masia-Warner et al., 2003) is a clinician-based rating scale for children ages 7–18 years and consists of 24 items rated on a 4-point scale. Each item has separate ratings of anxiety and avoidance, with separate subscales for Social Interaction situations and Performance situations. The scale has good psychometric properties, including internal consistency, test–retest reliability, and construct validity (Masia-Warner et al., 2003).

Assessment of Related Constructs

The *Child Automatic Thoughts Scale* (CATS; Schniering & Rapee, 2002) is an excellent 40-item scale for assessing the frequency of negative self-statements in children and adolescents. The CATS was developed and validated on a wide age range of youth (7–16 years old) and found to effectively discriminate between youth with and those without clinical anxiety, depression, and behavior disorders. Confirmatory factor analyses supported four distinct but strongly correlated factors relating to automatic thoughts regarding physical threat, social threat, personal failure, and hostility. Response options include a 5-point Likert scale from 0 ("not at all") to 5 ("all the time"). The CATS has demonstrated high internal consistency for the total score and subscales (alpha > .85), in addition to acceptable test–retest reliability at 1 and 3 months ($r = .91$).

The *Revised Children's Anxiety and Depression Scale—Child and Parent Form* (RCADS-C/P; Chorpita, Yim, Moffitt, Umemoto, & Francis, 2000) is a 47-item scale whose items corresponded closely to DSM-IV anxiety and major depressive disorders. Parallel parent and child versions can be used. Factor analysis has yielded subscales associated with DSM-IV diagnoses of SAD, social phobia, GAD, panic disorder, OCD, and major depressive disorder. The subscales have demonstrated good factorial validity, internal consistency, and 1-week test–retest reliability, in addition to reasonable convergent validity with other leading anxiety and depression measures (e.g., Revised Children's Manifest Anxiety Scale, Children's Depression Inventory; Chorpita et al., 2000).

The *Self-Efficacy Questionnaire for Children* (SEQ-C; Muris, 2001) is a 24-item self-report measure of youth self-efficacy. Factor analysis of the SEQ-C has revealed three factors: Social Self-Efficacy, Academic Self-Efficacy, and Emotional Self-Efficacy. The SEQ-C asks participants to indicate how well they believe they can perform a variety of activities. Response options are given on a 5-point Likert scale from 1 ("not at all") to 5 ("very well"). The SEQ-C has good reliability and internal consistency and correlates meaningfully with measures of depression and anxiety.

The *School Refusal Assessment Scale* (SRAS; Kearney & Silverman, 1993) assesses social anxiety and three other functional conditions maintaining school refusal behavior. The SRAS is administered to the child and separately to each parent (Kearney, 2001).

Idiographic Behavioral Assessment

The *Fear and Avoidance Hierarchy* (FAH) is a list of the 10 most anxiety-provoking situations as experienced by each child. Situations represented on the FAH are those most frequently avoided by the child or endured with the most distress. The FAH is generated by the child and the therapist based on situations endorsed in the ADIS or further elaborated in the early course of treatment. Children provide subjective units of distress (SUDs) ratings for each situation on a 9-point scale ranging from 0 ("not at all") to 8 ("very, very much"). The FAH is utilized as a framework for the implementation of behavioral exposures for socially anxious youth. Figure 2.1 presents a FAH for a 16-year-old female with SoD.

In addition to the FAH, behavioral approach tasks (BATs) are excellent for clinicians to use in an idiographic manner to assess the level of anxiety, subjective experience of physical sensations, cognitions, and behavioral limits of a youth in confronting social anxiety-provoking situations. Reading aloud, giving an impromptu talk, introducing oneself to an unfamiliar person, engaging in a conversation, and using a telephone are just some examples of BATs that can be conducted in a clinician's office. BATs allow the clinician to observe whether the child can attempt the task, how long he or she continues to engage in the situation, and what social skills and cognitions are observed (or absent) during a specific situation. The BAT provides observation of the youth and input into treatment planning and monitoring progress in addressing social anxiety over time.

Situation	Fear	Avoidance
1. Working with a group of classmates on a project	4	3
2. Stating my opinion when it's contrary to someone else's	4	4
3. Being wrong in front of my classmates	6	8
4. Interviewing for a summer job or internship	6	8
5. Talking to my teacher to dispute a grade that I was given or to ask for an extension on a paper	7	7
6. Asking to get together with friends/classmates who I haven't hung out with before	7	8
7. When there's silence in a conversation	7	7
8. Having a sleepover, sharing a room with someone on a class trip, or doing an overnight for a college visit with students I don't know	8	8
9. Taking important tests like the SAT	8	8
10. Being the one to have to entertain somebody or make the arrangements for a get together	8	8

FIGURE 2.1. Fear and avoidance hierarchy for social phobia from a 16-year-old female.

A CBT Model: Social Anxiety and Developmental Transitions

Recently, we proposed a CBT model that incorporates the stages and tasks of development in understanding the impairment resulting from SoD and related anxiety disorders, as well as overprotection and overinvolvement of parents (Detweiler et al., 2014; Guerry et al., 2015). This approach is an enhanced version of our CBGT-A (Albano, 1995; Albano & DiBartolo, 2007a, 2007b; Albano et al., 1995; Hayward et al., 2000). Development sets the stage for continual challenges and transitions from early childhood to adulthood. Consistent with a developmental and family-informed intervention approach, we integrate CBGT-A for SoD (e.g., self-monitoring, psychoeducation, cognitive restructuring, exposure) with developmentally informed interventions designed to promote age-related independent functioning, meet normative developmental tasks, and prepare for appropriate transition to the next life stage. CBT components are meant to increase self-sufficiency by targeting youth social anxiety, as well as delays or deficits in life skills (e.g., problem solving, self-soothing, increasing personal responsibilities in self-care), parental overinvolvement (parent psychoedu-cation, goal setting, family communication, proactive cognitive coaching), and transition of age-appropriate tasks to the youth. Given that social anxi-ety is maintained in part by parental behaviors that inadvertently allow the child or adolescent either active or passive avoidance of socially challeng-ing activities, parent inclusion in the treatment program is meant to iden-tify and critically evaluate parent–youth patterns of interaction to expose unhealthy relationships that may take the form of overprotection, overcon-trol, or lack of confidence in the patient by the parent and/or avoidance of taking on age-appropriate responsibility on the part of the patient (passive or active).

Overview of the Treatment Plan

The plan is a flexibly applied treatment model that is tailored for each youth and family and presented in four phases. Although we present a session-by-session guide below, clinicians can personalize the goals and interven-tions according to the youth's level of clinical impairment, degree needed of family involvement to achieve clinical and developmental goals, and ability of the youth and caretakers to participate in the treatment. Hence, within each phase there could be more or fewer sessions to meet the needs of the youth.

Phase I: Psychoeducation—Understanding Social Anxiety, Development, and CBT

Session 1: Introduction to Social Anxiety and Developmental Transitions

- *Goals.* In this first session, patients and parents together are intro-duced to the model of SoD and the goals and process of CBT. The three-component model of anxiety is emphasized to encourage patients and par-ents to examine their own responses to social anxiety-provoking triggers within each component. CBT is described and the rationale explained. Therapists begin work on realistic, age-appropriate goal setting with the patients and their parents.

- *Rationale.* Parents attend with patients to learn the model of SoD and to understand the interaction of thoughts, feelings, and behavior.

- *Interventions.* Patients and parents are provided with reading mate-rials about SoD. Goal setting and self-monitoring are taught and assigned. Specifically, patients and parents will be asked to identify both short-term (e.g., 1 week, 1 month, 3 months) and long-term goals for the patient. Patients are taught use of a daily diary to monitor social anxiety-provoking situations and responses in the three-component model. Caretakers are provided with a structure for reporting their observations of the patient's functioning in anxiety-provoking situations.

Session 2: Examine Patterns of Social Anxiety and Avoidance

• *Goals*. Current domains of social anxiety and patterns of avoidance are examined. The therapist uses patient experiences and parent observations to highlight examples of the functional relationship between social anxiety and avoidance. A subgoal is to bring initial attention to the ways in which social anxiety has shaped certain patient–parent relations.

• *Rationale*. Discussions of the patient's own experiences with social anxiety can help him or her begin to learn to identify triggers, his or her own responses, and the reinforcing cycle of avoidance that serves to maintain the social anxiety. Using the goals set in Session 1, therapists will discuss the ways in which social anxiety interferes with goal attainment. The patient and parents are encouraged to discuss ways that they interact in response to the patient's anxiety and avoidance.

• *Interventions*. Socratic questioning will help lead patients to identify their emotional and behavioral reactions to their anxiety triggers and parents to discuss their reactions to the patients' behavior. A social anxiety hierarchy is developed that incorporates personally relevant social situations that trigger excessive social anxiety and behavioral avoidance (see Figure 2.2).

Sessions 3 and 4: Developmental Origins of SoD and Maintaining Factors

• *Goals*. Together, patients and parents attend sessions 3 and 4, in which etiological factors are discussed within a developmental psychopathology perspective. Biological and environmental factors are discussed in terms of elevating risk or exacerbating the expression of SoD. Therapists will explain the reciprocal interaction of heightened child anxiety and the emergence of certain parental behaviors that can inadvertently maintain social anxiety, such as parental overprotection. Focus is on patient–parent interactions that are characterized by patient avoidance or dependence and parent overinvolvement and assistance in age- and stage-related tasks. A major goal of these sessions is to identify the patient's functioning in specific age-appropriate tasks and elucidate the ways in which parents have assumed responsibility for the patient, in efforts to protect him or her from excessive anxiety, failure, missed opportunities, or other negative outcomes. This will set the stage for identifying any deficits in problem solving, social skills, assertiveness, and related social problem-solving skills that may be absent or deficient. Ultimately, the therapist will facilitate, through graded exposure, a transfer of responsibility for various role-functioning tasks from the parent to the patient, as his or her skill deficits are remediated.

• *Rationale.* These are critical sessions whereby patient–parent interactions and relationship patterns are examined to assist the participants in understanding the ways that seemingly helpful behaviors on the part of parents become drawn into the cycle of anxiety and avoidance, as help seeking by the patient becomes entrenched through a negative reinforcement paradigm.

• *Interventions.* Therapists are instructed to reframe what may be interpreted by some as assigning responsibility ("I caused my child to be this way") as a rational and natural expression of parenting a younger child (i.e., "Parents are meant to protect, reassure, and comfort"). The role of child anxiety, repeated and unrelenting through childhood and early adolescence, should be understood as shaping the patient–parent interactions. The therapists and participants will discuss past occurrences of help seeking and avoidant behavior in response to anxiety that prompted parent overinvolvement. Elucidating these interactions and evaluating their impact in terms of short- and long-term cost–benefit outcomes will assist the patient in understanding how avoidant patterns are learned and maintained. A hierarchy of developmental tasks is created collaboratively between all parties as a first step in developing a plan to transition responsibility to the patient for both anxiety management and developmentally appropriate role transitions and tasks. Table 2.2 presents tasks that are the focus of the developmental hierarchy and chosen to reflect expected functioning for a youth's age and stage.

Once the hierarchy is developed, parents will be invited back for further sessions as needed. At this point, the burden of responsibility for treatment and focus of attention is shifted solely to the patient. Patients are responsible for setting and keeping their own appointments as a step toward shaping their acceptance of responsibility.

Phase II: Individual Skills Training in Cognitive Restructuring and Social Problem-Solving Skills

Sessions 5 and 6: Cognitive Restructuring Skills Training

• *Goals.* To teach patients to identify, evaluate, and refute thoughts and beliefs that impede their ability to function in social situations and effectively master age-related roles and tasks.

TABLE 2.2. Developmental Hierarchy Items

- Takes control of personal self-care (e.g., puts him- or herself to sleep at reasonable hour and wakes on his or her own, health care, exercise, diet, maintains clean clothing).
- Seeks information from available sources when needed (reference books, teacher, study guides, want ads, information sites online for summer activities or college).
- Displays appropriate emotional independence from parents (self-soothing, conflict resolution, managing difficult emotions).
- Takes action independent from parents as appropriate (assertiveness, task completion, shows initiative).
- Wakes up on his or her own and is on time to school and appointments.
- Able to navigate travel within community on his or her own using appropriate level of transportation (school bus, public transportation, arranging rides to outings).
- Takes care of basic household assigned tasks (chores, prepares own simple meals and snacks, runs errands as appropriate, does laundry).
- Asks for and manages basic health care as needed (e.g., by mid-teens will attend annual physical on his or her own, schedules and keeps own doctor and therapist appointments).
- Manages own choices for grooming and dressing (e.g., shopping for clothing, hair-care appointments).
- Takes driving lessons; attains license.
- Manages money responsibly.
- Initiates social activities, calls and sees friends outside of school.
- Engages in activities such as school clubs or other extracurricular programs.
- Engages in volunteer community or civic service as appropriate (e.g., registers to vote at age 18).

- *Rationale.* Negative, self-defeating self-talk arises from inaccurate beliefs about the potential dangers of social situations, negative predictions about the outcomes of social situations, and negative recall bias about one's performance in past social interactions. These biases result in negative self-appraisal of one's ability to manage social anxiety-provoking tasks, setting up avoidance patterns and a shifting of management of age-appropriate tasks and role responsibilities to others.

- *Interventions.* Using techniques from individual CBT and CBGT-A, therapists teach Socratic questioning to devise rational disputes for automatic thoughts and negative schema. Role plays and *in vivo* behavioral experiments assist the patient in engaging in activities that undermine their beliefs and provide evidence to refute their negative thinking. Systematic homework assignments assist in developing a healthy cognitive self-coaching style.

Sessions 7–9: Social Problem Solving and Behavioral Skills Training

• *Goals.* To provide concrete tools for managing difficult situations, remediating specific social and behavioral skill deficits, and/or promoting healthy and independent self-soothing behaviors that will enable patients to get their needs met and meet responsibilities in different life domains (e.g., school/work, friendships, self-care).

• *Rationale.* To address the anxiety-mediated behavioral avoidance that solidifies skill deficits by preventing the opportunity to experience, test, and refine skills that should naturally emerge throughout childhood and adolescence. Failure to develop effective behavioral skills furthers the dependence on others and interferes with effective role transitions.

• *Interventions.* Patients are taught to identify cues that activate their beliefs about insecurity and failure and the subsequent behaviors that result in self-defeating cycles of avoidance and escape. To provide patients with a broad tool for preventing negative spirals of anxiety and comorbid affective disturbance, problem-solving skills are taught and applied to a range of situations encountered in daily life. Examples include prioritizing time allocation when multiple tasks demand attention or approaching and negotiating with superiors (e.g., teachers, supervisors). Individual skills deficits identified during the assessment phase and early treatment sessions are addressed through the application of specific CBT techniques (e.g., assertiveness and social skills training, relaxation training, affect regulation). Patients learn to integrate cognitive restructuring into adaptive problem solving and/or specific areas of skills training to reduce their reliance on others and develop proactive, coping-focused independent solutions to daily issues and challenges. Didactic instruction, Socratic questioning, role play, and behavioral homework assignments are utilized to facilitate skill acquisition.

Session 10: Increasing Independent Functioning and Transfer of Responsibilities (Conjoint Session)

• *Goals.* Patients and parents attend this session (and additional sessions as needed) together to continue the process of building proactive, independent self-management skills and encourage positive role transitions.

• *Rationale.* Following the skills training sessions, parents are included in this session to address ongoing overprotective patterns and to further reinforce disengagement and transfer of responsibility to the patient.

- *Interventions.* Using the task hierarchy developed in Phase I, the therapist assists the patient and parents in uncovering interaction patterns that impede the patient's independent behavior. Communication skills training and family problem solving (Wells & Albano, 2005) are taught to facilitate this process. Parents and patients are encouraged to discuss their fears, expectations, and hopes for this process and for role transitions. Parents are provided with a model of a healthy, positive coaching style to support the patient and encourage the use of CBT skills. Cognitive restructuring, role plays, and behavioral experiments are used to progress through the task hierarchy and allow the patient to develop success experience in managing tasks.

Phase III: Integrated Therapeutic Exposure Groups

Group exposure sessions are offered in cycles of 10 sessions at the beginner (i.e., new to CBT and exposure), intermediate (i.e., prior participation in CBT and/or exposure groups), or advanced level. We also assign to level based on the patient's experience of distress and disability from the anxiety. An individual may repeat the beginner or intermediate groups as often as he or she needs to, as the advanced group is often focused on high-level and *in vivo* exposures in real-world settings (e.g., putting in applications for a job). These groups allow the youth to test and refine his or her cognitive and behavioral skills within the experience of the therapeutic exposure exercise.

- *Goals.* Exposure is the core behavioral component of CBT for social anxiety and phobic disorders, and its inclusion has a significant favorable impact on the trajectory of reducing symptoms (Peris et al., 2015). By this point, patients will have learned skills for cognitive restructuring and remediation of specific behavioral skill deficits. Also, patient–parent interactions involved in the maintenance of SoD are made explicit, and a gradual plan of transition to proactive, independent functioning is in progress. In this phase, patients engage in group exposure sessions composed of six to eight age-similar youth and following the exposure procedures outlined in CBGT-A (Albano & DiBartolo, 2007a, 2007b). Group-based exposure exercises allow an ecologically valid milieu in which patients can test out their skills, receiving and giving feedback to one another with the goal of facilitating the attenuation or tolerance of anxiety while increasing experience in coping mastery and proactive problem solving.

- *Rationale.* Habituation, or tolerance, to rises in anxiety occurs through the repeated exposure of the individual to feared and previously avoided situations. Exposure provides the patient with experience in confronting his or her fears while testing and refining his or her cognitive restructuring skills. Repeated exposure allows the patient to gather evidence to refute his or her automatic thoughts while building coping templates for similar situations as they occur. The cycle of negative reinforcement of escape or avoidance is extinguished through exposure, as the patient is able to learn that entering or staying in a situation may result in initial rises of anxiety but that the anxiety will naturally dissipate or can be tolerated as he or she stays with the situation and focuses his or her attention on what is actually transpiring, as opposed to focusing on his or her internal, anxious state.

• *Interventions.* The therapist and patient collaborate to define and develop exposure situations both within session and *in vivo*. Initial exposures begin with items from the social anxiety hierarchy that are rated at a moderate level and that can be reproduced in session with ecological validity. Therapists will follow the structure of exposures outlined in individual cognitive behavioral therapy (ICBT), or in CBT as usual, one-on-one with the therapist, and CBGT-A: (1) define the situation, (2) specify concrete and observable behavioral goals, (3) identify and challenge automatic thoughts, (4) conduct a 10- to 15-minute exposure, and (5) examine and process the exposure. Examining and processing the exposure involves guiding the patient through an analysis of what happened to his or her anxiety during the exposure while attending to the occurrence of and degree of success with challenging automatic thoughts. Initially, office-based exposures are developed with the goal to move the patient to *in vivo* exposures in relevant community-based settings. Concurrently, items from the developmental task hierarchy are assigned and eventually imbedded in these exposures to facilitate the acceptance of responsibility and development of independent role-related behaviors. Homework tasks are assigned to promote the generalization of exposure gains.

Phase IV: Solidifying Gains and Relapse Prevention

Follow-Up Family Session: Consolidating Independent Functioning and Acceptance of Role Responsibilities

• *Goals.* A final conjoint patient and parent session is scheduled toward the end of treatment. In a prior individual session, the therapist works with the patient to define the issues to be presented in this session and assist the patient in accepting responsibility for managing the session. The focus is on the patient's facilitating a discussion with his or her parents and collaboration over full acceptance of role responsibilities. A related goal is to assist the parents in letting go of control and in viewing their son or daughter as a responsible and capable adolescent or emerging adult.

- *Rationale.* Parents often maintain control for fear of their child's not following through with or mismanaging a responsibility. By putting the patient in control of the agenda and progress of the session, the parent gains experience with allowing the transfer of control to occur while also learning that errors or mistakes occur but that they also facilitate learning and problem solving.

- *Interventions.* While the therapist models confidence in the patient by giving over the session and using a healthy coaching style when indicated, the patient is encouraged to use family problem solving to work through final plans for transitioning responsibility for personally relevant tasks that the parent has managed (e.g., requesting an appointment to discuss a medication issue). Behavioral contracts are used as needed to specify upcoming role transitions and responsibilities that are not yet within the age-appropriate limit for the patient (e.g., looking for a part-time summer job, scheduling college interviews, working with an apartment locator service) but that are imminent. These contracts should specify each individual's responsibilities and operationally defined time limits for completion, along with a problem-solving plan for what to do if the task or transition is not completed.

Final Group and Individual Sessions (Roughly Sessions 20–22): Final Exposures, Relapse Prevention, and Termination

- *Goals.* Patient and therapist in these sessions discuss how to apply skills and self-guided exposure to promote continued anxiety management and acceptance of role responsibilities. A large focus in these sessions will be on preventing the patient from returning to old coping patterns (e.g., avoidance and escape behavior, forfeiting of responsibility) once therapy is terminated. Initial goals are reviewed to determine whether changes have occurred, and the patient's progress and ongoing issues are addressed. The patient's future goals and expectations for transitions to his or her next developmental stage are discussed.

- *Rationale.* Patients will continue to be confronted with social anxiety-provoking situations and developmental challenges after therapy ends. The patient and therapist will evaluate treatment progress and goal attainment to facilitate self-efficacy about anxiety management and acceptance of role-related responsibilities.

- *Interventions.* We encourage our patients to discuss their feelings associated with termination of therapy and working on their own. Thoughts and beliefs related to increasing responsibility for oneself and role transitions are processed, and this is very individualized for each patient.

The patient and therapist discuss methods for increasing exposure to more complex and challenging social anxiety situations (e.g., negotiating for a change in grade with a teacher, standing up to a peer who is rejecting of the patient, confronting a college roommate about substance use) that will emerge with role transitions. Skills and exposure exercises are utilized to examine these hypothetical situations, and written relapse prevention plans are developed with the patient. Patient and therapist maintain open discussion of termination while processing appropriate use of support systems such as parents or future therapy contacts posttreatment.

Case Example

Jackson was referred by a local psychiatrist for the treatment of long-standing social anxiety and attention-deficit/hyperactivity disorder (ADHD). At the time of referral, Jack was a sophomore in a private high school in New York City. Although Jack was an excellent student and liked by his teachers, Jack's parents were worried about his lack of participation in any extracurricular activities and his increasing avoidance of meeting up with longtime friends. Rather than getting together with friends to attend outings, parties, or school events, Jack spent most of his time alone, either reading, playing his guitar, or gaming online. He had been diagnosed with ADHD, primarily inattentive type, at age 7 and had responded well to a stimulant medication. Jack met with the child psychiatrist several times per year, and there were no adverse events or problems with his low dose of stimulant medication. His psychiatrist noted Jack's social reticence and timidity throughout his childhood and often commented to Jack and his parents about this. Through his sixth-grade year, Jack always had two or three good friends who would come over for playdates when arranged by his mother. With advancing adolescence, these playdates grew more infrequent, and Jack refused to attend the parties, baseball games, and sleepovers to which he was invited. Although Jack's friends still attended school with him, he saw them very rarely and usually on his birthday or when his parents also arranged to get together with the families of these boys. Hence, by sophomore year, his parents were increasingly concerned about his growing social isolation and contacted his psychiatrist, who referred him for a diagnostic consultation and for CBT through our anxiety specialty clinic.

Assessment Results

Social anxiety was Jack's most prominent anxiety concern. He reported being often "worried that I won't look happy enough" to others and that they would then feel uncomfortable around him. In response to the ADIS, Jackson reported that he was anxious and avoided giving talks or presentations; introducing himself to a group; performing in front of others; eating in public; most social interactions, including attending parties; speaking to unfamiliar persons; participating in class or meetings; talking with girls to whom he was attracted; talking to persons in authority positions, including teachers; taking any sort of test (despite doing well on exams); being assertive with peers or unfamiliar people; and initiating and maintaining conversations. Jack recognized that social anxiety interfered with his life and reported that he had had "a ton of friends" in elementary school, although he was quiet then, too. He played T-ball and then Little League but dropped out by sixth grade due to his discomfort. He struggled through his freshman year of high school and felt different from the other kids, who all seemed to be enjoying school and socializing. During the school year, Jackson was comfortable and at ease only from Friday afternoons through Sunday mornings or over holidays. Summers were much better, although there were struggles with his parents regarding how to fill his day, and the dread of school started to creep in during the first week of August. At 14, he could never recall a full school year being at ease and happy to be around others. He also reported much anticipatory anxiety about exams and presentations, so much so that he had "meltdowns" of irritability, panic sensations, and outbursts at his parents, most especially when they tried to help him in any way. Jack's parents confirmed his report, and they added that he also retreated to his room when family or friends came to visit and that he did not mix and speak to people when they were out as a family or vacationing. He did not order for himself in a restaurant, and his mother shopped for him to buy clothing, school supplies, and anything that he could not get for himself online. With the exception of ADHD, no other psychopathology was identified, although Jack was evidencing mild symptoms of depression that did not meet diagnostic significance but did need monitoring. Based on the ADIS, Jack was assigned a diagnosis of SoD, generalized subtype, at a clinician severity rating of 6 on the 0 ("none at all") to 8 ("severely disabling/disturbing") scale.

Phase I of Treatment

Treatment began with Jackson, his parents, and the therapist developing an agreement on the boundaries of confidentiality and that, outside of situations involving self-harm, suicidality, or intent to harm another, all that Jackson discussed would be kept private. The need for a collaborative working relationship between the therapist and Jack and, at specified times such as during this initial phase, also including the parents, was presented and agreed to by all the parties. As noted in the outline of sessions above, Jack and his parents were then engaged in a discussion about the nature of social anxiety, the ways that overprotection may contribute to maintaining the problem, and the plans for learning specific CBT skills to reduce anxiety and increase functioning. During our sessions, Jack and his parents were asked to describe their reactions to socially challenging situations according to the three components (what you think, feel, and do) so that all might understand how the emotion manifests. In this way, Jack's parents also were able to relate to various aspects of the three components and identified feelings of irritability and physical sensations within themselves when anxious. His parents were then asked to report on their treatment goals for Jack:

- Developing coping skills for independence
- Increasing self-confidence
- Lessening self-consciousness
- Experiencing more joy and happiness
- Decreasing fear of such things as buying clothes, answering the phone, and being wrong

Jack's goals were also identified and discussed:

- Feeling more comfortable joining conversations and less self-conscious
- Asking people to hang out with him outside of school
- Decreasing his fear of rejection
- Speaking up in class
- Reaching out to friends in school more than once per week
- Being OK with changing his mind about something
- Not replaying what he's done in his mind and judging himself negatively again and again
- Asking teacher and peers for help when he needed it

Specifying these goals allowed the family and the therapist to discuss setting realistic, observable goals and linking these to the process and role of exposure in helping to apply anxiety management skills in these situations. Through these sessions, it was also found that, in response to Jack's feeling stuck or about to "melt down" with anxiety, his parents engaged in any number of responses that all agreed were not often helpful. These included nagging, overidentifying with him, taking over for him and doing what he couldn't do, encouraging him, leaving him alone, yelling, getting angry, and trying to distract him. Mostly, and through tears, Jack's mother and father reported feeling increasingly helpless and guilty about Jack's anxiety and not sure how to respond to assist him. They reported feeling frustrated and at times responded in anger when they tried to do what was best when Jack was upset but found Jack to be unable or unwilling to accept their help. In response, Jack was asked to identify what he found helpful from his parents. This led to a discussion of his feelings of guilt and shame about imposing his anxiety on his parents; he said that he felt stuck and unable to accept his parent's help, then retreated, which, he recognized, made things worse. These honest discussions enabled Jack and his parents to discuss these feelings and come to an understanding of mutual respect for one another's perspectives, which led to their being able to communicate clearly and to find time for problem solving, as well as to respect boundaries and do relaxing things together. As we often have found, these sessions resulted in the family's talking through the anxiety and each other's reactions, with the result of agreeing to talk out their feelings rather than to retreat. Most of all, Jack received good support and reinforcement of his feelings, as well as an understanding of his parents' perspectives. As a result of these sessions, Jack and his parents devised a developmental hierarchy of age-appropriate tasks that he would start assuming that had been done by or with much prodding from his parents (Figure 2.2). These tasks, in addition to his social anxiety, were to be worked on by Jack and his therapist. The tasks themselves had some overlap with anxiety; however, it was mostly habit that kept him from doing these things or from trying to take them on. A total of four sessions were provided to Jack and his parents in this first phase of therapy.

Rate each task according to the degree of emotional challenge (e.g., 0 = "not at all"; 100 = "the most emotionally challenging") and degree of independence in completing the task (e.g., 0 = "I am never independent in completing this task"; 100 = "I am always independent in completing this task").

Task	Emotional Challenge	Independence
Looking for a summer internship	100	0
Meeting with my doctor alone	100	0
Buying my own clothes	100	0
Waking up to alarm clock on own	90	10
Preparing my own food	80	10
Doing my own laundry	70	25
Washing my dishes	50	40
Taking the subway/bus to get around	50	40
Exercising two to three times per week	40	35
Turning off computer by 11 P.M.	40	30
Getting 7 to 8 hours of sleep per night	30	45

FIGURE 2.2. Jack's developmental hierarchy.

Phase II of Treatment

Jack worked with the same therapist during this second phase of therapy, which focused on skills training and preparing for the exposure phase of treatment. First, Jack's individual fear and avoidance hierarchy was developed so that he could track his own progress over therapy and also define targets for the later exposure phase. Jack was a socially skilled young man who had developed habits of looking down instead of straight at someone when conversing, of talking himself out of engaging in situations through self-deprecating statements, and of retreating at the earliest physical sensation associated with anxiety. This resulted in Jack's not speaking up in class or volunteering to join in discussions, staying in study hall instead of eating lunch with his friends, and avoiding a wide range of social activities with peers. He reported that the last party that he had attended was in seventh grade, although he had been asked to go by his friends. He did not return text messages and never posted on his Facebook page, which was set up for him by his mother. Jack was upset with himself for not attending school dances or allowing himself to hang out with his friends after school, as he knew they were getting together, and yet he felt too anxious to join. Also, when a girl to whom he was attracted approached him, he felt shaky or nervous and beat a retreat down a different corridor at school or ducked into a restroom.

Therapy during this phase comprised six individual sessions in which Jack was first taught somatic management skills and self-monitoring. He found breathing exercises particularly helpful and was encouraged to use a downloadable app called "MindShift" to coach him in these skills and other "chill out" skills. Jack was instructed in using self-monitoring forms to track the three components of anxiety, and through this he was able to identify his automatic, negative self-talk. As an example, Jack had to reply to his school advisor about setting up a time to meet to discuss his electives for junior year. Despite having written a reply, he reported having left the email unanswered for over a week and endorsed feeling nervous "right before clicking 'send,'" so he just simply avoided his email. His specific thoughts were: "My spelling and grammar might not be good enough and he'll think I'm stupid"; "He might think I'm not interested in school because I don't know what I want to take." The therapist helped him identify these thoughts as examples of the "mind reading" thinking trap, pointing out that Jack couldn't know what the advisor was thinking unless he asked him or the advisor offered to give Jack some feedback. On another occasion, a long-standing friend had asked Jack to have lunch, and, although this was generally a positive experience for him, the friend had also invited some unfamiliar peers to sit with them. Jack reported that he attempted to go outside of his comfort zone and sit with the group; however, one young woman commented that Jack was "very quiet" and that she "never sees me outside of a classroom." Jack reported that he felt flushed and his heart was racing. He had the thought that she was not interested in his being a part of their lunch table and that she never would have spoken to him if she hadn't been stuck sitting next to him. He felt like leaving but, at the same time, felt frozen in place. Using the downward arrow technique, the therapist helped Jack to identify his core beliefs and fears associated with his thoughts that he was not likable nor able to have friends. Jack was encouraged to identify thinking traps, reappraise the situation, and generate alternative thoughts. In brainstorming alternatives to his negative thoughts, Jack admitted that she was kind and smiling at him and that she talked to him and not to the whole group. He did respond to her questions, and although he did not ask her any, this girl kept talking to him about school and her interests and asked about his. She also offered to share her dessert with him, which he accepted but "felt like the cookie was stuck in my throat." Jack was able to recognize that she was being kind, friendly, and maybe even flirtatious, and also that she was possibly giving a message that she would like to see him join the table at lunch more often. These types of cognitive restructuring exercises helped to loosen Jack's tendency to jump to negative conclusions. Role playing with the therapist, Jack practiced addressing these situations while engaging in rational responding to his negative thoughts. Problem-solving skills were used to address situations in which Jack felt stuck or behind on a task (e.g., reviewing options for next year's courses). And Jack began working on his developmental hierarchy, taking on getting up on his own in the morning, making his own meals when his parents were not at home, and doing his chores at home without needing his parents' prompting. Throughout these sessions, the therapist also prepared Jack for the next phase of treatment, group-based exposure therapy.

Phase III: Exposure Group

Jack entered a beginner social anxiety group with five other teenagers. Each group met for 90 minutes and was co-led by two therapists. Jack and the group members were told that in this phase they would feel anxious, as the goal was to expose them to the situations that they feared and avoided, while providing them with the opportunity to try out and refine their anxiety management skills. The first groups involved some classic group-process and engagement-building exercises to develop cohesion and to get used to being together in session. During the first few group sessions, therapists wove psychoeducation about social anxiety, with emphasis on the role of avoidance in solidifying anxiety, into the group session. Cognitive restructuring was conducted throughout the exposures. In the first group, Jack and each member had shared anxiety-provoking situations and the associated anxious thoughts, feelings, and behaviors that occurred over the previous week. As each of the members had individual CBT sessions to prepare for this phase, very quickly the group brainstormed the following anxiety-provoking exposures to attempt in the group: bothering others, asking for help, and maintaining a conversation when you don't have much in common with the other people. Individual group members engaged in exposures by initiating and maintaining conversations, while the rest of the group was "double exposed" by assisting as role players and giving feedback to the group members on their performances during the exposure.

An early exposure for Jack involved giving a speech in front of the group about the upcoming World Series and his thoughts on the Yankees' chances to win the title. He reported automatic thoughts, such as "I want to get out of here" and "I hope I don't make a bad impression." He was also able to come up with rational responses, such as "I will talk about what I know and give my best effort." Jack reported that his anxiety rating before the exposure was at a 90 on the 0–100 scale. His goals were to look at the audience when he spoke, be able to pause and read from his note card, and to talk for at least 5 minutes. Jack met his goals and reported decreasing anxiety ratings throughout the talk: 95, 90, 80, 80, 70, and 70 for each minute that he spoke. Also, in the minutes following the talk when he had to answer questions about his topic, he continued to look at the questioner, and his anxiety fell further, to a final rating of 50. Jack completed his goal and reported feeling good about having given the talk and looking at people. Various exposures were conducted targeting Jack's individual fears. In an exposure for "starting a conversation with several kids at lunch," Jack was able to be engaged and asked the three other youth who were role players in the exposure a lot of questions, and he even told some jokes and was able to maintain the conversation for 10 minutes. At the end of this exposure, group members gave Jack positive feedback on his great social skills. Jack had reported a baseline anxiety rating of 65, and at the end of exposure, this fell to 35.

As the group progressed, Jack was given a mixed *in vivo* exposure—mixed in that his anxiety and a developmental goal were challenged. One of Jack's developmental hierarchy items was to take public transportation to get around, rather than relying on his parents' driving him. There was no parental objection to this and no safety concerns, just that Jack had never traveled on his own to get around, and this also hampered his ability to get out with friends. Hence, Jack was sent an email for a "mission is possible" task stating that he was to take the subway to the group session on his own and providing him with a form to fill in and record his pre-exposure thoughts and anxiety ratings. Jack reported that the situation was initially "stressful" and that he had a "pit in his stomach" due to not having done this before and his thoughts that he would get lost and be late, resulting in looking foolish in front of the group. His coping thought was "If I can do this, I can go many places that I want to visit," and his initial anxiety was rated as a 75. Jack did arrive late, as the subway was stalled for a while (not unusual in New York City), but Jack coped well and arrived flushed but smiling, reporting that he had challenged his own anxiety and mastered a new task without help from his parents. He reported that upon arriving at the Columbus Circle subway station, his anxiety was by then a 20 and that he had thought, "I can't believe I haven't done this already, it's really not that bad, just a bit smelly in places."

Phase IV and Beyond

Jack and his parents met twice more to continue his progress in taking on responsibility and increasing his social interactions. He continued to push himself in group to address his social anxiety and took two more rounds of group through the following 2 years, during which time he increased the intensity and focus of his exposures to include traveling to a college interview on his own, volunteering to debate a fellow student in class about a political issue, and engaging in more activities with his friends outside of school. In relapse prevention, Jack was taught to recognize when anxiety was again rising, and this was readily apparent in a situation in which Jack found himself at a party, was anxious about how he'd present himself to others and how to fit in. Consequently, and not unlike other youth, Jack drank at this party, and despite not wanting to take shots of alcohol, he could not say no, wound up very drunk, and vomited in the taxi on his way home. Fortunately, his parents were awake and able to assist him. This was his first time drinking in this way, and it was dealt with in group as well as discussed with his primary therapist. Jack recognized that he was drinking to fit in and to reduce his anxiety in the moment. Peer refusal skills and harm reduction strategies were employed. Fortunately, this was an isolated incident, and, although Jack did drink again at times, he was careful not to drink on an empty stomach, to manage his anxious thoughts with skills, and not overindulge in alcohol. Jack's parents also handled this situation well by expressing their concern for him and listening to his feelings about the drinking and party scene and his plans for managing future situations involving alcohol. At the conclusion of his therapy, Jack had engaged in individual therapy, family work on his developmental milestones and anxiety, and three rounds of group exposure therapy (a total of 30 sessions) over a 2½-year period that eventually led to his graduation from high school and move to an out-of-state college. During the winter break of his freshman year of college, Jack came to our clinic for an intensive 2-week booster group and worked on several situations that prompted anxiety (speaking to the professors, dealing with his roommate's late-night work habits, advocating for extra time due to his ADHD) in the college setting. Both Jack and his parents were pleased with his progress and with his taking responsibility on his own to manage anxiety in a mature and independent manner.

Conclusion

Social anxiety is common, and SoD can be a chronic mental health condition that starts early in life and may extend well into adulthood. The distress experienced by individuals with SoD is real, uncomfortable, and alarming, resulting in interference in family and friend relationships, school progress, self-care, and meeting critical tasks of development. Advances in the CBT of SoD are examined in this chapter and provide hope for many who can access this form of psychotherapy in their community or by new and innovative means that are being developed in online approaches (e.g., Joyable) and via technology (e.g., see Camp Cope-A-Lot for younger children; Kendall & Khanna, 2008). Although not covered in this chapter, pharmacological treatments for social anxiety are also efficacious, especially when combined with CBT (e.g., Walkup et al., 2008), and are available for more moderate to severely impairing disability. Overall, the advances in the treatment of social anxiety gives hope to many youth who otherwise would suffer in silence but, like Jack, can go onto pursue their interests and lead a productive and full life.

References

Albano, A. M. (1995). Treatment of social anxiety in adolescents. *Cognitive and Behavioral Practice, 2*, 271–298.

Albano, A. M., Chorpita, B. F., & Barlow, D. H. (2003). Anxiety disorders. In E. J. Mash & R. A. Barkley (Eds.), *Child psychopathology* (2nd ed., pp. 279–329). New York: Guilford Press.

Albano, A. M., & DiBartolo, P. M. (2007a). *Stand up, speak out: Adolescent workbook*. New York: Oxford University Press.

Albano, A. M., & DiBartolo, P. M. (2007b). *Stand up, speak out: Therapist manual for cognitive behavioral therapy for social phobia in adolescents*. New York: Oxford University Press.

Albano, A. M., & Hayward, C. (2004). The developmental psychopathology approach to understanding and treating social anxiety disorder. In T. H. Ollendick & J. S. March (Eds.), *Phobic and anxiety disorders: A clinician's guide to effective psychosocial and pharmacological interventions* (pp. 198–235). New York: Oxford University Press.

Albano, A. M., & Kendall, P. C. (2002). Cognitive behavioural therapy for children and adolescents with anxiety disorders: Clinical research advances. *International Review of Psychiatry, 14*, 128–133.

Albano, A. M., Marten, P. A., Holt, C. S., Heimberg, R. G., & Barlow, D. H. (1995). Cognitive-behavioral treatment for social phobia in adolescents: A preliminary study. *Journal of Nervous and Mental Disease, 183*, 649–656.

Albano, A. M. (with Pepper, L.). (2013). *You and your anxious child: Free your child from fears and worries and create a joyful family life*. New York: Penguin Press.

Albano, A. M., & Silverman, W. K. (in press). *The Anxiety Disorders Interview Schedule for DSM-5—Child and Parent Versions*. New York: Oxford University Press.

American Psychiatric Association. (2013). *Diagnostic and statistical manual of mental disorders* (5th ed.). Arlington, VA: Author.

Asendorpf, J. (1994). The malleability of behavioral inhibition: A study of individual developmental function. *Developmental Psychology, 30,* 912–919.

Barlow, D. H. (2002). *Anxiety and its disorders* (2nd ed.). New York: Guilford Press.

Barrett, P. M., Dadds, M. R., & Rapee, R. M. (1996). Family treatment of childhood anxiety: A controlled trial. *Journal of Consulting and Clinical Psychology, 64*(2), 333–342.

Barrett, P. M., Duffy, A. L., Dadds, M. R., & Rapee, R. M. (2001). Cognitive-behavioral treatment of anxiety disorders in children: Long-term (6-year) follow-up. *Journal of Consulting and Clinical Psychology, 69*(1), 135–141.

Barrett, P. M., Rapee, R. M., Dadds, M. M., & Ryan, S. M. (1996). Family enhancement of cognitive style in anxious and aggressive children. *Journal of Abnormal Child Psychology, 24,* 187–203.

Beidel, D. C., Turner, S. M., & Fink, C. M. (1996). Assessment of childhood social phobia: Construct, convergent, and discriminative validity of the Social Phobia and Anxiety Inventory for Children (SPAI-C). *Psychological Assessment, 8*(3), 235–240.

Beidel, D. C., Turner, S. M., & Morris, T. L. (1999). "Psychopathology of childhood social phobia." *Journal of the American Academy of Child and Adolescent Psychiatry, 38*(6), 643–650.

Beidel, D. C., Turner, S. M., & Morris, T. L. (2000). Behavioral treatment of childhood social phobia. *Journal of Consulting and Clinical Psychology, 68*(6), 1072–1080.

Beidel, D. C., Turner, S. M., & Taylor-Ferreira, J. C. (1999). Teaching study skills and test-taking strategies to elementary school students: The Testbusters Program. *Behavior Modification, 23,* 630–646.

Burstein, M., He, J.-P., Kattan, G., Albano, A. M., Avenevoli, S., & Merikangas, K. R. (2011). Social phobia and subtypes in the National Comorbidity Survey—Adolescent Supplement: Prevalence, correlates, and comorbidity. *Journal of the American Academy of Child and Adolescent Psychiatry, 50,* 870–880.

Chorpita, B. F., Albano, A. M., & Barlow, D. H. (1996). Cognitive processing in children: Relation to anxiety and family influences. *Journal of Clinical Child Psychology, 25,* 170–176.

Chorpita, B. F., & Barlow, D. H. (1998). The development of anxiety: The role of control in the early environment. *Psychological Bulletin, 124,* 3–21.

Chorpita, B. F., Yim, L., Moffitt, C., Umemoto, L. A., & Francis, S. E. (2000). Assessment of symptoms of DSM-IV anxiety and depression in children: A Revised Child Anxiety and Depression Scale. *Behaviour Research and Therapy, 38,* 835–855.

Cohen, J., & Kendall, P. C. (2015). Peer victimization among children and adolescents with anxiety disorders. *Child Psychiatry and Human Development, 46,* 393–405.

Comer, J. S., Blanco, C., Grant, B., Hasin, D., Liu, S. M., Turner, J. B., et al. (2011). Health-related quality of life across the anxiety disorders: Results from the National Epidemiologic Survey on Alcohol and Related Conditions. *Journal of Clinical Psychiatry, 72,* 43–50.

Logsdon-Conradsen, S. (1998). *Family interaction patterns in adolescents with social phobia.* Unpublished doctoral dissertation, University of Louisville, Louisville, KY.

Detweiler, M. F., Comer, J., Crum, K. I., & Albano, A. M. (2014). Social anxiety in children and adolescents: Biological, psychological, and social considerations. In S. G. Hofmann & P. M. DiBartolo (Eds.), *Social anxiety: Clinical, developmental and social perspectives* (3rd ed., pp. 254–309). Amsterdam: Elsevier.

DiBartolo, P. M., Albano, A. M., Barlow, D. H., & Heimberg, R. G. (1998). Cross-informant agreement in the assessment of social phobia in youth. *Journal of Abnormal Child Psychology, 26,* 213–220.

Guerry, J., Hambrick, J., & Albano, A. M. (2015). Adolescent social phobia in clinical services. In K. Ranta, A. M. La Greca, L.-J. García-Lopez, & M. Marttunen (Eds.), *Social anxiety and phobia in adolescents* (pp. 201–223). Cham, Switzerland: Springer International.

Hayward, C., Killen, J. D., Kraemer, H. C., & Taylor, C. B. (1998). Linking self-reported childhood behavioral inhibition to adolescent social phobia. *Journal of the American Academy of Child and Adolescent Psychiatry, 37,* 1308–1316.

Hayward, C., Varady, S., Albano, A. M., Thieneman, M., Henderson, L., & Schatzberg, A. F. (2000). Cognitive behavioral group therapy for female socially phobic adolescents: Results of a pilot study. *Journal of the American Academy of Child and Adolescent Psychiatry, 39,* 721–726.

Higa, C. K., Fernandez, S. N., Nakamura, B. J., Chorpita, B. F., & Daleiden, E. L. (2006). Parental assessment of childhood social: Psychometric properties of the social phobia and anxiety inventory for children–parent report. *Journal of Clinical Child and Adolescent Psychology, 35,* 590–597.

Higa-McMillan, C. K., Francis, S. E., Rith-Najarian, L., & Chorpita, B. F. (2016). Evidence base update: 50 years of research on treatment for child and adolescent anxiety. *Journal of Clinical Child and Adolescent Psychology, 45,* 91–113.

Hofmann, S., Albano, A. M., Heimberg, R. G., Tracey, S., Chorpita, B. F., & Barlow, D. H. (1999). Subtypes of social phobia in adolescents. *Depression and Anxiety, 9,* 8–15.

Hollon, S. D., & Beck, A. T. (2013). Cognitive and cognitive-behavioral therapies. In M. J. Lambert (Ed.), *Handbook of psychotherapy and behavior change* (6th ed., pp. 393–442). Hoboken, NJ: Wiley.

Hudson, J. L., Rapee, R. M., Lyneham, H. J., McLellan, L. F., Wuthrich, V. M., & Schniering C. A. (2015). Comparing outcomes for children with different anxiety disorders following cognitive behavioural therapy. *Behaviour Research and Therapy, 72,* 30–37.

Kearney, C. A. (2002). Identifying the function of school refusal behavior: A revision of the School Refusal Assessment Scale. *Journal of Psychopathology and Behavioral Assessment, 24,* 235–245.

Kearney, C. A., & Albano, A. M. (2004). The functional profiles of school refusal behavior: Diagnostic aspects. *Behavior Modification, 28*, 147–161.

Kearney, C. A., & Silverman, W. K. (1993). Measuring the function of school refusal behavior: The School Refusal Assessment Scale. *Journal of Clinical Child Psychology, 22*, 85–96.

Kendall, P. C. (1994). Treating anxiety disorders in children: Results of a randomized clinical trial. *Journal of Consulting and Clinical Psychology, 62*(1), 100–110.

Kendall, P. C. (2012). Anxiety disorders in youth. In P. C. Kendall (Ed.), *Child and adolescent therapy: Cognitive-behavioral procedures* (4th ed., pp. 143–189). New York: Guilford Press.

Kendall, P. C., Choudhury, M., Hudson, J., & Webb, A. (2002a). *The C.A.T. Project workbook for the cognitive-behavioral treatment of anxious adolescents.* Ardmore, PA: Workbook.

Kendall, P. C., Choudhury, M., Hudson, J., & Webb, A. (2002b). *The C.A.T. Project therapist manual.* Ardmore, PA: Workbook.

Kendall, P. C., Flannery-Schroeder, E., Panichelli-Mindel, S. M., Southam-Gerow, M., Henin, A., & Warman, M. (1997). Therapy for youths with anxiety disorders: A second randomized clinical trial. *Journal of Consulting and Clinical Psychology, 65*(3), 366–380.

Kendall, P. C., & Hedtke, K. (2006a). *Coping Cat workbook* (2nd ed.). Ardmore, PA: Workbook.

Kendall, P. C., & Hedtke, K. (2006b). *Cognitive-behavioral therapy for anxious children: Therapist manual* (3rd ed.). Ardmore, PA: Workbook.

Kendall, P. C., Hudson, J. L., Gosch, E., Flannery-Schroeder, E., & Suveg, C. (2008). Cognitive-behavioral therapy for anxiety disordered youth: A randomized clinical trial evaluating child and family modalities. *Journal of Consulting and Clinical Psychology, 76*(2), 282–297.

Kendall, P. C., & Khanna, M. (2008). *Camp Cope-A-Lot: Computer-assisted Coping Cat.* Ardmore, PA: Workbook.

Kessler, R. C., Berglund, P., Demler, O., Jin, R., Merikangas, K. R., & Walters, E. E. (2005). Lifetime prevalence and age-of-onset distributions of DSM-IV disorders in the National Comorbidity Survey Replication. *Archives of General Psychiatry, 62*, 593–602.

La Greca, A. M. (1998). *Manual for the Social Anxiety Scales for Children and Adolescents.* Unpublished manuscript, University of Miami.

La Greca, A. M. (1999). The Social Anxiety Scales for Children and Adolescents. *The Behavior Therapist, 22*, 133–136.

La Greca, A. M., & Lopez, N. (1998). Social anxiety among adolescents: Linkages with peer relations and friendships. *Journal of Abnormal Child Psychology, 26*, 83–94.

La Greca, A. M., & Stone, N. (1993). Social Anxiety Scale for children—revised: Factor structure and concurrent validity. *Journal of Clinical Child Psychology, 22*, 17–27.

Lewis-Morrarty, E., Degnan, K. A., Chronis-Tuscano, A., Pine, D. S., Henderson, H. A., & Fox, N. A. (2015). Infant attachment security and early childhood behavioral inhibition interact to predict adolescent social anxiety symptoms. *Child Development, 86*, 598–613.

Lewis-Morrarty, E., Degnan, K. A., Chronis-Tuscano, A., Rubin, K. H., Cheah, C. S. L., Pine, D. S., et al. (2012). Maternal over-control moderates the association between early childhood behavioral inhibition and adolescent social anxiety symptoms. *Journal of Abnormal Child Psychology, 40*, 1363–1373.

Logsdon-Conradsen, S. (1998). *Family interaction patterns in adolescents with social phobia.* Unpublished doctoral dissertation, University of Louisville, Louisville, KY.

Masia-Warner, C., Storch, E. A., Pincus, D. B., Klein, R. G., Heimberg, R. G., & Liebowitz, M. R. (2003). The Liebowitz Social Anxiety Scale for Children and Adolescents: An initial psychometric investigation. *Journal of the American Academy of Child and Adolescent Psychiatry, 42*(9), 1076–1084.

Mendlowitz, M. V., & Stein, M. B. (2000). Quality of life in individuals with anxiety disorders. *American Journal of Psychiatry, 157,* 669–682.

Merikangas, K. R., He, J., Burstein, M., Swanson, S. A., Avenevoli, S., Cui, L., et al. (2010). Lifetime prevalence of mental disorders in US adolescents: Results from the National Comorbidity Study—Adolescent Supplement (NCS-A). *Journal of the American Academy of Child and Adolescent Psychiatry, 49,* 980–989.

Mesa, F., Beidel, D. C., & Bunnell, B. E. (2014). An examination of psychopathology and daily impairment in adolescents with social anxiety disorder. *PLoS ONE, 9,* 1–9.

Muris, P. (2001). A brief questionnaire for measuring self-efficacy in youths. *Journal of Psychopathology and Behavioral Assessment, 23,* 145–149.

Peris, T., Compton, S., Kendall, P. C., Birmaher, B., Sherill, J., March, J., et al. (2015). Trajectories of change in youth anxiety during cognitive-behavior therapy. *Journal of Consulting and Clinical Psychology, 83,* 239–252.

Rapee, R. M., & Heimberg, R. G. (1997). A cognitive-behavioral model of anxiety in social phobia. *Behaviour Research and Therapy, 35,* 741–756.

Ranta, R., La Greca, A. M., García-Lopez, L.-J., & Marttunen, M. (Eds.). (2016). *Social anxiety and phobia in adolescents.* Cham, Switzerland: Springer International.

Reeb-Sutherland, B. C., Williams, L. R., Degnan, K. A., Perez-Edgar, K., Chronis-Tuscano, A., Leibenluft, E., et al. (2015). Identification of emotional facial expressions among behaviorally inhibited adolescents with lifetime anxiety disorders. *Cognition and Emotion, 29,* 372–382.

Rubin, K. H., Nelson, L. J., Hastings, P., & Asendorpf, J. (1999). The transaction between parents' perceptions of their children's shyness and their parenting styles. *International Journal of Behavioral Development, 23*(4), 937–958.

Schniering, C. A., & Rapee, R. M. (2002). Development and validation of a measure of children's automatic thoughts: The Children's Automatic Thoughts Scale. *Behaviour Research and Therapy, 40,* 1091–1109.

Silverman, W. K., & Albano, A. M. (1996). *The Anxiety Disorders Interview Schedule for DSM-IV, Child and Parent Versions.* Albany, NY: Graywind Press.

Silverman, W. K., & Eisen, A. R. (1992). Age differences in the reliability of parent and child reports of child anxious symptomatology using a structured interview. *Journal of the American Academy of Child and Adolescent Psychiatry, 31,* 117–124.

Silverman, W. K., & Nelles, W. B. (1988). The Anxiety Disorders Interview Schedule for Children. *Journal of the American Academy of Child and Adolescent Psychiatry, 27,* 772–778.

Spence, S. H., Donovan, C., & Brechman-Toussaint, M. (2000). The treatment of childhood social phobia: The effectiveness of a social skills training-based, cognitive-behavioural intervention, with and without parental involvement. *Journal of Child Psychology and Psychiatry, 41*(6), 713–726.

Velting, O. N., & Albano, A. M. (2001). Current trends in the understanding and treatment of social phobia in youth. *Journal of Child Psychology and Psychiatry and Allied Disciplines, 42,* 127–140.

Walkup, J., Albano, A. M., Piacentini, J. P., Birmaher, B., Compton, S., Sherrill, J., et al. (2008). Cognitive behavioral therapy, sertraline, or a combination for childhood anxiety. *New England Journal of Medicine, 359,* 2753–2766.

Wells, K. C., & Albano, A. M. (2005). Parent involvement in CBT treatment of adolescent depression: Experiences in the Treatment for Adolescents with Depression Study (TADS). In J. Curry, P. Rohde, & A. M. Albano (Eds.), Treatments for adolescents with depression: Special issue. *Cognitive and Behavioral Practice, 12,* 209–220.

CHAPTER THREE

Treatment of Obsessive–Compulsive Disorder

Martin E. Franklin
Sarah H. Morris
Simone Budzyn

Theoretical Models

Behavioral Learning Models

Most cognitive-behavioral therapy (CBT) protocols used for obsessive–compulsive disorder (OCD) are based on principles derived from (1) conditioning models and/or (2) belief and appraisal models that are applied to the development and maintenance of OCD symptoms (Taylor, Abramowitz, & McKay, 2007). Exposure and response prevention (E/RP), the treatment approach with the most empirical support for treating OCD in children and adolescents, is most closely associated with early theoretical models involving learning. Proposed initially by Mowrer (1939, 1960), the two-factor model of fear describes a process in which unconditioned behavioral responses (e.g., unlearned escape responses such as behavioral avoidance and compulsions) occur in situations in which physiologically mediated anxiety is experienced (e.g., unwanted intrusive thoughts and situations that provoke such thoughts). If an individual then performs a behavior that succeeds in reducing anxiety, that behavior will be negatively reinforced (i.e., the unpleasant feeling goes away temporarily). Thus situations in which similar anxiety-provoking stimuli are presented will produce this same learned anxiety-reducing behavior. In addition, behaviors related to avoiding situations that evoke physiological fear in the first place will also be reinforced. From this initial work, operant conditioning models were developed more specifically for OCD (e.g., Rachman & Hodgson, 1980). An individual could be diagnosed with OCD when escape/avoidance behaviors involved learned, compulsive rituals and when this process produced functional impairment or meaningful distress.

Using this formulation, E/RP is said to work because it makes those learned connections between safety behaviors and the physiological experience of anxiety more ambiguous (see Foa & Kozak, 1986). In E/RP, a patient would likely be encouraged to begin by exposing him- or herself to an OCD-related trigger that elicits at least a low to moderate level of fearful arousal. If the patient does so and then refrains from performing the ritual, it is believed that the patient will experience a gradual decline of the physiological arousal. With successive E/RP trials, the physiological response to the exposed trigger will gradually reduce across trials (i.e., habituation). As a patient habituates to the OCD trigger, the extinction of OCD behaviors typically follows. Other formulations of why E/RP works are discussed below.

Cognitive Belief and Appraisal Models

Cognition-based theoretical models expanded on earlier efforts to explain the etiology of OCD—two-factor theory is more useful in accounting for symptom maintenance through negative reinforcement but is agnostic as to the cause of the intrusive thoughts in the first place. Accordingly, cognitively oriented theorists and researchers put forth a broader argument that most forms of psychopathology stem from individuals having and overvaluing dysfunctional beliefs (e.g., Beck, 1976). In further explicating this process for OCD specifically, cognitive theorists (e.g., Salkovskis, 1989, 1996) explain that intrusive thoughts, which occur routinely in most people, may become obsessions when these thoughts are interpreted as having serious consequences for which the individual is personally responsible. Compulsive urges are strengthened by negative reinforcement, as described in earlier learning models, because they serve to immediately reduce an individual's distress associated with such cognitions. Cognitive theorists also suggest that compulsions persist because they prevent individuals from encountering situations that test whether obsessions lead to their unrealistic predictions of harm (Salkovskis, 1989).

An enduring legacy of the early cognitive theorists includes articulating the various themes of dysfunctional beliefs found in OCD obsessions. Although it has been shown that using pure cognitive therapy techniques (e.g., Socratic questioning) in isolation is not effective over and above applying E/RP techniques (Abramowitz, Franklin, & Foa, 2002), the nomenclature of cognitive content is quite useful in deriving exposures that directly target the core fears of an individual. Advancing on Salkovskis's seminal ideas, a collaborative group of OCD treatment experts outlined additional cognitive domains involved in obsessive content. Combining the expert consensus of its members, the Obsessive Compulsive Cognitions Working Group (1997) outlined the most common cognitive domains involved in OCD. The final cognitive domains included inflated responsibility, overestimation of threat, thought–action fusion (i.e., the belief that a thought is morally equivalent to performing the action), superstitious/magical thinking, intolerance of uncertainty/doubt, perfectionism, and concerns with controlling thoughts. Although these cognitive constructs were not necessarily specified for OCD in youth, such cognitions have been found to be helpful to differentiate children with OCD from youth without the disorder and those with other anxiety disorders (Barrett & Healy, 2003).

Despite the distinctions in theoretical explanations of OCD, it should be emphasized that there is as yet no evidence that any one of these approaches can uniquely account for the symptom variability observed in patients with OCD (Himle & Franklin, 2009). The E/RP treatment approach emphasizes a neurobehavioral framework, which combines biological, developmental, learning, and family interpersonal models (Freeman et al., 2003; March & Mulle, 1998). However, techniques used in other treatment approaches (e.g., motivational interviewing, mindfulness-based treatments) are also invoked in the flexible implementation of E/RP, particularly to promote sustained practice in E/RP activities and reduce family involvement in escape/avoidance behaviors that also reinforce OCD. This approach to CBT is described in more detail in the remainder of this chapter.

Cognitive-Behavioral Model

Contemporary E/RP treatments are based largely on a blended cognitive-behavioral model (Foa & Kozak, 1986) known as emotional processing theory. E/RP typically includes prolonged exposure to obsessional cues, procedures aimed at blocking rituals, and informal discussions of mistaken beliefs conducted in anticipation of and following exposure exercises. Exposures are most often done in real-life settings (*in vivo*) and involve prolonged contact with the feared external (e.g., contaminated surfaces) or internal (e.g., images of harming a family member) stimuli that the patient reports as distressing. For those who report fear of specific consequences that could or will ensue if they refrain from performing rituals or avoidance, such fears can be addressed via "imaginal exposure": creating very detailed image scripts of the patient's own "worst-case scenario" and listening to or reading these scripts repeatedly until they are perceived as less anxiety provoking. Following on from Foa and Kozak's theory, *in vivo* and imaginal exposures are designed specifically to prompt obsessional distress. It is believed that repeated, prolonged exposure to feared thoughts and situations will provide opportunities to disconfirm mistaken associations and evaluations held by the patient, thereby promoting habituation (Foa & Kozak, 1986). Exposures are typically conducted gradually, with situations provoking moderate distress confronted before more upsetting ones; however, there are some presentations of OCD (e.g., intrusive and spontaneous disturbing images) in which the hierarchical approach is less effective because the internal stimuli cannot be presented in an ordered fashion. Exposure "homework" is assigned between sessions, and patients are asked to refrain from rituals to the extent possible. The stated goal of treatment is complete abstinence from rituals, yet therapists must be cognizant of the need to encourage patients, especially younger patients, to achieve this goal over time rather than simply insisting upon it immediately. Patients are reminded throughout treatment about the theoretical model— "ritualizing maintains fear, whereas refraining from rituals promotes fear reduction." Accordingly, they are given specific recommendations as to how best to refrain from rituals when urges do arise.

A Brief Review of the Outcome Literature

CBT involving E/RP has garnered enough research support to now be deemed an empirically supported treatment, with randomized studies from around the world attesting to its efficacy relative to various comparison conditions (e.g., pill placebo, relaxation) and to active pharmacotherapy (for recent reviews, see Franklin et al., 2015; Freeman et al., 2014). The beneficial treatment effects appear to be both robust and durable, with follow-up studies indicating that the effects of treatment last for up to 9 months after treatment has ended (e.g., Barrett, Healy-Farrell, & March, 2004). Intensive treatment regimens are effective, although weekly treatment for approximately 12–14 weeks appears to be sufficient for most patients (Franklin et al., 1998; Storch et al., 2007). With respect to making clinical judgments about whether a more intensive form of CBT is needed for a given patient, it may well be the case that symptom severity, comorbidity, readiness for change, and case complexity (e.g., family problems) could dictate whether a more intensive approach is needed; however, the literature examining the predictive value of such factors is limited. What is clear is that the treatment of very young children requires a family-based approach; indeed, the first randomized controlled trial (RCT) of such a protocol supported the use of family-based E/RP over family-based relaxation (Freeman et al., 2014).

Efforts in recent years to enhance CBT's efficacy and reach have identified several promising avenues for each. Augmentation of CBT with motivational interviewing (MI) appears to have potential benefit (Merlo et al., 2010); what has yet to be addressed is whether MI augmentation would be particularly helpful for patients who are reporting more than the typical amount of reluctance to engage in CBT or who are actively refusing to initiate this treatment. Web-based CBT may be efficacious for select patients (e.g., Storch et al., 2011). Such an approach may reduce some of the practical burdens that prevent some patients from accessing care, such as travel distance to expert clinics; associated costs, such as child care for siblings when attending treatment sessions; disruption of work and home schedules; and patient reluctance to spare the time commuting to sessions. Web-based treatment may also assist treatment providers in conducting home-based exposures that are not readily re-created in session, such as conducting exposures to completing bedtime routines without resorting to compulsions.

Both alone and in combination with selective serotonin reuptake inhibitors (SSRIs), CBT provides a viable treatment alternative to SSRIs alone (Ivarsson et al., 2015), although the paucity of trained CBT therapists continues to make it difficult in some geographic regions to heed the expert consensus guidelines recommendations (e.g., those of the American Academy of Child and Adolescent Psychiatry) to start with CBT alone or with a combination. Dissemination of CBT for pediatric OCD thus remains a pressing challenge to the field, although research supporting a "supervision of supervisors" model is promising. Data suggest that this model can yield impressive results that are comparable to those achieved in the academic medical settings that developed the CBT protocol for use with children and adolescents (e.g., Torp et al., 2015).

Assessment and Outcome Measures

A thorough assessment is necessary to determine whether OCD is present and whether it should be considered principal over comorbid conditions. Table 3.1 describes the assessment battery used in our collaborative studies and treatment clinic. In general, we use the Children's Yale–Brown Obsessive Compulsive Scale (CY-BOCS; Goodman, Price, Rasmussen, Mazure, Delgado, et al., 1989; Goodman, Price, Rasmussen, Mazure, Fleischmann, et al., 1989) and the Mini International Neuropsychiatric Interview for Children and Adolescents (MINI-KID; Sheehan, Shytle, & Milo, 2004) for most children and adolescents. However, at times, due to a patient's age or the need to rule out or characterize other conditions in greater detail, we also may utilize sections of the Yale Global Tic Severity Scale (YGTSS; Leckman et al., 1989) or the Anxiety Disorders Interview Schedule (ADIS; Silverman & Albano, 1997), as appropriate. We also routinely use the Multidimensional Anxiety Scale for Children (MASC; March, Parker, Sullivan, Stallings, & Conners, 1997), the Child Obsessive–Compulsive Impact Scale (COIS-R; Piacentini, Peris, Bergman, Chang, & Jaffer, 2007), and the Children's Depression Inventory (CDI; Kovacs, 1992) to screen for comorbidities and inform treatment planning. Because internalizing disorders are the most common comorbidity seen in patients with OCD, we tend to emphasize

TABLE 3.1. Typical Obsessive–Compulsive Disorder (OCD) Assessment Battery

Measure	Age (years)	Target	Notes
		Interviews	
MINI-KID	6–17	Full range of DSM-IV criteria	
ADIS	8–17	DSM-IV criteria for anxiety disorders	Preferred for ruling out anxiety comorbidities
CY-BOCS	5–17	OCD symptoms and severity	Score of 16 indicated clinically significant OCD
YGTSS	5–17	Motor and vocal tics and severity	
		Self-report	
MASC	8–19	Depression symptoms	Includes parent- and child-rated scales
COIS-R	7+	OCD-related functional impairment	Includes parent- and child-rated scales
CDI	7–17	Depression symptoms	Includes parent- and child-rated scales

Note. ADIS, Anxiety Disorders Interview for Children; CDI, Children's Depression Inventory; COIS-R, Child Obsessive–Compulsive Impact Scale—Revised; CY-BOCS, Children's Yale–Brown Obsessive Compulsive Scale; DSM-IV, *Diagnostic and Statistical Manual of Mental Disorders, Fourth Edition*; MASC, Multidimensional Anxiety Scale for Children; MINI-KID, Mini International Neuropsychiatric Interview for Children and Adolescents; YGTSS, Yale Global Tic Severity Scale.

those instruments in the assessment protocol. However, it is important to screen for less common comorbid conditions if information is uncovered that leads the clinician to suspect the presence of such disorders (e.g., psychosis, oppositional defiant disorder); the ADIS covers most of these, and by surveying these areas in detail, the clinician will be able to develop a comprehensive evaluation plan that takes such conditions into account.

CBT Involving E/RP

The treatment is typically 12–14 sessions delivered weekly, but this format can be tailored to the specific needs and motivation of the family. As discussed above, this treatment can be delivered efficaciously in either weekly or intensive (e.g., one session per weekday) outpatient formats with similar results; intensive residential programs with E/RP at their core have also yielded encouraging findings (e.g., Leonard, Jacobi, Riemann, Lake, & Luhn, 2014). Regardless of the visit schedule, the general structure of the program is the same: (1) psychoeducation, (2) mapping the OCD hierarchy and identifying family involvement in OCD, (3) engagement in "bossing back" strategies, and (4) graded E/RP and family disengagement from OCD. However, developmental considerations require protocol adjustments based on the child's age. For an older child or adolescent, the treatment focus will be primarily on the patient. In this format, typically there will be parental check-ins only at the beginning and end of sessions, as well as periodic family sessions when needed (see March & Mulle, 1998). For younger children or in families with extensive family involvement in rituals and avoidance of OCD triggers, parents should be involved in most sessions, with inclusion of techniques such as differential attention, appropriate modeling of CBT skills, and scaffolding assistance to the child in ways that do not reinforce OCD symptoms (Freeman & Garcia, 2009). Contingency management should also be developmentally appropriate for the child. Parents should be encouraged to provide appropriate rewards/privileges for attending sessions, for participating actively in discussions in treatment, for completing assigned homework, and for using CBT skills spontaneously in unplanned situations. It is important to emphasize that the plan should reward behaviors reflecting good effort toward CBT practice, not necessarily positive results alone.

Psychoeducation

The first task of the protocol is to ground the family in the neurobehavioral model for OCD and highlight elements of the treatment program. By the time a family comes to treatment, it is likely that they have already experienced excessive distress, conflict between family members, fears of stigma, and feelings of hopelessness. Accordingly, the initial treatment focus should involve presenting OCD as a neurobehavioral condition that is no one's fault, as well as providing hope that there are now proven tools to manage OCD's influence on the child and the larger family. It may be helpful to discuss the position that OCD is a condition in the brain, albeit influenced by how the individual and family interact with OCD behaviors. Using metaphors involving descriptions of "brain hiccups," ineffective "circuits," or broken "alarms" has been effective.

During the psychoeducation portion, it is helpful to tailor the neurobehavioral discussion to the family's interest and clinical needs. Some families are quite interested in a brief, focused discussion of the neural circuits in play. For clinicians, it is good to dwell a little more here if there are concerns that the child is just being manipulative or if a particular parent is being labeled as merely coddling the child. For example, describing hypothetical situations that parents and children can relate to with a touch of humor (walking in a park, tripping, and accidentally putting your hand in dog poop) can be an excellent way to describe how the cortical–thalamic–striatal–cortical circuit is activated for everyone and that excessive hand washing can have some adaptive merit in specific situations! The heritability of OCD can be described as being like having a "birthmark" near these circuits, which lead to OCD behaviors. After the biological components of OCD have been explained, it is then important to discuss how CBT and other behavior changes can influence these "loud and leaky" circuits. This should be tailored carefully to the amount of insight the child has.

At this point, the clinician should ask about any questions the family has about OCD as a neurobehavioral disorder and assess the overall treatment engagement of each participant. After these have been addressed, the discussion can continue with describing the nuts and bolts of OCD and how CBT can help.

After the initial introduction of obsessions and compulsions takes place, it's often helpful to illustrate how a typical OCD pattern works. OCD episodes typically involve a sawtooth pattern that begins with the child at low distress. Once a child encounters an OCD-relevant trigger, anxiety increases to the point where a compulsion is performed, which then leads to a repetitive pattern of compulsions and oscillating anxiety.

The transition from psychoeducation to the start of active treatment usually begins by introducing externalization from OCD. Externalization starts with giving OCD processes a "nasty" nickname for younger children or simply calling it "OCD" for older children. Even prior to bringing up externalization explicitly, the language referring to the child's specific issues should also be consistent with externalization from your first meeting onward. For example, if a child is worried that her own intrusive thoughts about death might actually kill her mother, this should be described as "[OCD/nickname] makes you worry that your mom will die if you don't perform your rituals properly."

Mapping the OCD Hierarchy and Identifying Family Involvement

Before the process of skill building and E/RP can begin, the family must learn about how OCD is working in their family and the specific hierarchy of the child's symptoms. Some of this might already be addressed through the assessment and initial psychoeducation portion of the program. However, a more detailed functional analysis of the child's triggers, the child's particular obsessive content, subsequent compulsions, and family accommodation of OCD will provide further guidance to structure the graded E/RP to be introduced later in the program. The use of an OCD fear thermometer (usually on a 0–10 scale) to build the fear hierarchy will help the child and family get a little insight into the relative distress each OCD symptom causes.

Several things going on at this point in treatment provide further information about the child's OCD and set the stage for future exposures. First, the open discussion of OCD with the child is a minor exposure in itself for youth who spend a great deal of time avoiding thoughts of OCD. Second, in this early phase of treatment, the therapist's stance with regard to OCD should be nonplussed about the content but curious about how the child's OCD works. Third, it is important to start introducing degrees of separation from the usual OCD triggers, particularly for children who rate most OCD triggers as very high. After summarizing and validating the child's anxiety about touching anything he or she normally sees (e.g., objects covered in dog drool can actually be gross), the therapist then curiously asks about things that could be safer. Notice that when this line of questioning leads to most things the child rated high (even things that were washed and not touched by anyone else), the therapist should switch gears (to things others never touch). Typically, the child will lower his or her fear ratings for these hypothetical targets that he or she has not thought about. Finally, once you get some targets, even if they are only hypothetical ones in the middle range of the thermometer, the therapist inquires about elements that might be manipulated in a future E/RP exercise (touching something clean that briefly touched a "dirty" item). Finding some gradients in these milder targets will allow the therapist to then go back and reassess these same gradients at the higher numbers. It's likely that finding anxiety gradients will be easier at the higher ranges if they can first be fleshed out in the lower ones.

Identifying family involvement in OCD symptoms should be approached with similar sensitivity as was done for externalizing OCD from the child's values. This will be particularly important for families with a history of OCD, as well as in families in which a parent has been accused of facilitating OCD behaviors. It is imperative to validate the parents' desire to reduce their child's suffering and be effective parents. Proper psychoeducation and mapping of OCD processes at home can allow the parents to view OCD as something that interferes with these two values. Using externalization language (e.g., "OCD has the whole family running in circles") and painting OCD as tricky, an enemy, or inconsistent with the family's values can all be useful in building rapport and getting everyone united against OCD processes.

"Bossing Back" Strategies

For active treatment components, this CBT program is separated into two major categories: E/RP and elements that facilitate engaging in E/RP. As already noted, clinical experience and meta-analytic reviews show that E/RP is the primary active component for symptom reduction in OCD. However, affected children and their families are unlikely to perform exposures effectively in the first session. An early misplaced E/RP exercise that is too ambitious can sabotage treatment, which is why the CBT model must be carefully established, symptom monitoring introduced, and other "bossing back" skills that will facilitate future E/RP adherence should be added. Within bossing-back strategies, the two major categories are (1) externalization of OCD and (2) cognitive training elements such as cognitive restructuring. Identifying OCD thoughts and feelings as external to the child and then subsequently interacting with them with on a level of nonattachment is at the heart of E/RP and the process leading to habituation. Although cognitive restructuring activities can be important for a family prior to a given E/RP exercise (e.g., "What is the likelihood we will contract swine flu if we touch this table?"), it is important not to emphasize them too strongly as a means to reduce stress beyond the first few sessions. For some patients, an overemphasis on talking back to OCD with coping thoughts during acute stress (e.g., reminding themselves that "I'm safe" or "These germs can't really kill me") can elicit OCD-reinforcing mental safety behaviors. At these times, emphasis is better placed on tolerating discomfort without additional efforts to promote safety. Accordingly, it is recommended that cognitive training and techniques are used to make the child's engagement in E/RP effective and to facilitate approaching activities the child was otherwise avoiding due to OCD-related triggers. For the most part, cognitive strategies should only be used before and after E/RP to maximize effectiveness; doing so during exposures may well provide temporary relief in the midst of distress, which serves the same function as reassurance and thus may compromise outcome.

Graded E/RP and Family Disengagement

E/RP training can be initiated only after building rapport, establishing OCD externalization with the child, mapping common OCD processes in the child and greater family, and setting up enough cognitive training to portray OCD compulsions as ineffective and unnecessary. The primary goal is to make the initial E/RP sessions relevant to the child's core fears but not so distressing that the child engages in safety behaviors. To do so, it is recommended that, first, a thorough discussion ensue on areas in which the child already has some success resisting rituals (at least 50% of the time) and then that an in-session exposure be set up that can elicit moderate distress. The first E/RP should focus on targets that are well fleshed out on the child's hierarchy, including targets on the low (1–3), medium (4–6), and high (7–10) levels on the child's fear thermometer. Once an E/RP trial begins, the youngster should be encouraged to maintain awareness or contact with the feared trigger and notice how much the discomfort dissipates over time. We find that children often report meaningful reduction in distress between 30 seconds and 10 minutes, which is useful information but not entirely necessary—the most important point to emphasize is that they are fighting back against OCD and showing OCD who's boss. When a child's anxiety begins to plateau or go down, then begins to go up again, it is important to explore later (not then) what was happening at that moment. Such a pattern could indicate the presence of behaviors ranging from losing detached focus on the distress (e.g., "This is taking too long") to overt experiential avoidance, including mental rituals. Subsequent E/RP targets should generally hit in moderate range of the fear thermometer at the child's pace. If, after some E/RP successes, the only remaining targets are in the high range, take some time to flesh out some gradients of separation from the very high targets (e.g., touch something clean that first touched something dirty). Once a child is successfully habituating to the initial targets, continue E/RP by moving up the hierarchy on that particular fear until the child achieves habituation to the core fear, perhaps over several weeks. Only then should you switch to the next OCD fear.

Use of imaginal exposure can be useful for obsessional content that cannot be addressed *in vivo* (fears involving going to hell, stabbing a sibling, etc.). Before imaginal exposure is proposed, however, the family should already have some E/RP success in the fear target area, and the rationale for doing so should be carefully explained and understood. It is important to flesh out the plot of the imaginal exposure collaboratively with the patient first. The arc of the story should begin with a typical trigger that elicits obsessions related to the feared consequence, eventually leading to an imagined catastrophic conclusion that results from not having performed rituals or avoided the situation. As the story unfolds, the child's language should be included as much as possible to maximize benefit. The story should also incorporate relevant details, involving as many sensory descriptors as possible. The imaginal exposure can be either taped in session and provided to the child to replay at home or presented in written form like a script. These exposures should then be listened to or read at home in a quiet place without other distractions.

For the therapist, it is important to adhere to several key principles that will facilitate effective E/RP in session. First, the therapist should demonstrate first and join into exposures as much as possible. There is nothing reasonably safe that should be avoided in the service of the patient—common examples include touching bathroom toilets and standing in front of a child on a subway platform and encouraging him or her to allow thoughts of pushing you to enter his or her mind without neutralizing them. Granted, there are some nonzero risks to doing things such as touching dirty surfaces or eating off the floor, but children do respond to these ways to fight their OCD, particularly if it is first demonstrated by a supportive therapist willing to do it with them. To do this seamlessly prior to an exposure, you can talk about the plan for the child while you demonstrate it concurrently (e.g., "So the first thing we can do against OCD is take your finger like this, touch the table, and then quickly touch it on your tongue"). Second, when planning in-session E/RP, it is crucial to discuss any proposed exposure matter-of-factly in front of the child. Third, unless the family has demonstrated several successes with E/RP that they do independently at home, it's best to first initiate any increase in exposure intensity in a treatment session.

Allow the family to practice these new exposures at home without escalating them, unless the child is no longer getting anxious at home when these E/RPs are attempted. In conjunction with E/RP work for the child, you must also be mindful of helping the families disengage from OCD accommodation and related behaviors. A seminal text from some of our colleagues describes a step-by-step process of how to systematically put this program into place for the parents while concurrently working with the child (Freeman & Garcia, 2009). Most of the skills taught are consistent with other parent training approaches involving differential attention and scaffolding, passing more responsibility to the child regarding distress management. Allowing parents to see how you conduct symptom monitoring, OCD mapping, and E/RP exercises will also provide them with a model of how to do similar behaviors at home instead of accommodating OCD.

Descriptions of Materials Used in Treatment

In addition to the assessment materials already described (e.g., structured clinical interviews, self-report questionnaires), exposure treatment for OCD requires access to stimuli that evoke distress. Given the heterogeneous nature of OCD, such stimuli cut across a very wide variety of content areas, and it is imperative to be able to think creatively about how to access such materials on the fly. One of the most important tools in the profession is a computer with Internet access, since YouTube and other such sites provide ample fodder for exposure. For example, for a patient with contamination fears and compulsions associated with vomiting, a hierarchy exists on the Internet that includes both verbal content (e.g., a website that contains very detailed accounts of "Great Vomits of the 20th Century," fake vomit recipes) and visual aides that include still shots (e.g., pictures of vomit) and moving pictures (e.g., movie vomit scenes, Milk Challenges). There is simply no shortage of useful content, and such content may serve treatment well in the psychoeducation phase, as well as in exposure itself. Exposure therapists are often scanning the environment for relevant stimuli for their work and thus are frequently on the lookout for particularly filthy bathrooms, dead animals, very bumpy streets (for those with fear of running over pedestrians in their cars), ambiguous stains on carpets that could have been derived from body fluids, sharp objects (for those with fears that they will lose control and use them on unsuspecting people), dog feces, and a host of other such items. Part of the preferred stance of the exposure therapist who treats OCD is a willingness, if not outright enthusiasm, for crossing over conventional boundaries in the service of their patients, as such willingness also serves as a model of how to seek out such stimuli intentionally rather than avoiding it. In our view, everyone who does this work well embodies this spirit and enthusiastically shares it with their far less bold patients, until such time as some of that same spirit can be engendered during the treatment process.

Developmental and Multicultural Issues

CBT may need to be adapted to be sensitive to the context of specific cultural backgrounds. Although reviews in the pediatric OCD literature find little support for race or ethnicity moderating treatment effects (i.e., it is equally effective for all groups), the reality is that OCD symptoms are often misdiagnosed or underdiagnosed in minority populations (Hatch, Friedman, & Paradis, 1996). More research is required on tailoring CBT interventions to minority populations before commenting further on how to better serve these populations. However, it is imperative for any therapist treating a patient from a background different from his or her own to take the time to understand the patient's experiences, perspectives, and viewpoint so as to ensure that a respectful connection is fostered. For example, when treating transgender patients who suffer from OCD, learning about and then using preferred pronouns is a way to convey respect for that person; a therapist who is unclear about such issues risks coming across as disrespectful, so it is also important for the therapist to ask questions when he or she does not have the necessary knowledge to proceed effectively.

One particular cultural consideration that routinely comes up in our clinic is treating children with scrupulosity, harm, or sexual obsessions in families that are deeply religious. These families may pose some unique challenges to clinicians trying to treat OCD symptoms (e.g., concerns about sinning) through exposure while continuing to be supportive and validating of the family's spiritual values. Some families may be skeptical of the therapist's motives, particularly if the therapist does not share the family's particular religious tradition.

Siev and Huppert (2016) recently discussed some approaches to treating religious individuals with scrupulosity obsessions that have also been successfully employed in treating children. The therapist's stance should be respectful and supportive of the child's wish to have a more fulfilling religious life at all times, regardless of personal beliefs. Once OCD has been established as the main presenting problem, it must be made clear to the family that the child's OCD is not a result of their religious beliefs. Rather, OCD typically preys on the core values of the individual, leading to scrupulosity in children who are religious. This concept can be explored in detail during psychoeducation and initial efforts to externalize OCD from the family's religious tradition. Painting OCD as opportunistically compromising the child's faith can allow a therapist to discuss some distinctions between the religious practices of devout peers and how OCD might be distorting the child's sincere attempts to live a religious life. Most older children can articulate a perceived distinction between the true joy or awe of being spiritually connected and the emptiness felt when doing compulsive rituals.

Exposures for scrupulosity need to be handled sensitively and explicitly discussed ahead of time with both the child and family. The therapist should protect sufficient time to discuss the rationale for engaging in exposures and collaboratively discuss how it can be done in a manner with which the family is comfortable. The family must provide guidance on the boundaries of what their faith considers intentionally sinning (e.g., worshiping the devil) as opposed to doing things that elicit anxiety because they increase the person's risk of sinning (e.g., saying out loud the word "devil"). For example, one mother once said it was OK to do exposures regarding sinful images because "OCD puts these in his head all day anyway." In some cases, collaborative discussions with the family's clergy could also be useful.

Case Example

Tyler, an 11-year-old boy, presented to the clinic with his parents after several years of subclinical OCD symptoms that had more recently begun to affect his functioning at school. Tyler's symptoms of OCD were evaluated using the CY-BOCS, which revealed several obsessional themes and associated compulsions centered around fear of harm befalling him or other people; the obsessions typically came in the form of intrusive visual images that would occur spontaneously. The resulting compulsions would involve either repeating what he had been doing in sets of three or seeking reassurance from parents or from trusted sources (e.g., WebMD). Tyler also had been avoiding leaving his parents and siblings, but these symptoms did not warrant a diagnosis of separation anxiety because they were better explained by the OCD fears pertaining to harm and to the desire to be around family members to perform compulsive reassurance rituals. Tyler's assessment (MINI-KID, CDI) also revealed significant comorbid depressive symptoms that warranted both a formal diagnosis and clinical attention in treatment formulation.

Discussion with Tyler and his family indicated that they all saw the OCD symptoms as primary and most in need of intervention, and they also shared the belief that if the OCD could be addressed successfully, then the depressive symptoms would also be reduced. Like many youth with OCD, Tyler was stuck in a cycle of having the intrusion, trying to get rid of it, having some temporary success, then experiencing another intrusion. This process would result in great frustration, anger, and sadness and, in recent months, would result in Tyler's giving up on trying to attend to what he was doing, which oftentimes was schoolwork. His parents tried to provide reassurance and would eventually grow frustrated as well, which led to tension in the family: "It's like I can't get a break from this thing, and then I get in trouble for it." It was emphasized in the psychoeducational process that everyone in the family would learn how to deal with OCD in such a way that the fight would be against it rather than with one another.

One of the key points to make early on in treatment is that efforts to make obsessions go away are likely to provide negative reinforcement, so such efforts must be reduced and ultimately eliminated. Developing a new relationship with intrusive thoughts was emphasized in the cognitive retraining sessions, as was teaching Tyler that it was crucial to let obsessions go rather than to make them go: By doing so they would hold less power over him, he would become more effective at going about his business rather than getting engaged in the compulsive process, and the intensity and frequency of his obsessions would likely go down in the long run. Further, Tyler also needed to learn that harm-related obsessions do not lend themselves readily to a hierarchy in that the spontaneous intrusions rarely allow for a systematic progression in treatment from low to medium to high anxiety, so this was discussed in detail. Tyler identified some degree of a hierarchy to his intrusions in that thoughts that pertained to harm befalling him were generally easier to manage than those involving his siblings, and the hardest ones involved harm befalling his father and then his mother. This information was useful in forming the response prevention instructions for Tyler, who was asked to try to focus at first on resisting compulsions whenever thoughts about harm befalling him presented themselves. Simultaneously Tyler was introduced to some low-level exposures in the form of writing down relatively minor harmful things that might happen to him—for example, "I will fall down in gym and sprain my ankle." Tyler was asked to hold these types of thoughts in his mind without making efforts to neutralize them. As he was engaged in these exposures, the therapist provided psychoeducation about this process—that the logical connection between thoughts of spraining an ankle and having that actually occur was indeed weak—but also left open the possibility that such things could occur. "I like your odds but you never know," was a common refrain from the therapist in the midst of these exercises. Tyler learned how to manage his affect in the process by not managing his affect, by allowing it to come and remain while he held steady to the strategy of not "feeding the beast," as he referred to his OCD. Success in session was associated with success between sessions in dealing with these thoughts and set the stage for higher-level exposures.

Exposures in session with thoughts pertaining to parental harm were initially attempted in the context of a game known as "Harm Hangman," in which the therapist came up with a word or phrase related to parental harm and Tyler was asked to guess the letters of such words and phrases. Terms such as "minor motor vehicle accident" were soon replaced with "mad cow disease," "flesh-eating bacteria," and, eventually, less obscure terms such as "terminal liver cancer" and "extended prison term." The procedure put Tyler in touch with the content that he feared, albeit in a somewhat obscure and slightly humorous way—he came to enjoy the games in a sense and became better able to accept the presence of such thoughts without trying to neutralize them. "The more I allow these thoughts to hang around, the less they seem to really grip me," Tyler said after a particularly grim series of unfortunate events was presented in treatment. The therapist recognized this observation as a good sign of Tyler's learning the core principle of E/RP and continued to reinforce his efforts to reduce and eliminate compulsions regardless of their level of intensity.

Throughout this process, family members were informed of progress and encouraged to provide support and encouragement, rather than reassurance, when Tyler was letting them know he was distressed. "You got this," became Tyler's dad's signature line when his son presented to him with a distressed look on his face. This short and simple line was effective in helping Tyler to disengage from the reassurance process and became a source of pride for both when Tyler would simply nod and go on to the next task rather than seeking guarantees of safety from his father. Tyler tended to persist a bit more in seeking reassurance from his mother, who was the primary source of such reassurance. Both were invited into treatment to role-play how to break this cycle, with Tyler playing the role of his mother and his mother playing him. The process interjected some humor as well as empathy into the process and also provided the therapist with an opportunity to define clear rules to be followed closely between sessions. Tyler was instructed not to ask for reassurance, and Tyler's mother would point out when he did and decline initially. Then she would make suggestions for alternative activities he could engage in if the urges remained, and she would finally offer to leave the situation herself if he continued to ask. This process took some time to commit to the norm, but eventually both parties were able to do so successfully. Not surprisingly, shutting off the valve of compulsion was also associated with reduction of the frequency and intensity of obsessions, which in turn made the process easier.

Moderators and Mediators of Outcome

Although there are many viable candidates for prediction or moderation of CBT response, there is as yet an insufficient empirical foundation upon which to make confident and fully informed predictions about which patients will and which will not respond fully to this form of treatment. Ultimately, it would be of great benefit to be able to use patient, therapist, intervention, and associated contextual factors to make such predictions. However, here again the field is plagued by too few clinical outcome studies and by sample sizes that were recruited specifically to permit hypothesis testing for primary aims regarding treatment efficacy rather than prediction or moderation. Given the paucity of CBT providers available in most communities and the often lengthy wait lists that accrue in clinical practice as a result, it would be especially helpful to be able to predict response to CBT in light of the limitation of these resources. For example, it would be valuable to know specifically which patients would be likely to respond well to a course of CBT alone as opposed to which might benefit more from CBT after an adequate trial of an empirically supported pharmacotherapy. Building the evidence base upon which to make such recommendations is one of the most important goals facing our field in the next decade.

In the ideal world, questions about which child will respond to which treatment delivered under which circumstances would already be answered, but the field of pediatric OCD is clearly not there yet. At the same time, some progress has been made at least in identifying factors that could inform clinical judgment regarding treatment selection. Ginsburg, Kingery, Drake, and Grados (2008) reviewed the data on prediction or moderation of outcome in pediatric OCD and identified baseline OCD symptom severity and family psychopathology as predictors of poorer response to CBT. In the Pediatric OCD Treatment Study (POTS) I trial (Pediatric OCD Treatment Study Team, 2004), the presence of comorbid tic symptoms served as a moderator of pharmacotherapy response, that is, it predicted poorer outcome to sertraline alone but not to the treatment conditions that included CBT (CBT alone or a combination; March et al., 2007). A more comprehensive examination of the POTS I dataset that was published after Ginsburg and colleagues' systematic review (Garcia et al., 2010) identified several predictors of response to all treatments: lower OCD symptom severity, less OCD-related impairment, greater insight, fewer comorbid externalizing symptoms, and lower levels of family accommodation were all associated with better outcomes. With respect to predicting response to specific treatments, only a family history of OCD emerged as a moderator: Although family history did attenuate outcome somewhat across all treatment conditions, those with a family history had a sixfold decrease in effect size for CBT monotherapy compared with those without such a history. The mechanism by which this moderation occurs has yet to be elucidated, although examination of family variables in another RCT may prove helpful in thinking about how this effect may have been realized: Peris and colleagues (2012) examined data from Piacentini et al.'s (2011) RCT and found that families with lower levels of parental blame and family conflict, as well as higher levels of family cohesion at baseline, were more likely to have a child who responded to family-focused cognitive-behavioral therapy (FCBT). These findings suggest that environment and family history of OCD are important considerations to take into account clinically when treating OCD.

References

Abramowitz, J. S., Franklin, M. E., & Foa, E. B. (2002). Empirical status of cognitive-behavioral therapy for obsessive–compulsive disorder: A meta-analytic review. *Romanian Journal of Cognitive and Behavioral Psychotherapies, 2*(2), 89–104.

Barrett, P. M., & Healy, L. J. (2003). An examination of the cognitive processes involved in childhood obsessive–compulsive disorder. *Behaviour Research and Therapy, 41*(3), 285–299.

Barrett, P., Healy-Farrell, L., & March, J. S. (2004). Cognitive-behavioral family treatment of childhood obsessive–compulsive disorder: A controlled trial. *Journal of the American Academy of Child and Adolescent Psychiatry, 43*(1), 46–62.

Beck, A. T. (1976). *Cognitive therapy and the emotional disorders.* Madison, CT: International Universities Press.

Foa, E. B., & Kozak, M. J. (1986). Emotional processing of fear: Exposure to corrective information. *Psychological Bulletin, 99*(1), 20–35.

Franklin, M. E., Kozak, M. J., Cashman, L. A., Coles, M. E., Rheingold, A. A., & Foa, E. B. (1998). Cognitive-behavioral treatment of pediatric obsessive–compulsive disorder: An open clinical trial. *Journal of the American Academy of Child and Adolescent Psychiatry, 37*(4), 412–419.

Franklin, M. E., Kratz, H. E., Freeman, J. B., Ivarsson, T., Heyman, I., Sookman, D., et al. (2015). Cognitive-behavioral therapy for pediatric obsessive–compulsive disorder: Empirical review and clinical recommendations. *Psychiatry Research, 227*(1), 78–92.

Freeman, J. B., & Garcia, A. M. (2009). *Family-based treatment for young children with OCD: Therapist guide.* New York: Oxford University Press.

Freeman, J. B., Garcia, A. M., Fucci, C., Karitani, M., Miller, L., & Leonard, H. L. (2003). Family-based treatment of early-onset obsessive–compulsive disorder. *Journal of Child and Adolescent Psychopharmacology, 13*(2), S71–S80.

Freeman, J., Sapyta, J., Garcia, A., Compton, S., Khanna, M., Flessner, C., et al. (2014). Family-based treatment of early childhood obsessive–compulsive disorder: The Pediatric Obsessive–Compulsive Disorder Treatment Study for Young Children (POTS Jr)—A randomized clinical trial. *Journal of the American Medical Association Psychiatry, 71*(6), 689–698.

Garcia, A. M., Sapyta, J. J., Moore, P. S., Freeman, J. B., Franklin, M. E., March, J. S., et al. (2010). Predictors and moderators of treatment outcome in the Pediatric Obsessive–Compulsive Treatment Study (POTS I). *Journal of the American Academy of Child and Adolescent Psychiatry, 49*(10), 1024–1033.

Ginsburg, G. S., Kingery, J. N., Drake, K. L., & Grados, M. A. (2008). Predictors of treatment response in pediatric obsessive–compulsive disorder. *Journal of the American Academy of Child and Adolescent Psychiatry, 47*(8), 868–878.

Goodman, W. K., Price, L. H., Rasmussen, S. A., Mazure, C., Delgado, P., Heninger, G. R., et al. (1989). The Yale–Brown Obsessive Compulsive Scale: II. Validity. *Archives of General Psychiatry, 46*(11), 1012–1016.

Goodman, W. K., Price, L. H., Rasmussen, S. A., Mazure, C., Fleischmann, R. L., Hill, C. L., et al. (1989). The Yale–Brown Obsessive Compulsive Scale: I. Development, use, and reliability. *Archives of General Psychiatry, 46*, 1006–1011.

Hatch, M. L., Friedman, S., & Paradis, C. M. (1996). Behavioral treatment of obsessive–compulsive disorder in African Americans. *Cognitive and Behavioral Practice, 3*(2), 303–315.

Himle, M. B., & Franklin, M. E. (2009). The more you do it, the easier it gets: Exposure and response prevention for OCD. *Cognitive and Behavioral Practice, 16*(1), 29–39.

Ivarsson, T., Skarphedinsson, G., Kornør, H., Axelsdottir, B., Biedilæ, S., Heyman, I., et al. (2015). The place of and evidence for serotonin reuptake inhibitors (SRIs) for obsessive–compulsive disorder (OCD) in children and adolescents: Views based on a systematic review and meta-analysis. *Psychiatry Research, 227*(1), 93–103.

Kovacs, M. (1992). *The Children's Depression Inventory* [Manual]. Toronto, Ontario, Canada: Multi-Health Systems.

Leckman, J. F., Riddle, M. A., Hardin, M. T., Ort, S. I., Swartz, K. L., Stevenson, J., et al. (1989). The Yale Global Tic Severity Scale: Initial testing of a clinician-rated scale of tic severity. *Journal of the American Academy of Child and Adolescent Psychiatry, 28*(4), 566–573.

Leonard, R. C., Jacobi, D. M., Riemann, B. C., Lake, P. M., & Luhn, R. (2014). The effect of depression symptom severity on OCD treatment outcome in an adolescent residential sample. *Journal of Obsessive–Compulsive and Related Disorders, 3*(2), 95–101.

March, J. S., Franklin, M. E., Leonard, H., Garcia, A., Moore, P., Freeman, J., et al. (2007). Tics moderate treatment outcome with sertraline but not cognitive-behavior therapy in pediatric obsessive–compulsive disorder. *Biological Psychiatry, 61*(3), 344–347.

March, J. S., & Mulle, K. (1998). *OCD in children and adolescents: A cognitive-behavioral treatment manual.* New York: Guilford Press.

March, J. S., Parker, J. D. A., Sullivan, K., Stallings, P., & Conners, C. K. (1997). The Multidimensional Anxiety Scale for Children (MASC): Factor structure, reliability, and validity. *Journal of the American Academy of Child and Adolescent Psychiatry, 36*(4), 554–565.

Merlo, L. J., Storch, E. A., Lehmkuhl, H. D., Jacob, M. L., Murphy, T. K., Goodman, W. K., et al. (2010). Cognitive-behavioral therapy plus motivational interviewing improves outcome for pediatric obsessive–compulsive disorder: A preliminary study. *Cognitive Behaviour Therapy, 39*(1), 24–27.

Mowrer, O. H. (1939). A stimulus–response analysis of anxiety and its role as a reinforcing agent. *Psychological Review, 46*(6), 553–565.

Mowrer, O. H. (1960). *Learning theory and behavior.* New York: Wiley.

Obsessive Compulsive Cognitions Working Group. (1997). Cognitive assessment of obsessive–compulsive disorder. *Behaviour Research and Therapy, 35*(7), 667–681.

Pediatric OCD Treatment Study Team. (2004). Cognitive-behavioral therapy, sertraline, and their combination for children and adolescents with obsessive–compulsive disorder: The Pediatric OCD Treatment Study (POTS) randomized controlled trial. *Journal of the American Medical Association, 292*(16), 1969–1976.

Peris, T. S., Sugar, C. A., Bergman, R. L., Chang, S., Langley, A., & Piacentini, J. (2012). Family factors predict treatment outcome for pediatric obsessive–compulsive disorder. *Journal of Consulting and Clinical Psychology, 80*(2), 255–263.

Piacentini, J., Bergman, R. L., Chang, S., Landley, A., Peris, T., Wood, J. J., et al. (2011). Controlled comparison of family cognitive-behavioral therapy and psychoeducation/relaxation training for child obsessive–compulsive disorder. *Journal of the American Academy of Child and Adolescent Psychiatry, 50*(11), 1149–1161.

Piacentini, J., Peris, T. S., Bergman, R. L., Chang, S., & Jaffer, M. (2007). The Child Obsessive–Compulsive Impact Scale—Revised (COIS-R): Development and psychometric properties. *Journal of Clinical Child and Adolescent Psychology, 36*(4), 645–653.

Rachman, S., & Hodgson, R. (1980). *Obsessions and compulsions.* Englewood Cliffs, NJ: Prentice Hall.

Salkovskis, P. M. (1989). Cognitive-behavioural factors and the persistence of intrusive thoughts in obsessional problems. *Behaviour Research and Therapy, 27*(6), 677–682.

Salkovskis, P. M. (Ed.). (1996). *Frontiers of cognitive therapy.* New York: Guilford Press.

Sheehan, D., Shytle, D., & Milo, K. (2004). *MINI-KID: Mini International Neuropsychiatric Interview for Children and Adolescents.* Tampa: University of South Florida.

Siev, J., & Huppert, J. D. (2016). Treatment of scrupulosity-related obsessive–compulsive disorder. In E. A. Storch & A. B. Lewin (Eds.), *Clinical handbook of obsessive–compulsive and related disorders: A case-based approach to treating pediatric and adult populations* (pp. 39–54). Cham, Switzerland: Springer International.

Silverman, W., & Albano, A. M. (1997). *The Anxiety Disorders Interview Schedule for Children (DSM-IV).* San Antonio, TX: Psychological Corporation.

Storch, E. A., Caporino, N. E., Morgan, J. R., Lewin, A. B., Rojas, A., Brauer, L., et al. (2011). Preliminary investigation of web-camera-delivered cognitive-behavioral therapy for youth with obsessive–compulsive disorder. *Psychiatry Research, 189*(3), 407–412.

Storch, E. A., Geffken, G. R., Merlo, L. J., Mann, G., Duke, D., Munson, M., et al. (2007). Family-based cognitive-behavioral therapy for pediatric obsessive–compulsive disorder: Comparison of intensive and weekly approaches. *Journal of the American Academy of Child and Adolescent Psychiatry, 46*(4), 469–478.

Taylor, S., Abramowitz, J. S., & McKay, D. (2007). Cognitive-behavioral models of obsessive–compulsive disorder. In M. M. Antony, C. Purdon, & L. J. Summerfeldt (Eds.), *Psychological treatment of obsessive–compulsive disorder: Fundamentals and beyond* (pp. 9–29). Washington, DC: American Psychological Association.

Torp, N. C., Dahl, K., Skarphedinsson, G., Thomson, P. H., Valderhaug, R., Weidle, B., et al. (2015). Effectiveness of cognitive behavior treatment for pediatric obsessive–compulsive disorder: Acute outcomes from the Nordic Long-Term OCD Treatment Study (NordLOTS). *Behaviour Research and Therapy, 64*, 15–23.

CHAPTER FOUR

Treatment of Generalized Anxiety Disorder

Elizabeth A. Gosch
Rachel Brookland
Megan Wolensky

Theoretical Foundations

Generalized anxiety disorder (GAD) is characterized by excessive, uncontrollable anxiety and worry about a wide variety of events and activities (Whitmore, Kim-Spoon, & Ollendick, 2014). The worry and anxiety associated with GAD are out of proportion to the feared event and typically, in youth, are accompanied by at least one physiological response such as restlessness, muscle tension, irritability, and difficulty sleeping (Whitmore et al., 2014). Worry in children is often conceptualized as repetitive thinking about threatening events happening in the future, the negative outcomes associated with those events, and their lack of ability to cope. Youth with GAD commonly worry about their health, the health of loved ones, school, personal harm, their family, dying, what others think, and social issues such as homelessness (e.g., Muris, Merckelbach, Meesters, & van den Brand, 2002; Weems, Silverman, & La Greca, 2000). DSM-5 has identified worries associated with competence and performance to be the most common among children with GAD (Whitmore et al., 2014). In our clinic, we often see children worrying about such things as taking tests, getting into trouble, or intruders breaking into their homes. Although worry and anxiety are common experiences in youth, those with GAD find that their worries interfere with their daily lives and cause significant distress, making it difficult for them to go to school, sleep at night, and enjoy time with friends. They often excessively seek reassurance from others or try to do things perfectly as a means to quell their worries. These children experience more somatic symptoms and sleep problems than other clinically anxious youth without GAD (Ginsburg, Riddle, & Davies, 2006; Alfano, Ginsburg, & Kingery, 2007).

GAD typically begins early in life, with prevalence rates estimated between 0.47% and 5.9% (Ford, Goodman, & Meltzer, 2003), but children with GAD are understudied, in part due to the internalizing nature of their symptoms. As a result, there is limited information about the specific etiological or maintaining factors (Kertz & Woodruff-Borden, 2011). Emerging evidence supports the applicability of a metacognitive model of GAD (Wells, 1995; Wells & Carter, 2009) as applied to children's worry and anxiety (Ellis & Hudson, 2010). This model emphasizes the role of metacognitive beliefs in the development and maintenance of GAD. Accordingly, children's positive beliefs about the benefit of the worry, along with negative beliefs about the danger and uncontrollability of worry, are factors that maintain the worry and anxiety (Ellis & Hudson, 2010). For example, children may initially believe that their worrying helps them cope, but as their worrying increases in intensity, they may see worry as harmful to them and feel powerless to influence it, which then leads them to experience more anxiety and distress. This model supports the importance of treatment targeting how children think about their worry in addition to the worry itself. Later in this chapter we illustrate how to approach "thinking about thinking" with youth who may have difficulty understanding such cognitive and abstract concepts.

Preliminary evidence suggests that children who engage in excessive worry also tend to have difficulty tolerating uncertainty, have a negative problem orientation, and attempt to avoid threatening cognitive stimuli (Holmes, Donovan, Farrell, & March, 2014). These factors are thought to play a role in the development and maintenance of GAD (Dugas & Robichaud, 2007). Cognitive-behavioral therapy (CBT) for children with GAD incorporates attention to these factors. In this treatment, children may repeatedly engage in exposure exercises in situations that provoke feelings of uncertainty, helping them to develop new beliefs about their ability to tolerate uncertainty. Children with a negative problem orientation may have the ability to solve problems but doubt their ability to do so because they see problems as threatening and difficult (D'Zurilla & Nezu, 1999). CBT helps children to develop their problem-solving skills, to more realistically appraise problems and their ability to cope, and to successfully implement a problem-solving approach in anxiety-provoking situations. Children further engage in exposures to threatening cognitive stimuli, such as images of harm, and conduct behavioral experiments to test their negative beliefs about worry.

More general theories of anxiety propose that early family influences and environmental events interact with temperamental vulnerabilities to strengthen or ameliorate children's maladaptive cognitive and behavioral strategies (Chorpita & Barlow, 1998). Some of the better known temperamental vulnerabilities associated with anxiety in youth include behavioral inhibition, negative affectivity, and harm avoidance (Mian, Wainwright, Briggs-Gowan, & Carter, 2011). Research has shown that children as young as 2 years of age who exhibit high levels of behavioral inhibition, a temperamental style characterized by fear and withdrawal in unfamiliar situations, are at risk for developing anxiety disorders (Kagan, Reznick, & Snidman, 1988; Biederman et al., 1990). Harm avoidance, a related temperamental trait, has been found to be associated with GAD in children and adults (Rettew, Doyle, Kwan, Stanger, & Hudziak, 2006). Negative affectivity, a temperamental trait characterized by difficulty being soothed, irritability, negative mood, and intense negative emotional reactions, has been linked to child psychopathology, including anxiety (Sanson, Hemphill, & Smart, 2004). CBT approaches to GAD provide psychoeducation to help children and families understand the role of temperament in their difficulties and how these tendencies can be affected by the use of more adaptive cognitive and behavioral strategies, environmental changes, and parenting practices.

A number of maladaptive behavioral and cognitive strategies have been identified in youth with anxiety disorders. From a behavioral perspective, children with anxiety disorders such as GAD experience anxiety as highly aversive and typically respond with avoidance of anxiety-evoking and related situations. Avoidance leads to short-term relief, but this relief (negative reinforcement contingency) increases the likelihood of future avoidance and future problems with anxiety (Gosch, Flannery-Schroeder, Mauro, & Compton, 2006). Anxious behavior, such as asking for reassurance or avoiding performance situations, may be positively reinforced, often unintentionally, by attention or rewards from significant others (e.g., parents, teachers). CBT for GAD in children incorporates relaxation training and cognitive strategies to help children manage their physiological arousal, providing an alternative to avoidance as a means to decrease arousal. Therapeutic exposure to anxiety-provoking situations provides children with the opportunity to habituate and develop more adaptive beliefs about threat and their ability to cope. A key component of CBT for child anxiety, contingency management (CM), provides positive reinforcement for approaching previously avoided situations and using adaptive coping strategies. In addition, efforts are made to stop reinforcing maladaptive behaviors such as reassurance seeking and avoidance.

Family influences associated with anxiety in children include parental psychopathology, parenting style or practices, and parental modeling of anxious behavior and attitudes (Rapee, Schniering, & Hudson, 2009). Children with anxiety are more likely to have a parent with an anxiety disorder than children without anxiety (Burstein, Ginsburg, & Tein, 2010). Parenting styles associated with anxiety in youth include high levels of parental control, particularly control that limits or threatens the child's autonomy (overprotection, overcontrol), and low levels of parental warmth (rejection, criticism, low involvement or emotional support; McLeod, Wood, & Weisz, 2007; Borelli, Margolin, & Rasmussen, 2015). Recent reviews recognize that both the parent and the child play a role in creating a shared dynamic of parenting and childhood anxiety (e.g., Negreiros & Miller, 2014). For example, withdrawn child behaviors may evoke parental overprotection, and parental overprotection may limit the child's independent development. Often related to overprotective parenting and parental anxiety, anxious rearing can be described as encouragement of anxious cognitions and avoidance behaviors in children (Brakel, Muris, Bogels, & Thomassen, 2006). In a study of children with GAD, separation anxiety, and social phobia, parents' expectation of the child's threat bias and child-reported family dysfunction significantly predicted the child's self-reported threat bias (Blossom et al., 2013). Manassis et al. (2014) identified several parenting-related obstacles to treatment success that we have also encountered in our clinic, including parental anxiety, anxiogenic parenting styles, parental frustration with the child, and parents' tendency to inadvertently encourage avoidant coping.

As a means to address these obstacles in CBT for GAD, parents facilitate children's practice of skills (e.g., positive problem orientation, relaxation, positive self-talk) and therapeutic exposure in real-world settings, promoting generalization of skills. Parents are coached by therapists about how to appropriately prompt, encourage, and reinforce the adaptive behaviors (e.g., "brave" behavior), as well as how to withhold reinforcement for maladaptive behavior (e.g., asking for reassurance). Parents are encouraged to model coping skills and positive problem orientation, thus providing a positive example of how to experience anxiety/worry and cope with it. In our work with families, we encourage parental autonomy granting, support for independence, and less parental involvement as a means to increase children's self-efficacy and adaptive functioning.

Assessment

In youth, the assessment of anxiety disorders can be complex. Assessment of GAD in children requires multiple methods (e.g., interview, report inventories) and various informants, such as the child, parents, and teachers. Important areas to emphasize include the nature and intensity of the anxiety symptoms, as well as the current socialization context (e.g., home and school). Functional behavioral assessment of situations in which the child struggles often yield valuable information as to conditions that trigger and maintain the child's anxiety. Particular antecedents and consequences may be associated with the child's adaptive and maladaptive responses. It is also critical to evaluate skill deficits (e.g., social skills, learning issues) that can underlie child anxiety, as these may need to be part of the focus of treatment. Specific to GAD, the child's perceived self-efficacy, sense of control, intolerance of uncertainty, and problem-solving orientation, as well as estimations about the probability of threat, the dangerousness of situations, and the magnitude of negative outcomes, should be evaluated.

A clear pretreatment picture can serve as the groundwork for effective treatment. Both structured and semistructured diagnostic interviews such as the Anxiety Disorders Interview for DSM-5, Parent and Child Versions (ADIS-5; Albano & Silverman, in press) allow clinicians to do a thorough assessment of mental health disorders. When time limitations preclude administration of the full ADIS-5, clinicians will still find the detailed diagnostic questions helpful in assessing particular disorders and symptoms associated with GAD.

In addition to diagnostic interviews, self-report inventories provide broad information but also information specific to anxiety symptoms. The present discussion will be limited to a few of the most well-known, standardized measures that possess sound psychometric properties. These inventories require only a short amount of time to administer and score, making them highly useful in clinical settings.

Several self-report scales can assist clinicians in discriminating between the various anxiety disorders, depression, and other disorders among children. Two well-respected measures for clinicians to consider include the Multidimensional Anxiety Scale for Children (MASC; March, Parker, Sullivan, Stallings, & Conners, 1997) and the Screen for Anxiety and Related Emotional Disorders (SCARED; Birmaher et al., 1999). The MASC, which has been evaluated favorably in several countries and cultures, offers a GAD index that differentiates children with anxiety disorders from those with depression or no disorders (Villabø, Gere, Torgersen, March, & Kendall, 2012). The MASC also provides information about specific factors of anxiety: physical symptoms, social anxiety, harm avoidance, and separation/panic anxiety. The SCARED is a child and parent report inventory that is consistent with the DSM-IV classification of anxiety disorders. Available for no cost online, this instrument measures several domains, including GAD, panic/somatic, separation anxiety, and school phobia.

In addition to assessing anxiety in general, it may be helpful to evaluate specific aspects of anxiety. The Severity Measure for Generalized Anxiety Disorder—Child Age 11–17 (10 items; Craske et al., 2013), the Penn State Worry Questionnaire for Children (14 items; Chorpita, Tracey,

Brown, Collica, & Barlow, 1997), and the Intolerance of Uncertainty Scale for Children (27 items; Comer et al., 2009; Read, Comer, & Kendall, 2013) enable clinicians to easily monitor key GAD symptoms over time, as they contain only a few items and are available online for no cost (for a fuller review of worry and intolerance of uncertainty measures, see Ginsburg & Affrunti, 2013). Another measure sensitive to change over time, the Coping Questionnaire (CQ; parent and child versions; Kendall, 1994), assesses the child's ability to manage three anxiety-provoking situations that are identified based on interview data. The child and parent rate the child's ability to cope with each on a 7-point scale (1 = "not at all able to help myself" to 7 = "completely able to help myself feel comfortable"). The Revised Fear Survey Schedule for Children—Child and Parent Versions (FSSC-R; Ollendick, 1983) allows clinicians to identify a child's specific fear sensitivities, providing information as to the focus of child worries. Another critical outcome measure is based on the development of a hierarchy of anxiety-provoking situations specific to each child. Standardized ratings of child anxiety and avoidance for each hierarchy item provide a means of monitoring improvement over the course of treatment.

Treatment

A strong research base supports the use of CBT for the treatment of anxiety, including GAD, in youth. Numerous randomized clinical trials (RCTs) have established the effectiveness of CBT for treating children with anxiety disorders, with 55–65% of treated youth no longer meeting criteria for an anxiety disorder following treatment (e.g., Dadds, Spence, Holland, Barrett, & Laurens, 1997; Kendall et al., 1997; Kendall, Hudson, Gosch, Flannery-Schroeder, & Suveg, 2008; Short, Barrett, & Fox, 2001; Walkup et al., 2008; Hudson et al., 2009). A few promising GAD-specific CBT protocols have been developed that place additional emphasis on the cognitive factors associated with worry, sleep problems, and perfectionism (e.g., Clementi & Alfano, 2013; Payne, Bolton, & Perrin, 2011). An RCT of the No Worries! Program, a group treatment for children with GAD, has provided evidence to support the efficacy of this approach (Holmes, Donovan, Farrell, & March, 2014; Holmes, Donovan, & Farrell, 2015), but there is need for further RCT evaluations.

Perhaps one of the most researched CBT protocols for treating anxiety in children, the Coping Cat program, combines a variety of behavioral strategies such as *in vivo* exposure tasks with cognitive strategies such as problem solving to help children cope with their anxiety (Podell, Mychailyszyn, Edmunds, Puleo, & Kendall, 2010). The program consists of 16 sessions that are described in a detailed therapist manual. The accompanying child workbook includes child-friendly activities for the child to complete during and between sessions. The Coping Cat Parent Companion (Kendall, Podell, & Gosch, 2010) provides parents with psychoeducation about anxiety and their child's treatment program. The goal of Coping Cat is to teach children to recognize signs of anxiety and learn strategies to cope with anxiety-provoking situations. The program focuses on building skills to cope with anxiety (e.g., coping self-talk, problem solving) followed by practice using the coping skills through exposure to anxiety-provoking situations.

We have found specific strategies helpful when applying the Coping Cat protocol to GAD. Given the abstract nature of the cognitive components of GAD in youth, we find it beneficial to externalize the cognitive process by helping children create a character that incorporates their maladaptive cognitions, such as a "worry bug" or the "what if? monster." We find that youth can better recognize "thinking traps" and "talk back" to their maladaptive cognitions in this form. *In vivo* exposures may target perfectionism (e.g., handing in homework half completed), dealing with uncertainty (e.g., changes in family plans), and breaking rules/getting in trouble (e.g., running in the halls). To modify worry schemas, children may create a story or picture of the feared event (e.g., someone breaking into their home) and then add a ridiculous twist generated by the child (e.g., the burglar transformed into a unicorn bringing jelly beans to the child). As the child repeatedly reviews the story or picture, the emotional state associated with the cognitive content of the worry shifts, and anxiety tends to dissipate. To address being consumed with worries all day, we have children set a special "worry time" of 10 minutes each day. They may make a "worry box" in which they place a list of their worries and spend 10 minutes each day reviewing the worries with a parent. When they have a worry during the day, they acknowledge it and either physically or mentally put it in the "worry box" for review during the designated worry time. Often, when worry time rolls around, they have forgotten the worry or find it less distressing. Thus we encourage some strategic use of attention modification and mindful awareness but not suppression or avoidance of the fears underlying the worry. In addition to *in vivo* exposures, children with GAD frequently benefit from imaginal exposures to target abstract worries and fears of harm. For example, children suffering from GAD may worry about a death in the family or family financial problems. In these types of situations, imaginal exposure tasks asking the child to describe the situation in detail and discuss the fear can be beneficial (Kendall et al., 2005). The following case example illustrates a number of the aforementioned strategies in treating GAD in children.

Case Example

Robert was a 7-year-old Caucasian boy who entered treatment after an assessment using the Anxiety Disorders Interview Schedule for DSM-IV

(ADIS-IV; Silverman & Albano, 1996) confirmed diagnoses of GAD, separation anxiety disorder, and major depressive disorder, past episode in full remission. GAD was identified as the problem area of most concern. At the time, he lived in a major metropolitan area with his mother, father, and younger sister. His main worries concerned harm to himself. Robert worried excessively about burglars, murderers, and crime at night and was fearful of the "downtown" city area because "bad people" lived there. He also expressed worry about the future. For example, whenever he saw graffiti, he worried that he would grow up to do graffiti and "other bad things." Robert would check the locks on the doors and the alarm system multiple times every night. Additionally, Robert worried excessively about world affairs and would become fearful upon overhearing crime stories on the news. His worries caused him difficulty concentrating and sleeping, as well as irritability.

At pretreatment screening, Robert's total MASC score of 56 fell in the high average range, and his mother's MASC rating of 47 fell in the average range. His score of 15 on the Children's Depression Inventory (CDI; Kovacs, 1992) indicated a mild level of symptoms. Consistent with GAD, he endorsed items related to trouble sleeping, as well as worrying about aches and pains. Of note, he indicated that he was sure that bad things would happen to him, that he hated himself, and that he was not sure if anyone loved him. Robert indicated on the Coping Questionnaire (Kendall, 1994) that he had difficulty helping himself cope when he worried about his parents going out at night, when he worried about burglars, or when he worried that he had done something "bad." Finally, on the Children's Global Assessment Scale (CGAS; Shaffer et al., 1983), a numeric 1–100 scale used by clinicians to rate overall functioning (with 100 as optimal functioning), Robert was assigned a CGAS of 52, indicating that he had noticeable problems in numerous areas.

Robert was treated using the Coping Cat protocol (Kendall & Hedtke, 2006). Skills taught included somatic management, relaxation training, cognitive restructuring, and problem solving, followed by graded exposure tasks to practice acquired coping skills in situations involving the feared stimuli. Throughout the program, Robert learned to recognize, manage, and effectively cope with his anxiety. During the first eight sessions, the Coping Cat protocol uses the acronym of FEAR to describe the plan that children are taught to better cope with their anxiety. Each letter represents a step in the program, described herein as they unfolded in the skill-building phase with Robert. In addition, Show-That-I-Can (STIC) tasks serve as between-session assignments to bridge what was learned in session to the outside world (and thus consolidate treatment gains). Studies have shown that therapeutic homework assignments, frequently used in CBT, facilitate significant improvements (Burns & Spangler, 2000; West, Dozois, & Marcus, 2007; Hudson & Kendall, 2005). Time is spent at the beginning of each session reviewing the STIC task and reinforcing its completion.

Skill-Building Phase (Sessions 1–9)

Session 1: Building Rapport and Treatment Orientation

The goals of the first session are to orient the child and parents to the program, introduce and assign the first STIC task, and build rapport while encouraging the child's participation. In the first session, Robert presented as energetic, talkative, and occasionally hyperactive. The therapist first discussed with Robert and his mother the goals and structure of therapy and invited an open dialogue regarding any questions, comments, or concerns. The therapist then met with Robert alone and encouraged him to play a game of reciprocal questions so that they could get to know one another. The therapist discussed with Robert his overall goals of not being so stressed at nighttime and feeling safer in general. As DiGiuseppe (1989) points out, discussing a child's end goals in the beginning of therapy, rather than focusing on more specific session goals, is one way to build rapport. Robert was then asked if he would like to pick out a game to play. Robert came up with a drawing game to teach the therapist that he would choose to play at the end of every session as a sort of tradition for the remainder of treatment. The drawing game represented a reward for his work in each session. Helping the child to identify and create rewards early on in treatment is beneficial later when conducting exposures.

Session 2: Identifying Anxious Feelings

Children suffering from anxiety lack awareness of their ability to alter their emotions and the confidence to manage anxious experiences (Southam-Gerow & Kendall, 2000; Suveg & Zeman, 2004). The second session of Coping Cat is dedicated to building this awareness by teaching the child to identify and recognize anxious feelings while continuing to normalize the experience. The therapist first talked with Robert about how different feelings have different expressions in our bodies that can serve as clues for when we begin to feel bad. The following discussion took place:

THERAPIST: OK, Robert, you mentioned your sister was feeling sick last week. If she didn't tell you she was sick, how could you tell?

ROBERT: Well, she was lying on the couch curled up.

THERAPIST: Hmm. So her body seemed very still and lazy. Why, do you think?

ROBERT: Because she didn't feel well and was probably tired or something.

THERAPIST: I think that's probably right! What did her face look like, Robert?

ROBERT: It looked sort of sad, I guess.

THERAPIST: So what her face and her body looked like told you a lot about how she was feeling, even if she didn't tell you out loud she was sick?

ROBERT: Yep.

THERAPIST: So could those things be like clues to how a person is feeling?

ROBERT: I think so.

THERAPIST: Great! Now let's pretend we are detectives, Robert, and use these clues. Do you have a dog at home?

ROBERT: Yeah, my dog Mickey!

THERAPIST: Great! When Mickey's tail is wagging and his ears are perked up and he is prancing around the kitchen, how do you think he feels?

ROBERT: Happy!

THERAPIST: Sure! And how can you tell when Mickey is scared?

ROBERT: His tail goes between his legs, and his ears go down sometimes, and if it's a person he's scared of he usually barks to tell us.

THERAPIST: That's exactly right, my dog does those things too when she is scared! Those are all good clues that tell us how they are feeling.

Following this discussion, the therapist helped Robert make a "feelings dictionary." Robert looked through magazines and cut out pictures of faces with various emotions on them. He then demonstrated an ability to identify different feelings by pasting them on a blank sheet of paper and labeling the emotion underneath. The therapist spent a few minutes with Robert beginning to construct his fear hierarchy, a chart that delineates and ranks his feared situations. Robert's hierarchy included items related to separation and safety fears (e.g., that mom or dad will be shot or stabbed when they are running an errand, that a serial killer will come into the house at night). Robert came up with his own Subjective Units of Distress (SUDs) scale (Wolpe, 1969) with numbers 1–1,000, using increments of 100 to rate his distress. The fear hierarchy and SUDs ratings were discussed throughout Sessions 1–9 to prepare for the exposure phase.

Session 3: Identifying Somatic Responses to Anxiety

The third session discusses specific somatic reactions to anxiety, practices identifying them, and introduces the "F" step in the FEAR plan. The therapist normalized Robert's experience of fears by using a false fire alarm analogy to help him understand that physical symptoms of anxiety can be clues to tell him when he is becoming worried or afraid.

THERAPIST: Has the fire alarm ever gone off at school before?

ROBERT: Yes.

THERAPIST: And was it loud?

ROBERT: It was so loud I thought my ears were going to fall off!

THERAPIST: Wow, that's loud! How were you feeling when the fire alarm went off? Were you feeling anything in your body?

ROBERT: Well it really surprised me at first and my heart started beating really, really fast, like bum-bum, bum-bum, like out of my chest!

THERAPIST: I bet! You know, the first step in the FEAR plan is what letter, do you think?

ROBERT: "F"?

THERAPIST: That's exactly right! The "F" step is first, and is stands for "Feeling frightened?" Sometimes when we are feeling frightened our bodies tell us first. The first alarm might make your heart go "bum-bum" because your body realizes there might be danger, even before you've had a chance to think about it! But fire alarms go off for all sorts of reasons, right? They might go off because someone pulled it, or because it's broken, or even for a fire drill just for practice, and is there danger in any of those situations?

ROBERT: Probably not.

THERAPIST: Right! But your body still reacts like there is, and it makes you feel really scared for a minute, right?

ROBERT: Right.

THERAPIST: So sometimes our worry or anxiety is the same way. We might feel scared even when there is no danger, sort of like a false alarm. We're going to practice in here how to figure out when the false alarm is happening so you don't think you're in danger when it's really safe. One way to tell a false alarm is by paying attention to those clues in your body.

The therapist then used a body cutout activity to assist Robert in identifying his own signals or clues for when he is feeling nervous. The therapist traced Robert's body and helped Robert identify and label the cutout. For example, Robert talked about how his heart raced sometimes when he thought about murderers. The therapist asked Robert to show this on the cutout, and he colored a heart where his chest was and wrote, "heart drumming-bum bum bum" next to it. The therapist then helped Robert practice how to use these somatic responses as clues to his worry by using role-playing techniques. Specifically, the therapist employed the "tag-along" procedure (Ollendick & Cerny, 1981) by first acting out her own example of being afraid of a big dog at the park. The therapist pretended to step out the front door and, as she was journeying to the park, identi-fied different clues (e.g., "I can feel my heart getting faster"). Robert used a recent example of a ride on a roller coaster; he acknowledged different parts of the experience during which he felt escalating bodily sensations (e.g., waiting in line with butterflies in his stomach, heart pounding on the ride). The therapist encouraged Robert to be aware of what his body was telling him in the coming week as part of his STIC task.

Session 4: First Meeting with Parents

The fourth session is a parent-only meeting dedicated to providing further information about treatment, addressing parents' questions and concerns, gathering additional information about the child's functioning, and discussing ways the parents can be involved in treatment. The therapist sensitively discussed common cycles of parent–child interactions that develop with anxious children and asked the parents if they had ever engaged in similar interactions. The parents were encouraged to monitor their behavior over the week to see whether they noticed inadvertent accommodations that might be playing a role in maintaining Robert's anxiety, worry, and avoidance. They were also asked to monitor their own modeling of anxiety and avoidance of anxiety-evoking situations, as well as other variables related to GAD (e.g., intolerance of uncertainty, worrying, overcontrol, rejection). Robert's parents were already implementing many positive and supportive techniques to help Robert manage his anxiety. However, it should be noted here that many parents of anxious children have anxieties themselves, and clinicians should be prepared to handle parents who are unaware that they are modeling poor coping strategies, are negativistic in parent–child interaction styles, or are simply conveying an excess amount of worry and accommodation regarding their child's anxiety. An important function of the parent sessions can be to teach parents how to effectively manage their child's anxiety and their own anxieties instead of inadvertently maintaining them through the avoidance cycle. Normalizing the tendency for all parents to want to protect their children from distressful situations can facilitate this conversation.

Session 5: Relaxation Training

The focus of the fifth session is on reviewing muscle tension as it relates to other somatic sensations of anxiety and on teaching relaxation. To begin, the therapist prompted Robert to imagine a time when he felt relaxed and to explore how his body felt. Then the therapist asked Robert to imagine again the roller coaster example used in the previous session and used imaginal techniques to help him remember how his body felt. A comparison was then made regarding how it felt to be relaxed rather than tense. The therapist also helped Robert externalize these bodily sensations of fear by helping him describe these feelings verbally, and he came up with "the

Incredible Hulk taking over" as a description of his feelings. Externalizing and labeling anxiety creates a common language between therapist and child and, as a result, might help children to better conceptualize these feelings and related cognitions. The therapist first introduced relaxation techniques by practicing some belly breathing with Robert. Robert had initial success with this and expressed that it helped his body feel calmer. The therapist then had Robert practice tensing and relaxing his body to further exaggerate the difference, using Koeppen's (1974) script for progressive muscle relaxation for children. The following is an excerpt from the script that was applied in this session with Robert:

THERAPIST: OK, Robert, we just talked about feeling tense versus feeling relaxed. We agreed that feeling relaxed is much better, and we usually feel tense when we are stressed out or afraid of something. Now that we know how to notice when the Incredible Hulk is taking over, we can use relaxing activities to make him go away so that you can feel relaxed again. It's hard to be afraid when we feel really relaxed, right?

ROBERT: Right. I wish I felt relaxed and happy all the time. That would be easy.

THERAPIST: Well, sometimes we just need to practice things so they can become easier for us, right? So let's practice relaxing our muscles. With enough practice, relaxing will just happen naturally, on its own!

ROBERT: OK.

THERAPIST: OK. Sit comfortable in your chair and take some deep, belly breaths. Plant both feet on the floor and let your arms hang loose. You can close your eyes if you'd like. Are you ready to begin?

ROBERT: I'm ready.

THERAPIST: OK, here we go. Remember to keep breathing and try to pay attention to your body. Pretend you have a whole lemon in your left hand. Now squeeze it hard. Try to squeeze all the juice out. Feel the tightness in your hand and arm as you squeeze. Now drop the lemon. Notice how your muscles feel when they are relaxed. Take another lemon and squeeze. Try to squeeze this one harder than you did the first one. That's right. Real hard. Now drop the lemon and relax. See how much better your hand and arm feel when they are relaxed.

The same process is repeated with the right hand and arm, followed by a section for arms and shoulders, jaw, face and nose, stomach, and legs and feet. The therapist then had a discussion with Robert about different times he could practice and use these new skills. He identified nighttime as when he felt the most stressed. Robert was given the opportunity at the end of the session to explain and show his mother these new skills, and the therapist gave Robert's mother a recording of the therapist reading the script so that Robert could continue to practice his relaxation skills at home each night.

Session 6: Identifying Anxious Self-Talk and Learning to Challenge Thoughts

Prior to beginning Session 6, relaxation was reviewed to consolidate gains, and Robert reported that he had done well with practicing along with the recording each night and that it had become a part of his bedtime routine. The goals of Session 6 are to introduce the concept of self-talk, to differentiate anxious self-talk from coping self-talk, and to introduce the "E" step in the FEAR plan.

To begin, Robert viewed cartoon characters in specific situations who were feeling different feelings and tried to guess what they were thinking (i.e., what was in their "thought bubble"). For example, one situation in the workbook involves two children who are going ice skating. One child has never skated before; the other is a skilled skater. Robert and the therapist discussed differences in the characters' feelings and thoughts to help Robert understand that "expecting that something bad is going to happen" is often associated with feeling anxious, while thinking that one can cope or have fun is often associated with positive feelings. The therapist explained that the next step in the FEAR plan, the "E" ("expecting") step, is to learn to feel better by changing anxious self-talk to coping self-talk. Utilizing the tag-along technique, the therapist practiced with her own example before guiding Robert through the process:

THERAPIST: Okay, Robert, let's try using one of your examples with the "E" step. We've been talking a lot about how it makes you nervous and scared when Dad goes out at night to run errands. Should we use that?

ROBERT: Sure.

THERAPIST: OK, great. So what happens when Dad gets ready to go out?

ROBERT: I get scared and, well, I usually ask him not to go, but it doesn't work. Then he goes out anyway, and I get upset.

THERAPIST: Would you say the Incredible Hulk takes over?

ROBERT: Oh, yeah.

THERAPIST: What would the Incredible Hulk's thought bubble say when Dad goes out?

ROBERT: He's thinking "Dad's going to get shot at the grocery store and die."

THERAPIST: OK, so you tried to get Dad to stay home, and he went out anyway. Are you feeling frightened? What's happening in your body?

ROBERT: Yes. My heart is pounding, and I'm crying.

THERAPIST: OK, so you did the "F" step and you know you're feeling frightened, maybe you're trying to take belly breaths and relax, but the Incredible Hulk is getting stronger, and you're starting to get more scared, and you keep thinking that Dad is going to get shot. Remember that the "E" step means "Expecting bad things to happen"? Let's go through the "E" step questions and pretend we are detectives gathering evidence. First, "Do I know for sure this is going to happen?"

ROBERT: Well, no, not for sure. I'm just afraid of it happening.

THERAPIST: OK, has it happened before, or has it happened to anyone you know?

ROBERT: Not to anyone I know, but I hear it in the news a lot, and I know it's happened near where I live.

THERAPIST: OK, but not to anyone you know.

ROBERT: No.

THERAPIST: So how likely do you think it is that it will happen to Dad?

ROBERT: Probably not that likely, but there's a lot of bad people and murderers out at night.

THERAPIST: Do you think we could try to use some coping thoughts and see if that helps the Incredible Hulk calm down? Who knows, maybe it might help.

ROBERT: I guess.

At this point the therapist helped Robert brainstorm different coping thoughts that he could believe in. He came up with "Dad will probably be fine and will be home soon." The therapist helped Robert make a coping card with this thought on it to remind him. Although Robert seemed to be able to come up with alternative coping thoughts to use, he did not feel confident regarding his ability to use them in stressful situations. The therapist helped Robert practice in situations that were likely to come up and encouraged him to try in the next week.

Session 7: Reviewing Anxious and Coping Self-Talk and Developing Problem-Solving Skills

The goals of Session 7 include introducing the "A" step and teaching problem-solving skills. At the beginning of Session 7, Robert said that he had continued to work on his relaxation skills at home and that he tried to use coping thoughts as well, although he was still experiencing significant distress at night. The therapist practiced the "F" and "E" steps with Robert in session before moving on, and he was encouraged to continue practicing these skills. Problem solving was taught through a red–yellow–green light game that the therapist created. The following transcript serves to illustrate the session:

THERAPIST: Do you remember what letter we are learning in the FEAR plan today?

ROBERT: The "A" step?

THERAPIST: That's right. The "A" step stands for "Action planning." Sometimes when we are feeling frightened, relaxation might help a little, and gathering the evidence might help, too, but we still might be scared after trying those things. That's what happened to you this week, right?

ROBERT: Yeah, I did everything we practiced, but it didn't really work.

THERAPIST: That's OK! We still have a couple more things to learn. So far we've learned to know how to do things with our feelings and thoughts. Today we're going to play a game to practice problem solving, so that when you feel stuck after trying those things, you know how to make a plan and do something about it. Sound good?

ROBERT: Sounds good.

THERAPIST: Cool, OK, so we're going to take a pretend problem to play the game with first. Pretend you wake up for school in the morning, and you can't find your shoes. The bus is coming, and your mom is yelling at you to hurry up. The first step in problem solving is to brainstorm— that means to think of all the possible things you could do, even if they seem silly or like a bad idea. Let's see how many we can think of together in the next 3 minutes. Ready? Go.

The therapist and Robert created a list that included items such as "wear different shoes," "go to school with no shoes," "go to school late," and "ask mom to help me look." Next, the therapist went through the list with Robert and asked, for each one, "What would happen if I did this?" and "How would I feel if that happened?" After that, Robert colored each one red, yellow, or green depending on whether he thought it was a bad idea, an OK idea, or a great idea. The green choices were combined to make an action plan, with the yellow being the backup plan. Afterward, Robert created an action plan using the same steps for his stressful situation of his dad going out at night. Once an action plan was created, it was added to his coping card for use over the following week.

Session 8: Introducing Self-Evaluation and Self-Reward and Reviewing Skills

Session 8 is spent reviewing skills already learned and explaining the "R" step ("ratings and rewards"), as well as preparing to transition into the exposure phase of treatment. The therapist summarized for Robert the first three steps of the FEAR plan: recognizing his fearful feelings, recognizing and replacing his anxious self-talk with coping self-talk, and taking action to help change the situation and get the power back. Then she introduced the idea of rating his performance and rewarding himself for effort and for staying in the situation even when he was afraid. The therapist used the example of teaching a dog to roll over on command by rewarding the dog for each little step he takes. The dog is rewarded for sitting, then lying down, then turning on his side, and then flipping over. Like us, dogs learn things in pieces and with practice. When we make a good effort, a reward can motivate us to try even harder next time. The therapist emphasized that rewards were for trying hard, not just for when we do things perfectly. The therapist then used different examples relevant to Robert's life to help him practice deciding whether or not he thought he should be rewarded in different situations and what rewards he might receive. The therapist and Robert made a "FEAR plan ID card" that summarized the steps so that he could carry it with him during exposures. They practiced the plan using several examples: riding a roller coaster, Robert's dad going out at night, and Robert sleeping in his own bed. The therapist discussed the process and rationale for upcoming exposure exercises. She explained that he would likely experience some fear or anxiety, much like he already did, but that with practice his anxiety would go down, and he would start to feel better. Prior to the end of the session, Robert expressed anxiety about not wanting therapy to end. After validating Robert's feelings, the therapist helped Robert label this "anxious thought," identify thinking traps (e.g., negative fortune telling), and problem-solve how to cope with the situation. At this time, Robert also continued to express harm-to-himself and harm-to-others concerns, but he seemed motivated to try exposure challenges to help decrease these fears.

Session 9: Second Meeting with Parents

The ninth session is a parent session focusing on preparation for the exposure tasks that come next in treatment. The therapist reviewed the rationale and process for the exposure phase, and then she and Robert's parents collaboratively developed a hierarchy of anxiety-provoking situations for upcoming exposures. She discussed what they might expect over the coming weeks, the things they could do at home to best support exposures (e.g., providing appropriate prompts, encouragement, and rewards), and problem-solved potential obstacles to treatment.

Exposure Phase (Sessions 10–16)

Exposure serves as the main focus of in-session and between-session work in Sessions 10–16. One potential therapeutic mechanism underlying exposures is habituation to the feared stimuli coupled with response prevention, which in turn leads to long-term corrective learning (Barlow, 2014; Foa & McNally, 1996). It is hypothesized that once the client repeatedly stays in the feared situation without being allowed to engage in known safety behaviors, a corrective experience occurs that helps the client realize that he or she is capable of coping and successfully dealing with the feared stimuli and that it is unlikely that the feared outcome will occur. Another theoretical slant focuses on the new learning that occurs following exposure: The child learns that the feared catastrophe doesn't happen. The Coping Cat protocol is flexible in that multiple areas of stress can be targeted at once, depending on therapist discretion. At the beginning of Robert's exposure phase, the therapist, Robert, and his mother collaboratively decided to first target Robert's fear of guns, as well as sleeping in his own bed. At the time, Robert was sleeping on the floor of his bedroom every night by the door, where he could see into his sister's room. He was fearful of sleeping in his own bed, which was next to a window, because he thought someone would point a gun through the window and shoot him. For Robert's first *in vivo* exposure, he looked at a picture of a gun for 10 seconds, then again for 15 seconds. During the exposure, he rated his fear using the SUDs rating scale that he previously created (100–1,000). His first week of at-home exposures involved continuing to look at this picture for increasing amounts of time, as well as lying in his bed for 1 minute the first night, adding a minute each night. The therapist explained to both Robert and his parents that exposures are meant to be flexible, emphasizing the importance of at least attempting to complete the exposures and of rewarding these attempts.

When beginning exposures, it can be helpful to assign easier exposures so that the child does not become overly fearful and overwhelmed by the process. Over sessions, the therapist and child move up the fear hierarchy, making exposures incrementally difficult. Encouraging the family to take initiative and be creative at home during this process can ensure that successes are strung together more quickly. In Robert's case, the family reported that Robert found the initial exposure plan easy, so they had altered the length of time Robert did each challenge to make them more difficult. In fact, Robert had a lot of initial success with sleeping in his own bed and with looking at different pictures of guns (the therapist had emailed the pictures to Robert's mom). During the next session, his SUDs ratings before, during, and after each exposure were charted so that Robert could identify for himself the pattern of fear: at its highest before the challenge and progressively going down until it was over. *In vivo* exposures included watching YouTube videos of guns being shot at a gun range and listening to the sound. The therapist expressed satisfaction with Robert's efforts and encouraged him to keep it up. In addition, the therapist consistently checked with Robert's mom to make sure that Robert was being rewarded for completing his challenges as planned. Robert's next challenge sheet was created collaboratively on the computer. They decided to keep building on prior exposures while adding in the challenge of his father going out for errands at night. For example, the first night, Robert would do an activity with his mom while his dad went out for 5 minutes, then 10 minutes the next night, then 20 minutes the next, followed by playing with his sister (not bothering his mom) while his dad went out for 10, then 15, then 20 minutes.

During the exposure phase, we continued to practice examining Robert's thoughts and how they related to his anxiety. More and more, Robert developed adaptive thoughts along with his new relaxation skills to help him cope successfully with anxiety. Robert quickly stopped checking the locks on the doors and the alarm system. Robert began to experience success with his exposures and was rewarded for his efforts. He displayed less intense reaction to guns, graffiti, and people living in the city and thus did not become as upset by them or think of them as harmful. His avoidance and associated safety behaviors of clinging to his mom and engaging in behavioral outbursts or crying decreased. By the time therapy terminated, Robert was sleeping in his own bed every night. He reported that he no longer believed the world was a dangerous place but more realistically expressed feeling that he and members of his family would be safe as long as they were careful and looked out for each other.

At posttreatment, Robert's total MASC score of 39 and his mother's rating of 28 both fell in the low range. His CDI score of 8 suggested that he was experiencing minimal depressive symptoms. Posttreatment data on the coping questionnaire suggested that both Robert and his mother felt that Robert was much more in control of his coping abilities. They indicated that he was very much able to help himself cope if he worried about his parents going out at night, if he worried about burglars, or if he worried that he had done something "bad." At posttreatment assessment, Robert was assigned a CGAS of 80, which means he was experiencing no more than minor impairment in functioning in school, at home, and with peers. He expressed normal emotional distress in response to life stressors, which occasionally resulted in behavioral outbursts, but these were brief and transient, and, in general, Robert was functioning well.

Mediators and Moderators of Outcome

As CBT has been found helpful in treating children with anxiety, researchers are beginning to explore potential moderators and mediators of outcomes. Studies to date indicate that race, ethnicity, and gender do not appear to differentially influence outcome (Treadwell, Flannery-Schroeder, & Kendall, 1995). A few studies suggest that children who are more active and involved with the treatment tend to have better outcomes (e.g., Chu & Kendall, 2009). Some studies have found a relationship between treatment response, decreases in negative automatic thoughts, and increased perceived control over anxiety, consistent with the CBT model (e.g., Kendall & Treadwell, 2007; Muris, Mayer, den Adel, Roos, & van Wamelen, 2009). Gains in coping efficacy have been found to mediate treatment improvement in anxiety symptoms (Kendall et al., 2016). In our experience, involvement can be fostered by helping the child learn through activities and play—teaching through discovery versus didactic instruction. There is evidence that therapists who are more collaborative and empathic, who follow the Coping Cat manual, and who implement the treatment in a developmentally appropriate way have better treatment outcomes (Podell et al., 2013). Such findings speak to the need to maintain fidelity with treatment procedures being sensitive to children's emotional and developmental needs when implementing treatment for child GAD.

References

Albano, A. M., & Silverman, W. K. (in press). *The Anxiety Disorders Interview Schedule for DSM-5—Child and Parent Versions*. New York: Oxford University Press.

Alfano, C., Ginsburg, G., & Kingery, J. (2007). Sleep-related problems among children and adolescents with anxiety disorders. *Journal of the American Academy of Child and Adolescent Psychiatry, 46*(2), 224–232.

Barlow, D. H. (Ed.). (2014). *Clinical handbook of psychological disorders: A step-by-step treatment manual* (5th ed.). New York: Guilford Press.

Biederman, J., Rosenbaum, J. F., Hirshfeld, D. R., Faraone, S. V., Bolduc, E. A., Gersten, M., et al. (1990). Psychiatric correlates of behavioral inhibition in young children of parents with and without psychiatric disorders. *Archives of General Psychiatry, 47*, 21–26.

Birmaher, B., Brent, D. A., Chiappetta, L., Bridge, J., Monga, S., & Baugher, M. (1999). Psychometric properties of the Screen for Child Anxiety Related Emotional Disorders (SCARED): A replication study. *Journal of the American Academy of Child and Adolescent Psychiatry, 38*(10), 1230–1236.

Blossom, J., Ginsburg, G., Birmaher, B., Walkup, J., Kendall, P., Keeton, C., et al. (2013). Parental and family factors as predictors of threat bias in anxious youth. *Cognitive Therapy Research, 37*, 817–819.

Borelli, J., Margolin, G., & Rasmussen, H. (2015). Parental overcontrol as a mechanism explaining the longitudinal association between parent and child anxiety. *Journal of Child and Family Studies, 24*, 1559–1574.

Brakel, A., Muris, P., Bogels, S., & Thomassen, C. (2006). A multifactorial model for the etiology of anxiety in non-clinical adolescents: Main and interactive effects of behavioral inhibition, attachment and parental rearing. *Journal of Child and Family Studies, 15*(5), 568–578.

Burns, D. D., & Spangler, D. L. (2000). Does psychotherapy homework lead to improvements in depression in cognitive-behavioral therapy or does improvement lead to increased homework compliance? *Journal of Consulting and Clinical Psychology, 68*(1), 46–56.

Burstein, M., Ginsburg, G., & Tein, J. (2010). Parental anxiety and child symptomatology: An examination of additive and interactive effects of parent psychopathology. *Journal of Abnormal Child Psychology, 38*, 897–909.

Chorpita, B. F., & Barlow, D. H. (1998). The development of anxiety: The role of control in the early environment. *Psychological Bulletin, 124*(1), 3–21.

Chorpita, B. F., Tracey, S. A., Brown, T. A., Collica, T. J., & Barlow, D. H. (1997). Assessment of worry in children and adolescents. *Behavior Research and Therapy, 35*(6), 569–581.

Chu, B., & Kendall, P. (2009). Positive association of child involvement and treatment outcome within a manual-based cognitive-behavioral treatment for anxious youth. *Journal of Consulting and Clinical Psychology, 72*, 821–829.

Clementi, M., & Alfano, C. (2013). Targeted behavioral therapy for childhood generalized anxiety disorder: A time-series analysis of changes in anxiety and sleep. *Journal of Anxiety Disorders, 38*, 215–222.

Comer, J. S., Roy, A., Furr, J., Gotimer, K., Beidas, R., Dugas, M., et al. (2009). The Intolerance of Uncertainty Scale for Children: A psychometric evaluation. *Psychological Assessment, 21*, 402–411.

Craske, M., Wittchen, U., Bogels, S., Stein, M., Andrews, G., & Lebeu, R. (2013). Severity Measure for Generalized Anxiety Disorder—Child Age 11–17 [Measurement instrument]. Retrieved from *www.psychiatry.org/practice/dsm/dsm5/online-assessment-measures*.

Dadds, M. R., Spence, S. H., Holland, D. E., Barrett, P. M., & Laurens, K. R. (1997). Prevention and early intervention for anxiety disorders: A controlled trial. *Journal of Consulting and Clinical Psychology, 65*, 627–635.

DiGiuseppe, R. (1989). Cognitive therapy with children. In A. Freeman, K. Simon, L. Beutler, & H. Arkowitz (Eds.), *Comprehensive handbook of cognitive therapy* (pp. 515–533). New York: Springer.

Dugas, M. J., & Robichaud, M. (2007). *Cognitive-behavioral treatment for generalized anxiety disorder: From science to practice.* New York: Routledge.

D'Zurilla, T., & Nezu, A. M. (1999). *Problem-solving therapy: A social competence approach to clinical intervention* (2nd ed.). New York: Springer.

Ellis, D. M., & Hudson, J. L. (2010). The metacognitive model of generalized anxiety disorder in children and adolescents. *Clinical Child and Family Psychology Review, 13*(2), 151–163.

Foa, E. B., & McNally, R. J. (1996). Mechanisms of change in exposure therapy. In R. Rapee (Ed.), *Current controversies in the anxiety disorders* (pp. 329–343). New York: Guilford Press.

Ford, T., Goodman, R., & Meltzer, H. (2003). The British Child and Adolescent Mental Health Survey 1999: The prevalence of DSM-IV disorders. *Journal of the American Academy of Child and Adolescent Psychiatry, 42*(10), 1203–1211.

Ginsburg, G., & Affrunti, N. (2013). Generalized anxiety disorder in children and adolescents. In R. Vasa & A. Roy (Eds.), *Pediatric anxiety disorders: A clinical guide* (pp. 71–90). New York: Springer.

Ginsburg, G. S., Riddle, M. A., & Davies, M. (2006). Somatic symptoms in children and adolescents with anxiety disorders. *Journal of the American Academy of Child and Adolescent Psychiatry, 45*, 1179–1187.

Gosch, E., Flannery-Schroeder, E., Mauro, C., & Compton, S. (2006). Principles of cognitive behavioral therapy for anxiety disorders in children. *Journal of Cognitive Psychotherapy, 20*(3), 247–262.

Holmes, M., Donovan, C. L., & Farrell, L. J. (2015). A disorder-specific, cognitively focused group treatment for childhood generalized anxiety disorder: Development and case illustration of the No Worries! Program. *Journal of Cognitive Psychotherapy: An International Quarterly, 29*(4), 275–301.

Holmes, M., Donovan, C., Farrell, L., & March, S. (2014). The efficacy of a group-based, disorder-specific treatment program for childhood GAD: A randomized controlled trial. *Behaviour Research and Therapy, 61,* 122–135.

Hudson, J., & Kendall, P. C. (2005). Children. In N. Kazantzis, F. Deane, K. R. Ronan, & L. L'Abate (Eds.), *Using homework assignments in cognitive-behavior therapy* (pp. 63–78). New York: Routledge.

Hudson, J. L., Rapee, R. M., Deveney, C., Schniering, C., Lyneham, H., & Bovopoulos, N. (2009). Cognitive-behavioral treatment versus an active control for children and adolescents with anxiety disorders: A randomized trial. *Journal of the American Academy of Child and Adolescent Psychiatry, 48,* 533–544.

Kagan, J., Reznick, J. S., & Snidman, N. (1988). Biological bases of childhood shyness. *Science, 240,* 167–171.

Kendall, P. C. (1994). Treating anxiety disorders in children: Results of a randomized clinical trial. *Journal of Consulting and Clinical Psychology, 62,* 100–110.

Kendall, P., Cummings, C., Villabo, M., Narayanan, M., Treadwell, K., Birmaher, B., et al. (2016). Mediators of change in the Child/Adolescent Anxiety Multimodal Treatment Study. *Journal of Consulting and Clinical Psychology, 84*(1), 1–14.

Kendall, P. C., Flannery-Schroeder, E., Panichelli-Mindel, S. M., Southam-Gerow, M., Henin, A., & Warman, M. (1997). Therapy for youths with anxiety disorders: A second randomized clinical trial. *Journal of Consulting and Clinical Psychology, 65*(3), 366–380.

Kendall, P. C., & Hedtke, K. A. (2006). *Cognitive-behavioral therapy for anxious children: Therapist manual.* Ardmore, PA: Workbook.

Kendall, P. C., Hudson, J., Gosch, E., Flannery-Schroeder, E., & Suveg, C. (2008). Cognitive-behavioral therapy for anxiety disordered youth: A randomized clinical trial evaluating child and family modalities. *Journal of Consulting and Clinical Psychology, 76,* 282–297.

Kendall, P. C., Podell, J., & Gosch, E. (2010). *The Coping Cat Parent Companion.* Ardmore, PA: Workbook.

Kendall, P. C., Robin, J. A., Hedtke, K. A., Suveg, C., Flannery-Schroeder, E., & Gosch, E. (2005). Considering CBT with anxious youth?: Think exposures. *Cognitive and Behavioral Practice, 12*(1), 136–150.

Kendall, P. C., & Treadwell, K. H. (2007). The role of self-statements as a mediator in treatment for youth with anxiety disorders. *Journal of Consulting and Clinical Psychology, 75*(3), 380–389.

Kertz, S. J., & Woodruff-Borden, J. (2011). The developmental psychopathology of worry. *Clinical Child and Family Psychology Review, 14*(2), 174–197.

Koeppen, A. S. (1974). Relaxation training for children. *Elementary School Guidance and Counseling, 9,* 14–21.

Kovacs, M. (1992). *Children's Depression Inventory*. North Tonawanda, NY: Multi-Health Systems.

Manassis, K., Lee, T. C., Bennett, K., Zhao, X. Y., Mendlowitz, S., Duda, S., et al. (2014). Types of parental involvement in CBT with anxious youth: A preliminary meta-analysis. *Journal of Consulting and Clinical Psychology, 82*, 1163–1172.

March, J. S., Parker, J. D., Sullivan, K., Stallings, P., & Conners, C. K. (1997). The Multidimensional Anxiety Scale for Children (MASC): Factor structure, reliability, and validity. *Journal of the American Academy of Child and Adolescent Psychiatry, 36*(4), 554–565.

McLeod, B. D., Wood, J. J., & Weisz, J. R. (2007). Examining the association between parenting and childhood anxiety: A meta-analysis. *Clinical Psychology Review, 27*(2), 155–172.

Mian, N. D., Wainwright, L., Briggs-Gowan, M. J., & Carter, A. S. (2011). An ecological risk model for early childhood anxiety: The importance of early child symptoms and temperament. *Journal of Abnormal Child Psychology, 39*(4), 501–512.

Muris, P., Mayer, B., den Adel, M., Roos, T., & van Wamelen, J. (2009). Predictors of change following cognitive-behavioral treatment of children with anxiety problems: A preliminary investigation on negative automatic thoughts and anxiety control. *Child Psychiatry and Human Development, 40*(1), 139–151.

Muris, P., Merckelbach, H., Meesters, C., & van den Brand, K. (2002). Cognitive development and worry in normal children. *Cognitive Therapy and Research, 26*, 775–785.

Negreiros, J., & Miller, L. D. (2014). The role of parenting in childhood anxiety: Etiological factors and treatment implications. *Clinical Psychology: Science and Practice, 21*, 3–17.

Ollendick, T. H. (1983). Reliability and validity of the Revised Fear Survey Schedule for Children (FSSC-R). *Behaviour Research and Therapy, 21*, 685–692.

Ollendick, T. H., & Cerny, J. (1981). *Clinical behavior therapy with children*. New York: Plenum Press.

Payne, S., Bolton, D., & Perrin, S. (2011). A pilot investigation of cognitive therapy for generalized anxiety disorder in children aged 7–17 years. *Cognitive Therapy and Research, 35*(2), 171–178.

Podell, J., Kendall, P., Gosch, E., Compton, S., March, J., Albano, A., et al. (2013). Therapist factors and outcomes in CBT for anxiety in youth. *Professional Psychology: Research and Practice, 44*(2), 89–98.

Podell, J. L., Mychailyszyn, M., Edmunds, J., Puleo, C. M., & Kendall, P. C. (2010). The Coping Cat Program for anxious youth: The FEAR plan comes to life. *Cognitive and Behavioral Practice, 17*(2), 132–141.

Rapee, R., Schniering, C., & Hudson, J. (2009). Anxiety disorders during childhood and adolescence: Origins and treatment. *Annual Review of Clinical Psychology, 5*, 311–341.

Read, K., Comer, J., & Kendall, P. C. (2013). The Intolerance of Uncertainty Scale for Children (IUS-C): Discriminating between primary anxiety diagnoses. *Psychological Assessment, 25*, 722–729.

Rettew, D. C., Doyle, A. C., Kwan, M., Stanger, C., & Hudziak, J. J. (2006). Exploring the boundary between temperament and generalized anxiety disorder: A receiver operating characteristic analysis. *Journal of Anxiety Disorders, 20*(7), 931–945.

Sanson, A., Hemphill, S., & Smart, D. (2004). Connections between temperament and social development: A review. *Social Development, 13*(1), 142–170.

Shaffer, D., Gould, M. S., Brasic, J., Ambrosini, P., Fisher, P., Bird, H., et al. (1983). A Children's Global Assessment Scale (CGAS). *Archives of General Psychiatry, 40*(11), 1228–1231.

Short, A. L., Barrett, P. M., & Fox, T. L. (2001). Evaluating the FRIENDS program: A cognitive-behavioral group treatment for anxious children and their parents. *Journal of Clinical Child Psychology, 30*, 525–535.

Silverman, W. K., & Albano, A. M. (1996). *The Anxiety Disorders Interview Schedule for Children for DSM-IV (Child and Parent Versions)*. San Antonio, TX: Psychological Corporation.

Southam-Gerow, M. A., & Kendall, P. C. (2000). A preliminary study of the emotion understanding of youths referred for treatment of anxiety disorders. *Journal of Clinical Child Psychology, 29*(3), 319–327.

Suveg, C., & Zeman, J. (2004). Emotion regulation in children with anxiety disorders. *Journal of Clinical Child and Adolescent Psychology, 33*(4), 750–759.

Treadwell, K. H., Flannery-Schroeder, E. C., & Kendall, P. C. (1995). Ethnicity and gender in relation to adaptive functioning, diagnostic status, and treatment outcome in children from an anxiety clinic. *Journal of Anxiety Disorders, 9*(5), 373–384.

Villabø, M. A., Gere, M. K., Torgersen, S., March, J. S., & Kendall, P. C. (2012). Diagnostic efficiency of the child and parent versions of the Multidimensional Anxiety Scale for Children (MASC). *Journal of Clinical Child and Adolescent Psychology, 41*, 75–85.

Walkup, J. T., Albano, A. M., Piacentini, J., Birmaher, B., Compton, S. N., Sherrill, J. T., et al. (2008). Cognitive behavioral therapy, sertraline, or a combination in childhood anxiety. *New England Journal of Medicine, 359*, 2753–2766.

Weems, C. F., Silverman, W. K., & La Greca, A. M. (2000). What do youth referred for anxiety problems worry about?: Worry and its relation to anxiety and anxiety disorders in children and adolescents. *Journal of Abnormal Child Psychology, 28*, 63–72.

Wells, A. (1995). Meta-cognition and worry: A cognitive model of generalized anxiety disorder. *Behavioural and Cognitive Psychotherapy, 23*(3), 301–320.

Wells, A., & Carter, K. (2009). Maladaptive thought control strategies in generalized anxiety disorder, major depressive disorder, and nonpatient groups and relationships with trait anxiety. *International Journal of Cognitive Therapy, 2*(3), 224–234.

Westra, H. A., Dozois, D. J., & Marcus, M. (2007). Expectancy, homework compliance, and initial change in cognitive-behavioral therapy for anxiety. *Journal of Consulting and Clinical Psychology, 75*(3), 363.

Whitmore, M. J., Kim-Spoon, J., & Ollendick, T. H. (2014). Generalized anxiety disorder and social anxiety disorder in youth: Are they distinguishable? *Child Psychiatry and Human Development, 45*(4), 456–463.

Wolpe, J. (1969). *The practice of behavior therapy*. New York: Pergamon Press.

CHAPTER FIVE

Treatment of Depression

John F. Curry
Allison E. Meyer

By age 18, approximately 1 in 10 adolescents will have experienced an episode of major depression (11%; Avenevoli, Swendsen, He, Burstein, & Merikangas, 2015). Depression during childhood and adolescence predicts higher likelihood of a depressive episode and associated impairment during adulthood (Reinherz, Giaconia, Hauf, Wasserman, & Silverman, 1999). A number of psychotherapies, particularly cognitive-behavioral therapy (CBT) and interpersonal therapy (IPT), are each effective in the treatment of child and/or adolescent depression (David-Ferdon & Kaslow, 2008) and the combination of CBT with the selective serotonin reuptake inhibitor fluoxetine shows the highest rate of short-term efficacy to date (71% response at 3 months; Treatment for Adolescents with Depression Study [TADS] Team, 2004).

In this chapter, the focus is on CBT for youth depression. We discuss the symptoms of depression and provide a brief review of the theoretical foundations and the evidence for efficacy of CBT for youth depression. We review methods of assessment and core treatment strategies and consider cultural and developmental issues and the role of parents in treatment. We place relatively more emphasis on adolescent depression because it is much more prevalent than its childhood counterpart. However, the principles of treatment are the same for children as for adolescents, with some developmental adaptations as needed.

Overview of Depressive Disorders

Symptoms

Nine symptoms constitute the diagnostic criteria for a major depressive episode, the defining characteristic of major depressive disorder (MDD). These include the core (required) symptoms of mood disturbance and/or anhedonia. In addition, there are the biological symptoms of disturbances in weight (or appetite), sleep, energy, or psychomotor functioning; trouble concentrating or making decisions; worthlessness or inappropriate guilt; and suicidal or morbid ideation, suicide plans, or suicide attempts. At least five of these symptoms must occur most days during the same 2-week period, accompanied by a decline in functioning (American Psychiatric Association, 2013). Given the presence of two potential core symptoms, the positive or negative direction of most of the biological symptoms (e.g., insomnia or hypersomnia), and the "five of nine" rule, the diagnosis pertains to a very heterogeneous clinical presentation. In fact, two adolescents with MDD may not overlap on even one symptom.

Dysthymia (now designated *persistent depression*) is a less severe but more chronic depressive disorder, in which depressed mood and at least two other symptoms are present most days for at least 1 year in children and adolescents. Most recent psychological treatment studies have focused on MDD, but some have included youths with dysthymia, or with depressive reactions to stressful events that fall short of MDD criteria (adjustment disorder).

Age, Gender, Comorbidity, and Course

Boys and girls are equally likely to experience depression prior to about age 13, when prevalence rates are relatively low (2–3%; Costello, Erkanli, & Angold, 2006). In adolescence, the prevalence rate doubles; girls are two to three times more likely than boys to experience MDD and four times more likely to have severe MDD. More often than not, depression co-occurs with other disorders, especially anxiety, disruptive behavior, or substance use disorders (Avenevoli et al., 2015; for a review, see Cummings, Caporino, & Kendall, 2014). The course of depression is quite variable: Some adolescents experience a single lifetime episode, whereas others experience multiple episodes. Duration of episodes is positively skewed, centering around 4–9 months in clinical samples and 3–6 months in community samples (Birmaher, Arbelaez, & Brent, 2002). In a sample treated for moderate to severe MDD, two-thirds of adolescents recovered fully within 1 year, and almost

90% within 2 years. However, almost half (46%) of those who recovered had a recurrent episode over a 5-year period (Curry et al., 2011). A subset of youth with depression will develop bipolar disorder (5–20% across various community, outpatient and inpatient samples; Kovacs, 1996), indicating the need to assess for mania or hypomania.

Theoretical Foundations of CBT for Depression

Early behavioral models of depression posited that low levels of positive reinforcement contingent on a person's behavior were a key antecedent of depression and found some support in that individuals with depression reported engaging in fewer pleasant activities (Ferster, 1973; Lewinsohn & Graf, 1973). More recent research has identified both deficits in social skills (Segrin, 2000) and generally low availability of environmental reinforcement (Sheeber, Hops, & Davis, 2001) as contributors to low reinforcement rates. Behavioral theory has been broadened to include stressful events as precipitants and maladaptive coping responses as maintaining factors for depression. For those vulnerable to depression, stressful events create negative affect, which then leads to a constriction of normal behavioral responses (e.g., reduced effort in school), followed by a decrease in positive reinforcement and an increase in aversive experiences (e.g., poor grades; Lewinsohn, Hoberman, Teri, & Hautzinger, 1985). Consequently, behavioral treatments focus on developing strategies to encourage patients with depression to experience reinforcing events, for example, scheduling pleasant activities, and on improving skills for coping with stress.

Parallel to the development of behavioral models, cognitive theories of depression were elaborated by Beck and others (Beck, Rush, Shaw, & Emery, 1979). Cognitive theory focuses on errors that occur during information processing, leading to negative views of oneself, the world, and the future. Individuals with depression focus on negative aspects of events and have negative automatic thoughts ("That was stupid of me") and dysfunctional attitudes ("Unless I am perfect, I am worthless") that form and maintain negative self-schemas (e.g., "I am unlovable" or "I am incompetent/helpless"). A primary component of cognitive therapy for depression is teaching clients to recognize and correct errors in thinking and to develop a more comprehensive and balanced self-schema. In addition, CBT can address other cognitive processes, such as depressive attributional style (Curry & Craighead, 1990), the tendency to ruminate unproductively (Burwell & Shirk, 2007), and unrealistically low beliefs about competence or control (Auerbach, Eberhart, & Abela, 2010).

A third theory of depression that informs contemporary CBT is linked to perceived competence or control, Nezu's (1987) social problem-solving model. Problem solving involves a systematic approach whereby a problem is identified and approached (not avoided), potential solutions are generated, and relatively more effective solutions are implemented. Ineffective problem solving raises the likelihood of depression, decreased positive reinforcement, decreased motivation, and an increase in social problems. In sum, at least three theoretical models have guided efficacious CBT for youth depression, and all current versions of CBT include aspects of each model.

Efficacy

CBT for youth depression emerged in the 1980s, was applied to clinical cases in the 1990s, and was tested in multisite randomized clinical trials in the first decade of this century. Strategies that make up the CBT interventions have varied to some extent across this time period. The earliest studies were conducted in schools, with elementary to middle school-age children who were experiencing depressive symptoms. Strategies characterizing these early cognitive-behavioral interventions included training in social skills, problem solving, self-modeling, and relaxation, often delivered in a group, rather than individual, format. Sample sizes were small, leading to very limited statistical power. Nevertheless, almost all of the studies showed that CBT was more effective than a wait-list condition (Curry, 2001).

Stark and his colleagues (Stark, Reynolds, & Kaslow, 1987) found that a primarily cognitive intervention (self-control training) led to somewhat better outcomes 2 months after brief treatment than a behavioral problem-solving intervention with fourth to sixth graders. Later, Weisz, Thurber, Sweeney, Proffitt, and LeGagnoux (1997) showed that a brief (eight sessions) CBT focused on primary and secondary control training was superior to wait list, with a similar age group. Essentially, primary control involves strategies for behavioral change in circumstances in which the child can actually effect change, whereas secondary control involves changing the way the child perceives or reacts to circumstances that cannot be changed. More recently, Weisz's model influenced the modular approach of Project MATCH, the Modular Approach to Therapy for Children with anxiety, depression, or conduct problems (Weisz et al., 2012). Strategies to alleviate depression in MATCH include scheduling pleasant activities, problem solving, relaxation, and cognitive restructuring.

Lewinsohn and colleagues (Clarke, Rohde, Lewinsohn, Hops, & Seeley, 1999; Lewinsohn, Clarke, Hops, & Andrews, 1990) were the first to treat adolescents with diagnosed depressive disorders (MDD, dysthymia) using CBT. Their behavioral group treatment model, Adolescent Coping with Depression Course, emphasized multiple skills for coping with stress and proved superior to a wait-list condition. Subsequently, Brent et

al. (1997) demonstrated that individual cognitive therapy was more efficacious after 12–16 weeks than supportive therapy or behavioral family therapy with adolescents with clinical depression. Based on component analyses of these and other studies, McCarty and Weisz (2007) concluded that
effective youth depression treatments, regardless of theoretical approach,
included psychoeducation, goal-setting to enhance perceived competence,
self-monitoring, social or communication skills, behavioral activation,
problem solving, and cognitive restructuring.

Considering combined treatment, two of three studies have demon-
strated that the addition of CBT to fluoxetine (or another antidepressant)
leads to better results than those obtained with medication alone (TADS
Team, 2004; Brent et al., 2008). But see also the Adolescent Depression
Antidepressants and Psychotherapy Trial (ADAPT) (Goodyer et al., 2007).
The Treatment for Adolescents with Depression Study (TADS Team, 2004)
is the only study to compare CBT to active medication and pill placebo.
The findings showed that CBT added significantly to the efficacy of fluoxetine alone, but as a stand-alone treatment, it did not surpass placebo. It is
unclear whether this result was attributable to characteristics of the sample,
the comparative conditions, challenges in multisite implementation, or features of the TADS CBT. The most parsimonious criticism of the TADS
model is that it included many diverse strategies that study therapists felt
compelled to include in the treatment (Curry et al., 2000; Hollon, Garber,
& Shelton, 2005). This hypothesis has not been tested, but it can serve as
a useful guide for clinicians. Indeed, recent advances in CBT for adolescent
depression, such as behavioral activation (McCauley et al., 2016), represent
relatively less complex treatment packages.

In light of the theoretical roots and efficacy evidence of CBT for youth
depression and the need for parsimonious and flexible intervention models,
we propose that there are three core strategies in CBT for youth depression:
behavioral activation, problem solving, and cognitive restructuring. Each
has been shown, as a defining component or as part of a broader treatment
package, to be an effective strategy for youth depression (Brent et al., 1997;
Clarke et al., 1999; Kennard et al., 2009; Lerner & Clum, 1990; McCauley
et al., 2016). Clinicians may decide to emphasize one or another and will
have to take into account preliminary and supplementary strategies. We
discuss the key strategies below, after describing assessment methods for
youth depression.

Assessment

Adequate assessment requires determination of diagnostic status; onset,
severity and duration of symptoms; and functional impairment. Assessing severity of current (e.g., past week or 2 weeks) symptoms is critical

for treatment planning and monitoring, whether or not the young person meets full criteria for a diagnosed disorder. Optimally, assessment methods include a diagnostic interview, clinician ratings and self-report of current symptoms, and a rating of functional impairment. In order to understand the individual, family, social, and developmental factors contributing to or maintaining depression for any given youth, these methods will need to be supplemented with assessment of such factors.

Diagnostic Interviews

The diagnostic interview can determine symptom onset and duration, diagnostic status, and the presence of other possible disorders, including bipolar, anxiety, behavior, substance use, and eating disorders. Leffler, Riebel, and Hughes (2015) recently provided an excellent review of several diagnostic interviews in terms of their suitability for clinical use. Considerations in choosing an interview include age range, breadth of coverage, cost, administration time, and required training.

In our work we have relied on the Kiddie Schedule for Affective Disorders and Schizophrenia for School-Age Children—Present and Lifetime (K-SADS-PL; Kaufman et al., 1997). An advantage of this instrument is the initial screening section, which covers the most salient symptoms of almost all child and adolescent disorders. Following the screen, only those disorders suggested by the screen are further explored. The K-SADS-PL is administered separately to the adolescent or child and the parents, with the interviewer then making best estimate conclusions. Interview time can be reduced by prescreening with a comprehensive parent- and/or youth-report measure to identify the most likely problem areas.

Clinician Severity Ratings

Clinician severity ratings, unlike diagnostic interviews, take a snapshot of current symptoms, typically using a time frame of 1 week. These ratings are useful in monitoring response if they are administered at intervals during treatment. They have advantages over self-report scales in taking into account information from the parent as well as the youth and in allowing the clinician to judge the significance of reported changes. In our work, we have used the Children's Depression Rating Scale—Revised for this purpose (CDRS-R; Poznanski & Mokros, 1996). The CDRS-R has been used extensively in medication and psychotherapy treatment studies, has excellent reliability, and is very sensitive to change (Mayes, Bernstein, Haley, Kennard, & Emslie, 2010). There are 14 interview-based items and 3 observational items. Each item is rated on a 1–7 or a 1–5 Likert-type scale, based on separate interviews with the young person and a parent.

Self-Report Scales

Self-report scales have the advantage of requiring only basic assessment training and a few minutes of the clinician's time. They can be completed as often as weekly during treatment, typically just before sessions. They monitor level of and fluctuations in symptom severity and may yield material to be incorporated immediately into sessions. Several reliable and valid scales are available, including the Reynolds Adolescent Depression Scale—Second Edition (RADS-2; Reynolds, 2004) and the Beck Depression Inventory—Second Edition (BDI-2; Beck, Steer, & Brown, 1996) for adolescents and the Children's Depression Inventory–2 (CDI-2; Kovacs, 2004) for children or adolescents. Stockings and colleagues (2015) have recently reviewed the psychometric properties of these instruments in the assessment of major depression. They are reliable measures of symptom severity but not adequate to determine a diagnosis.

Functional Impairment Ratings

The Children's Global Assessment Scale (CGAS; Shaffer et al., 1983) is a 0–100 rating that depicts the extent to which the young person's symptoms are affecting functioning in the "real world." CGAS functional ratings provide an index of comparison with treatment study samples, and, when repeated over time, the ratings assess broader improvement with treatment. The CGAS is rated by the clinician at the end of the diagnostic process.

Description of Treatment Strategies

Table 5.1 depicts our conceptualization of CBT for youth depression, and we discuss the application of this model for adolescents. In addition to the three core strategies, we propose necessary conditions, preliminary strategies, and optional (supplemental) strategies. From the outset, and continuing throughout treatment, it is necessary for the therapist to establish and maintain a therapeutic relationship with the adolescent and a parallel relationship with the parents. A component of the relationship, introduced at the outset of treatment and further specified as behavioral and cognitive strategies are introduced, is a shared understanding of the nature of the problem and the rationale for the overall treatment and for each strategy (psychoeducation). A major component of treatment relationship is collaborative goal setting and tracking. Before moving into the core skills of CBT for depression, the adolescent must learn how to monitor his or her mood. Only in this way can the adolescent know whether the strategies are having their intended effect. For some adolescents, mood monitoring must be preceded by further preliminary work on emotion recognition and labeling.

While helping the adolescent to learn the three core strategies and developing a more complete understanding of the individual case, the therapist may decide to work with the adolescent on related supplemental strategies, such as relaxation or other affect regulation methods, assertion, social interaction, or communication skills. Sleep disruption can be addressed by sleep hygiene strategies. However, the therapist should in no way feel compelled to "cover" all possible strategies, relying instead on a case conceptualization to guide the selection of treatment components.

The Therapeutic Relationship

The therapeutic relationship includes an emotional bond, as well as a working alliance involving agreement on goals and on the nature of the therapeutic tasks (Shirk, Karver, & Brown, 2011). Both an alliance with the youth and one with the parent(s) are needed. The alliance with the youth is associated with clinical improvement; the alliance with the parent is associated with greater attendance, family participation, and consensus on when to end treatment (Hawley & Weisz, 2005). Beck et al. (1979) emphasized "rapport" in the therapeutic relationship: creating an atmosphere in which the client feels accepted and free to express his or her thoughts and feelings.

Psychoeducation

The essence of psychoeducation is the creation of a shared understanding among the adolescent, the parents, and the therapist about the nature of the young person's depression and how it will be addressed in this treatment. Psychoeducation should be conducted as a dialogue rather than a lecture. Handouts can be used to describe the CBT model of depression and of treatment. In most cases, the initial psychoeducation can be conducted in

TABLE 5.1. Strategies for CBT for Youth Depression

Necessary conditions	Preliminary skills	Core skills	Optional supplemental skills
• Therapeutic relationship with youth • Working relationship with parent(s) • Psychoeducation about depression and CBT	• Goal setting • Mood monitoring	• Behavioral activation • Problem solving • Cognitive restructuring	• Social skills • Communication • Assertion • Affect regulation • Sleep regulation

a conjoint session, which models the kind of teamwork advocated in the treatment model. However, the therapist may make a clinical judgment to conduct psychoeducation in separate sessions, for example, if there is a high level of parent–adolescent conflict.

It is important to distinguish depression from ordinary sadness, to label it as a disorder that represents a change from what is typical for the adolescent, with symptoms and functional impairment that the young person cannot "snap out of" but that can be treated effectively. A handout listing symptoms of depression can be reviewed with the adolescent and parents to determine which symptoms are currently present and how these have affected the teenager's functioning at school, with friends, or in the family.

By drawing a "triangle" with thoughts, emotions, and behaviors represented on the three sides, the therapist can help the adolescent and parents to see how depression involves all three aspects of personality. Examples might include reacting to school failure by behavioral withdrawal, emotional sadness, and cognitive self-criticism. This triangular description leads readily to the explanation of CBT as a treatment for depression: By modifying the way he or she acts and thinks when stressed, the adolescent can become more resilient and reduce depressed mood.

The role of the parents in treatment is also part of CBT psychoeducation. Depending on the case, the parents may be involved primarily as supportive of the adolescent in learning new skills or more directly as participants in sessions designed to address parent–adolescent dysfunctional interactions.

Goal Setting

For most adolescents, initial treatment goals can be identified simply by asking what the adolescent would like to work on during treatment or how he or she would like things to improve in the family, at school, or with friends. If the adolescent has difficulty with the concept of goals, it may be helpful to inquire about past experiences he or she has had in making intentional positive changes or developing new skills, such as meeting new people, learning how to play a new sport or game, or improving performance in school.

Once general goals have been set, the therapist should then work with the youth to break them down into smaller incremental steps. For example, "getting along better with my parents" may be a major treatment goal. By focusing on what the adolescent can do before the next session that would be in line with this goal, the therapist can model the process of working toward goals. Once goals have been set, the therapist and youth should review progress toward these goals at regular intervals during treatment, to enhance the sense of self-efficacy.

Mood Monitoring

We begin teaching the adolescent how to monitor mood simply by asking how he or she has been feeling over the past week and whether there have been times when he or she has felt particularly bad or has felt better. If there has been some range of mood, we ask about what was happening or what the situation was at the time of the different feelings. The time frame for inquiry can be extended to ask about emotionally significant events at any point. We then introduce an "emotions thermometer" (Figure 5.1), which is labeled with numbers ranging from 0 (representing the worst the adolescent has felt) to 10 (representing the best the adolescent has felt). Working together, the therapist helps the adolescent to generate several examples of

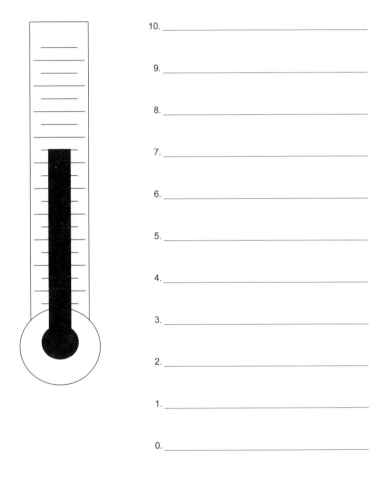

FIGURE 5.1. Emotions thermometer.

situations in which the adolescent's mood has fallen at various points on the thermometer. The therapist then explains that learning how to monitor mood will enable the adolescent to figure out what situations, activities, and thoughts are connected with feeling better or worse. This exercise will also help the adolescent to see that, in all likelihood, he or she does not feel equally depressed at all times.

Once the adolescent learns how to estimate mood on the thermometer, the daily mood monitor can be introduced (Figure 5.2). At least at the outset of treatment, we recommend using a mood monitor that can be easily filled out each day, with the opportunity to recall different times during the day when mood changed in either direction. As treatment progresses, the mood monitor can be modified to focus more on the associations between mood and activities or between mood and thoughts.

Core Strategy 1: Behavioral Activation (Activity Scheduling)

The key skill for the adolescent to learn through activity scheduling is that engaging in activities, especially pleasant activities and social activities, *whether or not one is in the mood to do so,* is a powerful tool to combat depression. Scheduling and increasing pleasant activities is a change that adolescents can make along the "behavior" side of the "triangle." To make this link come alive, the mood monitor should be incorporated into the homework tasks, so that the adolescent can learn the connection between engaging in activities and feeling better. When selecting pleasant activities as targets of behavior change, the therapist should take care to include some that are social. Although solitary activities can also improve mood, social activities may be particularly powerful in doing so, and they serve to combat the social isolation characteristic of many adolescents with depression. As is true for any of the CBT strategies, the therapist should explain the rationale for activity scheduling to the adolescent. Then the therapist can work with the adolescent to generate a list of pleasant activities—activities that either are, or used to be, enjoyable for the adolescent. To help the teen generate activities, the therapist can inquire about any of these (or other) areas:

1. Arts or hobbies (music, writing poetry or stories, crafts, drawing/painting, cooking, photography, mechanics)
2. Outdoor or athletic activities (sports, camping, driving)
3. Social connections (texts, phone calls, visits, or games with friends; shopping or going to a movie with friends)
4. Religious or spiritual activities (meditation, prayer, religious services, mindfulness)
5. Service activities (volunteering, tutoring)
6. Simple everyday tasks (bathing, showering, dressing)

	Morning	Afternoon	Evening
Sunday			
Monday			
Tuesday			

FIGURE 5.2. Daily mood monitor.

After the adolescent has chosen a number of activities, the therapist should then ask him or her to choose a few (two or three) to try to increase in the following week. These should be active, harmless, inexpensive, and feasible. Sleeping fails the "active" criterion, and drug use fails the "harmless" criterion! The therapist can help the adolescent to set realistic goals for the frequency of the target activities and point out the importance of monitoring mood during or after the activity. The form shown in Figure 5.3 can be used to record target activities in the left column and then their occurrence, retroactively over the past 3 days and prospectively during the next week.

In subsequent sessions, the therapist reviews with the adolescent how involvement in specific activities affected the adolescent's mood and works with the adolescent to problem-solve barriers to completion of scheduled activities. Such barriers might include unrealistic expectations, hopeless thinking, and other negative thoughts that interfere with here-and-now enjoyment of an activity. By problem solving in this way and looking at negative cognitions, the therapist models use of the other two core strategies for treating depression.

	Baseline			Days						
	Yesterday			Today						
				1	2	3	4	5	6	7
Date										
1										
2										
3										
4										
5										
6										
7										
8										
9										
10										
Total Number/ Mood										

FIGURE 5.3. Activity log.

Core Strategy 2: Problem Solving

The key skill for the adolescent to learn through problem solving is that she or he can successfully manage many life challenges through taking active steps to cope with problems. Problem solving serves to counter hopeless thinking and social withdrawal. Many approaches to problem solving can be found in the CBT literature, as it has been incorporated into the treatment of almost all child and adolescent disorders. When addressing depression, the therapist should locate this strategy on both the behavioral and cognitive sides of the "triangle," since it involves both increasing cognitive flexibility and taking action. As treatment progresses, the therapist can work with the adolescent to identify situations in which problem solving is likely to be helpful as opposed to those in which the adolescent has such limited control that cognitive restructuring is more likely to be appropriate.

Prior to active problem solving, two factors are important to consider.

First, it is critical to allow adolescents to express the strong emotions they may have when faced with a frustrating, sad, unfair, or challenging problem. To move too quickly into solving problems before the adolescent has the opportunity to express emotions and to have those emotions validated is to invite failure and threaten the success of the treatment. Second, a problem-solving approach requires acceptance that problems are an expected part of life, an opportunity for growth, and not things primarily to be avoided. Thus some adolescents will require preliminary work focused on their attitudes toward or expectations about problems.

By this point in treatment, the adolescent will invariably have brought up some interpersonal, academic, or family problem that is likely to be contributing to stress or depression. The therapist may want to begin problem-solving training by referring to such examples, if they are not highly challenging. Alternatively, the therapist can present examples of problems experienced by other adolescents to allow the client some emotional distance while engaged in learning the approach to problem solving.

Using didactic instruction, modeling, and role playing, the therapist then explains a stepwise problem-solving method. We use the acronym RIBEYE to delineate steps of problem solving: first, Relax, then Identify the problem, Brainstorm possible solutions, Evaluate each one, say "Yes" to one, and finally Encourage yourself for having completed this process. As the adolescent learns to apply these steps, it may become clear that there are certain barriers to successful implementation. These could include difficulty managing emotions (relaxing), a tendency to evaluate options too quickly, hopelessness, or depressive attributions or expectancies that block the adolescent's cognitive flexibility.

After completing one or more problem-solving exercises in the session, the therapist and adolescent can collaboratively identify a problem to be addressed before the next session. As treatment progresses, problem solving should be applied as frequently as possible to ensure the adolescent's incorporation of this basic and broadly generalizable skill.

Core Strategy 3: Cognitive Restructuring

Whereas problem solving can be viewed as a method to enhance behavioral and cognitive flexibility in stressful situations, cognitive restructuring focuses on enhancing cognitive flexibility. The key skill for the adolescent to learn through this strategy is that changing the way he or she thinks about a situation or event is a powerful way to combat depression. The therapist illustrates this by using the triangle of thoughts, behaviors, and emotions and using examples that have already arisen during treatment. Just as negative thoughts are associated with depressed mood, more realistic or positive thoughts can lift mood.

It is likely that the therapist will have had opportunities to encourage some cognitive restructuring earlier in treatment. In particular, it is often notable how adolescents with depression attribute negative outcomes to personal flaws, while failing to recognize their own contributions to positive outcomes. When this occurs in sessions, the therapist should point it out to the adolescent and thus begin the process of attribution restructuring. For example, if the adolescent reports that things have gone better recently, at home or in school, the therapist can ask what he or she did to contribute to that improvement. As treatment progresses and focuses more specifically on negative thinking, the therapist can help the adolescent to see that patterns of thinking that contribute to depression might have some degree of accuracy but are likely to be exaggerated, incomplete, or unrealistic.

There are three elements of cognitive restructuring that we emphasize at this later point in treatment: (1) identifying and challenging automatic thoughts; (2) countering individual tendencies to construct depressive interpretations of events ("cognitive distortions"); and (3) creating a more comprehensive and positive self-schema (Stark, Curry, Goldman, & Integrated Psychotherapy Consortium, 2004). It is optimal to identify the adolescent's current negative automatic thoughts in the context of in-session expressions of emotion by asking what went through the adolescent's mind as he or she was feeling the emotion. In other instances, exercises can be constructed to illustrate automatic thoughts. For example, the therapist might give an example of an event—for example, an automobile accident in which no one gets hurt—and have the adolescent say what his or her initial feeling would be. Then ask whether there were other possible feelings, and show the link between those different emotions and distinct thoughts. The classic cognitive therapy questions can be used to work with the adolescent to restructure depressive thoughts: "What is the evidence for and against that thought?" "Is there any other way to look at it?" "What if it were true?" As alternative thoughts are generated, their corresponding emotions are identified and linked to the mood monitor.

Careful attention to the adolescent's description of events and interpersonal interactions is likely to reveal characteristic ways of processing information that narrow or distort it and thus maintain depression. Again, it is optimal to identify and label these cognitive distortions or "dark glasses" in the here-and-now of the session. Alternative methods can include using short written descriptions of problems that demonstrate a cognitive distortion, for example, advice-seeking letters from hypothetical adolescents; giving examples of depressing thoughts that other adolescents might have following a negative event; or listing and defining several cognitive distortions (including ones that the adolescent has demonstrated in sessions) and asking the teenager to see whether any seem characteristic of his or her thinking. Once the adolescent's most typical cognitive distortions are identified, they can be incorporated into cognitive restructuring exercises in and between sessions.

In their work with depressed children, Stark et al. (2004) balances cognitive restructuring of negative thoughts with enhancement of a more complex and balanced self-image. The technique used for this purpose is a self-map, a single sheet of paper with a large circle representing the overall self and attached smaller circles representing areas of life (e.g., in school, as a friend, as a family member, after school). Self-mapping proceeds across several sessions as the young person is asked to identify and write in personal strengths in each circle, including any unique strengths that cut across domains (Stark et al., 2004). Inability to identify strengths can then be addressed by reference to attributional or perceptual blocks, furthering the process of cognitive restructuring.

Supplemental Strategies

Numerous additional strategies are consistent with a CBT framework and may be helpful to individual clients working to overcome depression. For those with emotion regulation challenges that interfere with learning new skills, relaxation training or elements from dialectical behavior therapy should be considered. For those who are socially isolated or overly passive in interpersonal interactions, social interaction or assertion strategies can be incorporated into treatment. Likewise, communication training may help adolescents to cope with family, parent, or peer conflict. Sleep disturbance is such a powerful influence on adolescents with depression that it merits being directly addressed in cases in which it does not improve with use of other strategies.

General Considerations

Differing CBT strategies should be embedded within a consistent session structure. We recommend agenda setting, review of goals, practice (homework) review, and safety check (for youths with suicidal ideation) as standard elements at the start of sessions. Session summaries and collaborative development of new practice tasks are standard elements at the end of sessions. It is critical that CBT strategies be presented and enacted in an active, experiential manner. Thus the therapist should rely on here-and-now learning in sessions, use role plays, and ensure that the adolescent is engaged in sessions rather than passively listening. Therapists may think that a strategy has been "taught," but this is of little importance unless it has been "learned."

Case Example

Joanna was a 16-year-old African American female in her junior year of high school. She lived with both parents and two younger brothers. Her parents brought her to the clinic because of concerns about her low mood, declining grades, and social withdrawal. Joanna expressed concerns about school performance, fatigue, and anxiety in social interactions.

Initial Assessment

Joanna was a likable and kind girl with a past history of diverse hobbies (e.g., reading, writing, singing). She easily took others' perspectives and, despite social anxiety, had developed a small network of friends at school. The diagnostic interview indicated that she had been depressed for about 4 months. The precipitant seemed to be a change in her planned class schedule due to the need to accommodate a required course. She had to drop an ongoing choral elective, which she had taken in previous years with her closest friends.

At the start of treatment, Joanna was moderately depressed, with anhedonia, initial insomnia, increased eating and weight gain, suicidal ideation without intent, fatigue, and guilt about being a burden for her parents. These symptoms resulted in impairment in school (declining grades) and with peers (withdrawal).

Course of Treatment

Treatment for depression took place over 10 weeks, after which focus shifted to treatment for social anxiety. Treatment included psychoeducation about depression, goal setting, mood monitoring, problem solving, behavioral activation, and sleep hygiene. As the focus shifted from depression to social anxiety, relaxation was introduced. The RADS was administered at three points. Joanna reported declining depressive symptoms across administrations.

Necessary Conditions

Alliance with Teen and Relationship with Parents

The therapist and Joanna's parents seemed to develop good rapport quickly. Although Joanna and her parents initially approached the therapist as an authority figure, the relationship became more collaborative over time. Joanna warmed quite quickly to the therapist and was amenable to assessment and recommendations.

Psychoeducation

During the initial two sessions, Joanna and her parents were provided psychoeducation about symptoms of depression and the availability of effective treatments (with a focus on CBT), as well as information on depression's course and duration. This information was particularly valuable for Joanna's mother, who was anxious about her prognosis. The therapist described the "downward spiral" of negative thoughts, feelings, and actions that contribute to depression and also how positive thoughts, feelings, and behaviors could disrupt the downward spiral and contribute toward alleviating Joanna's depression (Rohde, Feeny, & Robins, 2005).

In addition to psychoeducation about depression, we discussed components of good sleep hygiene. We adopted a collaborative problem-solving approach to identify ways to improve her sleep habits.

Preliminary Skills

Goal Setting

At intake, Joanna identified two goals for treatment. First, she wanted to experience less guilt. Second, she identified wanting to become more comfortable around people, particularly peers. The therapist conceptualized the second goal as an area that could be addressed through pleasant social activities and then treatment for social anxiety following the primary emphasis on depression. The first goal could be addressed through cognitive restructuring, possibly accompanied by supplemental parent or family sessions.

Mood Monitoring

During the second session, the skill of mood monitoring was introduced, using the 0–10 mood thermometer (Figure 5.1). High and low points were anchored using Joanna's observations about her mood (as recommended by Rohde et al., 2005). Joanna identified that she experienced her best moods when writing fiction stories or singing and her lowest moods when she was struggling to complete classwork. For homework, Joanna was assigned to complete a daily mood monitoring form. Like many adolescents, she did not complete this assignment during the week, but it was completed retrospectively at the next session. The concept of mood monitoring was repeatedly referenced throughout treatment as a means of assessing and reinforcing progress.

Behavioral Activation

After providing psychoeducation and teaching mood monitoring, we began to focus on ways to increase pleasant activities. The therapist placed particular emphasis on developing opportunities to spend times with peers, an activity that had dropped off significantly during her depressive episode. At first, the therapist asked Joanna to engage in one or two of the generated activities each week. However, these few activities, when she followed through, were not associated with an appreciable difference in her mood. It seemed that a more intensive and structured approach was required. Thus, in the next session, we used an activity scheduling form and worked together to plan for a couple of activities each day that she might be able to enjoy—with a pragmatic eye toward activities short in duration and requiring little to no planning. For Joanna, these included walking on a treadmill in her home, reading, and regularly participating in family activities. Following this homework assignment, Joanna noticed that her mood particularly improved after socializing with friends and exercise. Behavioral activation continued to be an important treatment component but became increasingly self-directed.

Problem Solving

A collaborative problem-solving approach was woven into many of the sessions and particularly used to brainstorm with Joanna ways to widen her social engagement. In Joanna's treatment, the skill was taught across two sessions; the first time occurred when Joanna came in feeling upset after she was told by a friend that her former classmates had forgotten about her. Using the RIBEYE acronym, we identified the problem as needing to find ways to renew contact with these friends. Together, we were able to generate a number of solutions—for example, texting one or more of the friends, attending that month's choral presentation, saying hello to these classmates at school. As each solution was identified, Joanna tended to evaluate the possibilities before completing the brainstorming, typically identifying logistic challenges. The therapist helped her to generate as many potential solutions as possible before embarking on evaluation. In this session, she proceeded only to the fourth step, but this itself represented progress, and we returned again to a similar problem in the next session.

In that session, problem solving focused on how to arrange for socializing outside of school. During the brainstorming, options included texting one or two friends, hanging out with a family friend at a gathering, or making plans with a friend she saw frequently at school. Joanna again raised a number of objections—some of which were genuine barriers (e.g., inability to arrange transportation), whereas others were suggestive of comorbid anxiety (e.g., worry about what she would say). She decided to make plans with a friend for the upcoming weekend. The therapist and Joanna then role-played this interaction several times until Joanna felt comfortable with a number of variations in the course of the conversation. This role play doubled as a mild exposure for social anxiety.

At the next session, Joanna proudly reported that she had asked the friend over and the friend had accepted. This instance marked the first time in treatment that Joanna had followed through on initiating social activity and a turning point in the course of her depression. Further, tying mood monitoring in with problem solving, Joanna observed that the social interactions were associated with a several-day-long elevation in her mood.

Relaxation

As Joanna's mood improved and she became more socially active, she began to encounter more anxiety-provoking social situations. With the goal of allowing her to engage more readily in these contexts, the therapist incorporated the relaxation into treatment. Specifically, we discussed the practice of diaphragmatic breathing as a means of relaxing and subsequently being able to reengage in the anxiety-provoking situations. At the session immediately after Joanna learned this skill, she reported that she had practiced the skill at a large social gathering and was able to return to the day's activities without a panic attack.

Cognitive Restructuring and Comorbid Anxiety

As Joanna's mood began to improve, she was ready to engage in cognitive restructuring related to her sense of being a burden on the family. This thought of being a burden was identified as an automatic thought, which came to the fore whenever her parents seemed upset. Through a supplemental parent meeting, it became clear that they were not, in fact, feeling burdened by her, so the thought appeared to be maintained by "jumping to conclusions" based on little or no evidence. We addressed this tendency by using examples of other common adolescent experiences that are open to either innocuous or negative interpretations—for example, passing a friend in the hallway at school who does not notice you. Looking for the evidence and discussing the alternative ways that such an event could be interpreted led to application of cognitive restructuring of Joanna's guilt-inducing interpretation related to her parents.

As suggested above, many of the CBT strategies to address Joanna's depression also addressed her social anxiety. During the sixth session, Joanna asked to practice a class presentation for the therapist. The therapist praised her for her willingness and provided genuine positive feedback about her presentation—noting that she seemed confident, poised, and knowledgeable. Joanna was surprised at this feedback, observing her negative self-talk ("I'm not doing a good job," "I must have looked nervous," "No one will understand what I'm saying"). The discrepancy between the therapist's observations and Joanna's self-talk was used as an opportunity to discuss common cognitive errors. At the eighth session, taking feedback from a RADS score in the normal range, as well as Joanna's and her parents' reports, we began to address social anxiety more directly by identifying bodily cues of anxiety and developing an anxiety hierarchy. The tenth session marked the transition point between depression-focused and anxiety-focused sessions.

The Role of the Parents, Developmental Issues, and Multicultural Issues

Parents

The role of the parents (or other caregivers) in CBT for youth depression varies according to characteristics of the family and the case. At a minimum, parents should be included in the psychoeducational aspects of treatment, so that there is a shared understanding of the problem and the treatment. Parents can then support their adolescent in efforts to implement new strategies. In cases in which parent or family factors are contributing to the youth's depression, parent or conjoint parent–adolescent sessions may be incorporated into the treatment plan. As reviewed by Wells and Albano (2005), a number of parental and family factors can be associated with adolescent depression. These include low frequency of parental reward, ineffective family problem solving, and interactions that are high in expressed emotion and criticism. Based on this research, Wells and Curry (2000) developed a manual with optional parent and family sessions that was used in TADS and later in the Treatment of SSRI-Resistant Depression in Adolescents (TORDIA) randomized controlled trial (Brent et al., 2008). These sessions address problems of family communication, compromise, excessively high parental expectations or low positive reinforcement, and emotional reattachment in cases of highly disrupted parent–adolescent relationships. Stark et al. (2004) also included parent sessions to enhance positive reinforcement, family problem solving and conflict resolution, and parental support of efforts to restructure negative thinking. There is no empirical evidence at present to guide the clinician in how best to incorporate parent or family sessions into youth CBT. It is important that such sessions not disrupt the alliance with the youth or the flow of individual CBT but rather serve to provide supplemental strategies.

Developmental Issues

Some variation is shown across childhood and adolescence in the presentation of depression. Adolescents are more likely to experience hypersomnia, weight and/or appetite loss, anhedonia, hopelessness, substance use, and suicide attempts. Compared with adults, children and adolescents with severe depression are less likely to experience delusions (Kovacs, 1996). Otherwise, depression looks similar across the developmental span.

With regard to treatment, it has been hypothesized that behavioral activation might be more developmentally appropriate for preadolescents than treatments that include a more substantial cognitive component (Ritschel, Ramirez, Cooley, & Craighead, 2016), although to our knowledge this hypothesis has not been tested. In the treatment of adolescent suicidal ideation, Daniel and Goldston (2009) describe developmental adaptations of therapy. Despite their capacity for abstract thinking, distressed adolescents, like younger children, may require more concrete materials, such as coping cards or other written reminders. Developmentally, adolescents may not wish to be in therapy given the social pressure for conformity and the potential fear that therapy marks them as different from their peers.

Multicultural Issues

In the United States, ethnic minorities are less likely to receive treatment for their depression (Alegría et al., 2008; Cummings & Druss, 2011), and, if they do receive treatment, the process (clinician diagnoses, modality, and duration) is often different from that given nonminorities (Cuffe, Waller, Cuccaro, Pumariega, & Garrison, 1995; Kilgus, Pumariega, & Cuffe, 1995). Some evidence suggests that the likelihood of experiencing particular symptoms of depression varies across racial and ethnic groups. In a nationwide study of treatment-seeking adolescents with major depression, Asian Americans more often reported inability to concentrate or make decisions compared with European Americans. African Americans were more likely to report anhedonia but less likely to report feelings of worthlessness (Cummings, Case, Ji, Chae, & Druss, 2014). In the TADS sample, minority (African American or Latino) adolescents did not differ from European American adolescents on any reported symptoms but had higher levels of observed signs of depression (e.g., sad appearance or slowed movements; Stein et al., 2010). Further, cultural idioms may be used by minority adolescents to describe the experience of depression and anxiety. These and other potential cultural issues can affect the accurate assessment of depression and influence the content of sessions, but CBT has been shown to be effective with minority youth with depression (Huey & Polo, 2008).

Incorporating parents and other family members flexibly and effectively into treatment for adolescent depression will likely require different emphases for different family systems. For example, clinicians may need to consider including members of the extended family in the treatment plan. Acculturation is another important process to assess in minority youth, particularly those in families that have immigrated in recent generations. The degree of acculturation of children may differ from that of their parents, an incongruence that often results in discord or stress in the parent–child relationship (Sweeney, Robins, Ruberu, & Jones, 2005).

Finally, youth may be considered minorities in terms of sexual orientation (lesbian, gay, bisexual, or transgender; LGBT). For young adults who identify as LGBT, rejection by family or friends during adolescence is associated with a greater risk of depression and suicide attempts, whereas family connectedness and feeling cared for are protective factors against suicidal ideation and attempts (D'Augelli, 2002; Eisenberg & Resnick, 2006), suggesting that social support is a key predictor of mental health outcomes among LGBT youth.

Predictors and Mediators of Outcome

Emslie, Kennard, and Mayes (2011) reviewed the three major multisite studies of CBT and medication for adolescent depression (TADS, TOR-DIA, and ADAPT) and reported that several characteristics predicted better outcome across treatments. Most were markers of episode severity: Less severe symptoms and shorter episode duration, better functioning, and less hopeless or suicidal thinking were associated with better outcomes. Absence of comorbid anxiety disorders and lower family stress or conflict predicted better outcome in two of three studies. Nilsen, Eisemann, and Kvernmo (2013) reviewed psychological treatment studies and found that baseline depression severity predicted poorer short-term outcome. They noted that pretreatment patient variables (age, gender) were not predictors and that comorbid anxiety yielded inconsistent results. At present the most reliable findings indicate that clinicians, youths, and parents can expect slower results in cases of more severe or prolonged depressive episodes.

Very little evidence exists on the processes that account for positive change in adolescent depression treatment. Webb, Auerbach, and DeRubeis (2012) reviewed the few mediator studies and found that cognitive change does mediate CBT outcome. However, studies are inconsistent regarding which cognitive variable mediates change: automatic thoughts or dysfunctional attitudes. Cognitive distortions have also been shown to improve with CBT, but mediation has not yet been tested.

Conclusion

Depression occurs in about 1 out of 10 adolescents and disproportionately affects girls after age 13. CBT for adolescent depression has been found to be efficacious in a number of clinical trials and to enhance outcomes when used in conjunction with antidepressant medication. Effective treatment requires alliances with the youth and his or her parent(s). The core strategies of CBT for youth depression include behavioral activation, problem solving, and cognitive restructuring. Preliminary strategies such as goal setting and mood monitoring pave the way for the core strategies, whereas supplemental strategies may be indicated based on the clinical presentation and case conceptualization. Further investigation is needed to determine why CBT works for adolescents with depression. Identification of key mediators will serve to sharpen the focus of future treatment models.

References

Alegría, M., Chatterji, P., Wells, K., Cao, Z., Chen, C., Takeuchi, D., et al. (2008). Disparity in depression treatment among racial and ethnic minority populations in the United States. *Psychiatric Services, 59*(11), 1264–1272.

American Psychiatric Association. (2013). *Diagnostic and statistical manual of mental disorders* (5th ed.). Arlington, VA: Author.

Auerbach, R. P., Eberhart, N. K., & Abela, J. R. Z. (2010). Cognitive vulnerability to depression in Canadian and Chinese adolescents. *Journal of Abnormal Child Psychology, 38*(1), 57–68.

Avenevoli, S., Swendsen, J., He, J.-P., Burstein, M., & Merikangas, K. R. (2015). Major depression in the National Comorbidity Survey—Adolescent Supplement: Prevalence, correlates, and treatment. *Journal of the American Academy of Child and Adolescent Psychiatry, 54*(1), 37–44.

Beck, A. T., Rush, A. J., Shaw, B. F., & Emery, G. (1979). *Cognitive therapy of depression*. New York: Guilford Press.

Beck, A. T., Steer, R. A., & Brown, G. (1996). *The Beck Depression Inventory—Second Edition*. San Antonio, TX: Psychological Corporation.

Birmaher, B., Arbelaez, C., & Brent, D. A. (2002). Course and outcome of child and adolescent major depressive disorder. *Child and Adolescent Psychiatric Clinics of North America, 11*(3), 619–637.

Brent, D. A., Emslie, G., Clarke, G., Wagner, K. D., Asarnow, J. R., Keller, M., et al. (2008). Switching to another SSRI or to venlafaxine with or without cognitive behavioral therapy for adolescents with SSRI-resistant depression: The TORDIA randomized controlled trial. *Journal of the American Medical Association, 299*(8), 901–913.

Brent, D. A., Holder, D., Kolko, D., Birmaher, B., Baugher, M., Roth, C., et al. (1997). A clinical psychotherapy trial for adolescent depression comparing cognitive, family, and supportive therapy. *Archives of General Psychiatry, 54*, 877–885.

Burwell, R. A., & Shirk, S. R. (2007). Subtypes of rumination in adolescence: Associations between brooding, reflection, depressive symptoms, and coping. *Journal of Clinical Child and Adolescent Psychology, 36*(1), 56–65.

Clarke, G. N., Rohde, P., Lewinsohn, P. M., Hops, H., & Seeley, J. R. (1999). Cognitive-behavioral treatment of adolescent depression: Efficacy of acute group treatment and booster sessions. *Journal of the American Academy of Child and Adolescent Psychiatry, 38*(3), 272–279.

Costello, E. J., Erkanli, A., & Angold, A. (2006). Is there an epidemic of child or adolescent depression? *Journal of Child Psychology and Psychiatry, 47*(12), 1263–1271.

Cuffe, S. P., Waller, J. L., Cuccaro, M. L., Pumariega, A. J., & Garrison, C. Z. (1995). Race and gender differences in the treatment of psychiatric disorders in young adolescents. *Journal of the American Academy of Child and Adolescent Psychiatry, 34*(11), 1536–1543.

Cummings, C. M., Caporino, N. E., & Kendall, P. C. (2014). Comorbidity of anxiety and depression in children and adolescents: 20 years after. *Psychological Bulletin, 140*(3), 816–845.

Cummings, J. R., Case, B. G., Ji, X., Chae, D. H., & Druss, B. G. (2014). Racial/ ethnic differences in perceived reasons for mental health treatment in US adolescents with major depression. *Journal of the American Academy of Child and Adolescent Psychiatry, 53*(9), 980–990.

Cummings, J. R., & Druss, B. G. (2011). Racial/ethnic differences in mental health service use among adolescents with major depression. *Journal of the American Academy of Child and Adolescent Psychiatry, 50*(2), 160–170.

Curry, J. F. (2001). Specific psychotherapies for childhood and adolescent depression. *Biological Psychiatry, 49*(12), 1091–1100.

Curry, J. F., & Craighead, W. E. (1990). Attributional style in clinically depressed and conduct disordered adolescents. *Journal of Consulting and Clinical Psychology, 58*(1), 109–115.

Curry, J. F., Silva, S., Rohde, P., Ginsburg, G., Kratochvil, C., Simons, A., et al. (2011). Recovery and recurrence following treatment for adolescent major depression. *Archives of General Psychiatry, 68*(3), 263–270.

Curry, J. F., Wells, K. C., Brent, D. A., Clarke, G. N., Rohde, P., Reinecke, M. A., et al. (2000). *Treatment for Adolescents with Depression Study (TADS) cognitive behavior therapy manual: Introduction, rationale, and adolescent sessions.* Unpublished manual, Duke University Medical Center, Durham, NC.

Daniel, S. S., & Goldston, D. B. (2009). Interventions for suicidal youth: A review of the literature and developmental considerations. *Suicide and Life-Threatening Behavior, 39*(3), 252–268.

D'Augelli, A. R. (2002). Mental health problems among lesbian, gay, and bisexual youths ages 14 to 21. *Clinical Child Psychology and Psychiatry, 7*(3), 433–456.

David-Ferdon, C., & Kaslow, N. J. (2008). Evidence-based psychosocial treatments for child and adolescent depression. *Journal of Clinical Child and Adolescent Psychology, 37*(1), 62–104.

Eisenberg, M. E., & Resnick, M. D. (2006). Suicidality among gay, lesbian and bisexual youth: The role of protective factors. *Journal of Adolescent Health, 39*(5), 662–668.

Emslie, G. J., Kennard, B. D., & Mayes, T. L. (2011). Predictors of treatment response in adolescent depression. *Pediatric Annals, 40*(6), 300–306.

Ferster, C. B. (1973). A functional analysis of depression. *American Psychologist, 28*(10), 857–870.

Goodyer, I., Dubicka, B., Wilkinson, P., Kelvin, R., Roberts, C., Byford, S., et al. (2007). Selective serotonin reuptake inhibitors (SSRIs) and routine specialist care with and without cognitive behaviour therapy in adolescents with major depression: Randomised controlled trial. *British Medical Journal, 335*(7611), 142.

Hawley, K. M., & Weisz, J. R. (2005). Youth versus parent working alliance in usual clinical care: Distinctive associations with retention, satisfaction, and treatment outcome. *Journal of Clinical Child and Adolescent Psychology, 34*(1), 117–128.

Hollon, S. D., Garber, J., & Shelton, R. C. (2005). Treatment of depression in adolescents with cognitive behavior therapy and medications: A commentary on the TADS project. *Cognitive and Behavioral Practice, 12*(2), 149–155.

Huey, S. J., Jr., & Polo, A. J. (2008). Evidence-based psychosocial treatments for ethnic minority youth. *Journal of Clinical Child and Adolescent Psychology, 37*(1), 262–301.

Kaufman, J., Birmaher, B., Brent, D. A., Rao, U., Flynn, C., Moreci, P., et al. (1997). Schedule for Affective Disorders and Schizophrenia for School-Age Children—Present and Lifetime Version (K-SADS-PL): Initial reliability and validity data. *Journal of the American Academy of Child and Adolescent Psychiatry, 36*(7), 980–988.

Kennard, B. D., Clarke, G. N., Weersing, V. R., Asarnow, J. R., Shamseddeen, W., Porta, G., et al. (2009). Effective components of TORDIA cognitive-behavioral therapy for adolescent depression: Preliminary findings. *Journal of Consulting and Clinical Psychology, 77*(6), 1033–1041.

Kilgus, M. D., Pumariega, A. J., & Cuffe, S. P. (1995). Influence of race on diagnosis in adolescent psychiatric inpatients. *Journal of the American Academy of Child and Adolescent Psychiatry, 34*(1), 67–72.

Kovacs, M. (1996). Presentation and course of major depressive disorder during childhood and later years of the life span. *Journal of the American Academy of Child and Adolescent Psychiatry, 35*(6), 705–715.

Kovacs, M. (2004). *Children's Depression Inventory–2.* Toronto, Ontario, Canada: Multi-Health Systems.

Leffler, J. M., Riebel, J., & Hughes, H. M. (2015). A review of child and adolescent diagnostic interviews for clinical practitioners. *Assessment, 22*(6), 690–703.

Lerner, M. S., & Clum, G. A. (1990). Treatment of suicide ideators: A problem-solving approach. *Behavior Therapy, 21*(4), 403–411.

Lewinsohn, P. M., Clarke, G. N., Hops, H., & Andrews, J. (1990). Cognitive-behavioral treatment for depressed adolescents. *Behavior Therapy, 21*(4), 385–401.

Lewinsohn, P. M., & Graf, M. (1973). Pleasant activities and depression. *Journal of Consulting and Clinical Psychology, 41*(2), 261–268.

Lewinsohn, P. M., Hoberman, H., Teri, L., & Hautzinger, M. (1985). An integrative theory of depression. In S. Reiss & R. R. Bootzin (Eds.), *Theoretical issues in behavior therapy* (pp. 331–359). Cambridge, MA: Academic Press.

Mayes, T. L., Bernstein, I. H., Haley, C. L., Kennard, B. D., & Emslie, G. J. (2010). Psychometric properties of the Children's Depression Rating Scale—Revised in adolescents. *Journal of Child and Adolescent Psychopharmacology, 20*(6), 513–516.

McCarty, C. A., & Weisz, J. R. (2007). Effects of psychotherapy for depression in children and adolescents: What we can (and can't) learn from meta-analysis and component profiling. *Journal of the American Academy of Child and Adolescent Psychiatry, 46*(7), 879–886.

McCauley, E., Gudmundsen, G., Schloredt, K., Martell, C., Rhew, I., Hubley, S., et al. (2016). The adolescent behavioral activation program: Adapting behavioral activation as a treatment for depression in adolescence. *Journal of Clinical Child and Adolescent Psychology, 45*(3), 291–304.

Nezu, A. M. (1987). A problem-solving formulation of depression: A literature review and proposal of a pluralistic model. *Clinical Psychology Review, 7*(2), 121–144.

Nilsen, T. S., Eisemann, M., & Kvernmo, S. (2013). Predictors and moderators of outcome in child and adolescent anxiety and depression: A systematic review of psychological treatment studies. *European Child and Adolescent Psychiatry, 22*(2), 69–87.

Poznanski, E., & Mokros, H. (1996). *Children's Depression Rating Scale—Revised manual.* Los Angeles: Western Psychological Services.

Reinherz, H. Z., Giaconia, R. M., Hauf, A. M. C., Wasserman, M. S., & Silverman, A. B. (1999). Major depression in the transition to adulthood: Risks and impairments. *Journal of Abnormal Psychology, 108*(3), 500–510.

Reynolds, W. M. (2004). *Reynolds Adolescent Depression Scale—Second Edition (RADS-2): Professional manual.* Odessa, FL: Psychological Assessment Resources.

Ritschel, L. A., Ramirez, C. L., Cooley, J., & Craighead, W. E. (2016). Behavioral activation for major depression in adolescents: Results from a pilot study. *Clinical Psychology: Science and Practice, 23*(1), 39–57.

Rohde, P., Feeny, N. C., & Robins, M. (2005). Characteristics and components of the TADS CBT approach. *Cognitive and Behavioral Practice, 12*(2), 186–197.

Segrin, C. (2000). Social skills deficits associated with depression. *Clinical Psychology Review, 20*(3), 379–403.

Shaffer, D., Gould, M. S., Brasic, J., Ambrosini, P., Fisher, P., Bird, H., et al. (1983). A Children's Global Assessment Scale (CGAS). *Archives of General Psychiatry, 40*(11), 1228–1231.

Sheeber, L., Hops, H., & Davis, B. (2001). Family processes in adolescent depression. *Clinical Child and Family Psychology Review, 4*(1), 19–35.

Shirk, S. R., Karver, M. S., & Brown, R. (2011). The alliance in child and adolescent psychotherapy. *Psychotherapy, 48*(1), 17–24.

Stark, K. D., Curry, J. F., Goldman, E., & Integrated Psychotherapy Consortium. (2004). *Project Liberty enhanced services: Depressive Symptoms Intervention Manual.* New York: New York State Office of Mental Health.

Stark, K. D., Reynolds, W. M., & Kaslow, N. J. (1987). A comparison of the relative efficacy of self-control therapy and a behavioral problem-solving therapy for depression in children. *Journal of Abnormal Child Psychology, 15*(1), 91–113.

Stein, G. L., Curry, J. F., Hersh, J., Breland-Noble, A., Silva, S. G., Reinecke, M. A., et al. (2010). Ethnic differences at the start of treatment: An examination of the Treatment for Adolescents with Depression Study (TADS). *Cultural Diversity and Ethnic Minority Psychology, 16*(2), 152–158.

Stockings, E., Degenhardt, L., Lee, Y. Y., Mihalopoulos, C., Liu, A., Hobbs, M., et al. (2015). Symptom screening scales for detecting major depressive disorder in children and adolescents: A systematic review and meta-analysis of reliability, validity and diagnostic utility. *Journal of Affective Disorders, 174,* 447–463.

Sweeney, M., Robins, M., Ruberu, M., & Jones, J. (2005). African-American and Latino families in TADS: Recruitment and treatment considerations. *Cognitive and Behavioral Practice, 12*(2), 221–229.

Treatment for Adolescents with Depression Study Team. (2004). Fluoxetine, cognitive-behavioral therapy, and their combination for adolescents with depression: Treatment for Adolescents with Depression study (TADS) randomized controlled trial. *Journal of the American Medical Association, 292*(7), 807–820.

Webb, C. A., Auerbach, R. P., & DeRubeis, R. J. (2012). Processes of change in CBT of adolescent depression: Review and recommendations. *Journal of Clinical Child and Adolescent Psychology, 41*(5), 654–665.

Weisz, J. R., Chorpita, B. F., Palinkas, L. A., Schoenwald, S. K., Miranda, J., Bearman, S. K., et al. (2012). Testing standard and modular designs for psychotherapy treating depression, anxiety, and conduct problems in youth: A randomized effectiveness trial. *Archives of General Psychiatry, 69*(3), 274–282.

Weisz, J. R., Thurber, C. A., Sweeney, L., Proffitt, V. D., & LeGagnoux, G. L. (1997). Brief treatment of mild-to-moderate child depression using primary and secondary control enhancement training. *Journal of Consulting and Clinical Psychology, 65*(4), 703–707.

Wells, K. C., & Albano, A. M. (2005). Parent involvement in CBT treatment of adolescent depression: Experiences in the Treatment for Adolescents with Depression Study (TADS). *Cognitive and Behavioral Practice, 12*(2), 209–220.

Wells, K. C., & Curry, J. F. (2000). *Treatment for Adolescents with Depression Study (TADS) cognitive behavior therapy manual: Parent and conjoint parent–adolescent sessions.* Unpublished manual, Duke University Medical Center, Durham, NC.

CHAPTER SIX

Treatment of Oppositional Defiant Disorder

Qshequilla P. Mitchell
Dustin A. Pardini
John E. Lochman

The conceptualization of oppositional defiant disorder (ODD) and its etiology have become more refined in recent years, while growing research documents many successful family- and child-based interventions. Most of these interventions introduce empirically supported procedures, including treatment strategies that address parenting and familial factors, maladaptive social-cognitive processes, and deficits in problem solving in children with ODD. We provide an overview of the etiology of ODD and discuss relevant evidence-based interventions, including factors that predict, moderate, and mediate differential outcomes. Specific treatment strategies, with a special emphasis on the role of parents and developmental and multicultural issues, are discussed. Finally, a case example and recommendations for working with children with ODD are provided.

Theoretical Foundations

ODD is characterized by a pattern of angry, defiant, or vindictive behavior occurring over a period of 6 months. It is one of the most common disorders among youth in mental health settings, and children with ODD are often disrespectful and disruptive and exhibit recurrent resentment and hostility (American Psychiatric Association, 2013). Described by the *Diagnostic and Statistical Manual of Mental Disorders* (DSM-5; American Psychiatric Association, 2013), ODD behaviors must be a departure from what is normally expected and at a level that is abnormal for the child's age or developmental level—and the symptoms must cause either distress to the child or others or impairment in social or academic functioning. There are several developmental theories that help to explain the development of ODD (Lahey et al., 1994; Lahey, Loeber, Quay, Frick, & Grimm, 1992), and mounting empirical evidence suggests that specific parenting and familial factors, deficits in social and cognitive processes, and problems with interpersonal problem solving place children at risk for antisocial behavior (Frick et al., 1992; Speltz, DeKlyen, Greenberg, & Dryden, 1995). We provide a review of the literature and a brief overview describing the etiology of oppositional and defiant symptoms.

Parenting and Familial Factors

Scientific evidence links various parenting and familial characteristics to the development of ODD in children (Boyle & Pickles, 1998; Frick et al., 1992). Oppositional and defiant symptoms are related to increased levels of familial dysfunction and lower levels of family income among adolescents diagnosed with ODD; these adolescents report higher levels of authoritarian parenting and lower levels of parental warmth when compared with normal control children (Rey & Plapp, 1990). Similarly, families of children with ODD report lower levels of parental supervision and consistent discipline and exhibit insecure attachment to their maternal caregivers (Speltz et al., 1995). Other investigations reveal that several characteristics of parents and other adult caregivers are associated with ratings of aggressive and deviant behavior in children (O'Brien & Chin, 1998; Lochman & Lenhart, 1993; Lochman & Craven, 1993). Parents of aggressive boys tend to use physical and verbal aggression to discipline their children and reported higher levels of marital hostility than parents of nonaggressive children (Lochman & Lenhart, 1993; Forgatch et al., 2016; Dishion, 2016). Additionally, parents of aggressive children tended to use unclear commands, rigid and controlling parenting strategies, and ineffective monitoring and to exhibit low levels of parental warmth and support (Lochman & Lenhart, 1993).

Genetic inheritance has also been linked to aggressive behavior and child deviancy. Data from a twin study (Simonoff et al., 1998) indicated general genetic liability for conduct problems such as property violations, oppositional behavior, and aggression. Results from a similar study suggest that ODD symptoms during adolescence represent an early expression of genetic liability for adult antisocial personality in males (Langbehn, Cadoret, Yates, Troughton, & Stewart, 1998). Frick et al. (1992) linked childhood conduct problems and parental criminality and also revealed that having a biological parent with antisocial personality disorder may be a risk factor for ODD (Frick et al., 1992).

Multicultural Issues

Race has not been extensively studied among children with disruptive behavior problems (McNeil, Capage, & Bennett, 2002); however, available data suggest that the experiences of minority children differ from those of nonminorities (Canino & Spurlock, 1994). For example, adult expectancies for child behaviors such as submissiveness, language acquisition, motor skills, and dependence differ from culture to culture (McNeil et al., 2002), and ethnicity affects children's presentation of symptoms, types of defenses, and how they cope with anger, fear, and anxiety (Gibbs & Huang, 1989). African American children are most likely to live in low-income homes, and statistics reveal that almost half of all African American children live in poverty (DeNavas-Walt & Proctor, 2014). Due to the strong relationship between race and poverty, it has been difficult to separate their impacts on diagnosis and treatment of ODD. Moreover, socioeconomic disadvantage continues to be linked to course of treatment (McNeil et al., 2002).

Social–Cognitive Processes

Children with oppositional and deviant behaviors have problems with social-cognitive processing and deficits in interpersonal problem solving. Research reveals that children with ODD have difficulties at six different stages of social-information processing: (1) encoding social cues, (2) making interpretations and attributions about social information, (3) identifying goals to be addressed in the social situation, (4) generating possible solutions to interpersonal problems, (5) deciding which plan to enact based on the perceived consequences, and (6) enacting the chosen plan (Matthys, Vanderschuren, Schutter, & Lochman, 2012). An accumulation of research reveals that children with conduct problems exhibit maladaptive social-cognitive processes at each of these stages (Pardini, Lochman, & Wells, 2004; de la Osa, Granero, Domenech, Shamay-Tsoory, & Ezpeleta, 2016; Noordermeer, Luman, & Oosterlaan, 2016).

Antisocial behavior in children is associated with hostile cues and intentions, and children with ODD are more likely to expect and value the positive consequences rather than the negative consequences associated with violent behavior (Matthys et al., 2012; Pardini et al., 2004). Several studies have found that antisocial children are also more likely to support social goals that are harmful to interpersonal relationships when compared with normal peers (Lochman, Wayland, & White, 1993) and lack perspective-taking skills and emotional empathy during social interactions (Cohen & Strayer, 1996). Moreover, youth with conduct problems have greater difficulty generating alternative methods for resolving social conflicts (Lochman, Meyer, Rabiner, & White, 1991) and are less skillful at exhibiting positive interpersonal behaviors than children without conduct problems (Dodge, Pettit, McClaskey, Brown, & Gottman, 1986).

Recent studies indicate that children with ODD have substantial difficulties with social problem-solving skills (Matthys et al., 2012; Ellis, Weiss, & Lochman, 2009; Matthys & Lochman, 2010). Specifically, children with ODD tend to have severe challenges encoding social cues and generating solutions to problems, and they are more confident enacting aggressive responses across a variety of different problematic social situations in comparison with normal control children (Ellis et al., 2009; Schutter, Van Bokhoven, Vanderschuren, Lochman, & Matthys, 2011). Furthermore, when provided the opportunity to choose from a group of responses in common problem conditions, they are also more likely to choose an aggressive response and less likely to choose a prosocial response in comparison with normal control children (Pardini, Lochman, & Frick, 2003). Children with ODD are more likely to generate a smaller number of positive problem-solving strategies to resolve imaginary conflicts in comparison with normal controls (Webster-Stratton & Lindsay, 1999). During play interactions with peers, children with ODD engage in parallel play, display fewer positive social skills, and exhibit aggressive problem-solving skills more often than normal control children (Webster-Stratton & Lindsay, 1999).

Evidence-Based Interventions

There are several empirically supported interventions for children with oppositional and defiant behaviors. Many of these programs apply a multicomponent approach that targets a variety of risk factors for antisocial behavior (Lochman, Powell, Boxmeyer, Young, & Baden, 2010; Hawkins, Catalano, & Miller, 1992). Interventions can be grouped by age (preschool to early elementary school; late elementary school; early adolescence) and include classroom prevention programs, as well as treatment programs. Both the treatment and the prevention programs described in this chapter include programs that are child and parent or family directed. Universal prevention programs are presented first, followed by indicated prevention and treatment programs for oppositional youth. Brief summaries of intervention research findings describing the rationale for the programs and relevant example programs for developmental periods of early childhood through adolescence are described.

Intervention in Preschool and Early Childhood

Universal Prevention Programs

Promoting Alternative THinking Strategies (PATHS)

The Promoting Alternative THinking Strategies (PATHS) program is an example of a universal prevention program that is aimed at promoting general social-emotional competencies and cognitive skill-building in elementary school children (Greenberg & Kusché, 2006). Greenberg and colleagues train teachers to use PATHS, a social-emotional curriculum, to instruct children in emotion awareness and regulation and social problem-solving skills. Although this curriculum has been implemented mostly with children in regular education classrooms, PATHS has also been used with children with special needs (e.g., behaviorally at-risk and deaf children). Overall program results at 1- and 2-year follow-ups indicated that children receiving the PATHS intervention were better able to understand emotions and independently problem-solve. Additionally, children who received PATHS reported reduced conduct problems and impulsivity when compared with children in a control group (Greenberg, 2006; Greenberg, Domitrovich, & Bumbarger, 2001). Likewise, children who received multiyear versions of the PATHS program, across first through third grades, when compared with control children, exhibited reduced aggression, increased prosocial behavior, and increased academic functioning (Dodge, Godwin, & Conduct Problems Prevention Research Group, 2013). PATHS effects were strongest in less disadvantaged schools and among more at-risk children, and the intervention effects for aggression were stronger for boys. Domitrovich, Cortes, and Greenberg (2007) also developed a preschool version of PATHS; findings revealed that preschool children exposed to PATHS had higher emotion knowledge and were more socially competent in comparison with control preschool students.

Linking the Interests of Families and Teachers

The Linking the Interests of Families and Teachers (LIFT) program is an example of a multicomponent universal preventive intervention designed to prevent conduct problems (Reid & Eddy, 2002). The program begins in first grade and continues until the end of the elementary school period. The LIFT program targets elementary-age schoolchildren and their families living in high-risk neighborhoods and includes a 10-week intervention that addresses (1) parent training in consistent limit setting, effective discipline practices, and active involvement in children's school and social activities; (2) a 20-session classroom-based social skills program designed to increase children's social problem-solving skills and to help children resist negative peer groups; (3) a behavioral program to reduce playground aggression based on the Good Behavior Game (Embry & Straatemeier, 2001); and (4) systematic communication between teachers and parents regarding schoolwork and classroom behavior, via a phone and answering machine installed in each classroom. In a randomized trial with 671 families, Reid, Patterson, and Snyder (2002) found significant improvements in family problem solving and playground aggression following LIFT. Likewise, in their middle school years, children in the intervention group were significantly less likely to have been arrested by the police and to have used alcohol 30 months following the intervention. Additionally, as adolescents, later in high school, effects on substance use were evident for the LIFT program; the intervention significantly reduced youths' self-reported substance use, and there was a significant reduction of the growth rate in girls' use of tobacco and illicit drugs. The LIFT program had an overall impact on the average levels of use of tobacco, alcohol, and illicit drugs (DeGarmo, Eddy, Reid, & Fetrow, 2009). The LIFT program's effects in improving family problem solving mediated mean reductions in tobacco use; similarly, the intervention's effects on reducing playground aggression had indirect effects on reducing growth in substance use.

Treatment and Targeted Prevention Programs

The Incredible Years

The Incredible Years Training Series was initially developed as a parent training intervention for the treatment of ODD in young children. This series included a child training program, the Dinosaur School, and a teacher component (Webster-Stratton, 2005). The Dinosaur School was developed to address common issues that young children with conduct problems regularly endured: social skills problems, an inability to emotionally empathize or engage in perspective taking, effective conflict resolution, and dealing with feelings of loneliness, stress, and anger. Similarly, the teacher curriculum for the Incredible Years program consists of various strategies for strengthening home–school partnerships, improving teachers' behavior management skills, fostering teachers' use of effective discipline techniques, reinforcement of prosocial child behaviors, and increasing teachers' ability to teach and reinforce social-emotional skills in the classroom setting. Analysis of treatment groups found that the Dinosaur School child training led to a significant reduction in the number of conduct problems reported in the home and increased social problem-solving skills in comparison with control groups (Webster-Stratton & Hammond, 1997). Additionally, at 1-year follow-up, nearly two-thirds of children in the child treatment group had parent ratings of behavioral problems in the normal rather than clinically significant range. The Dinosaur School has been examined as one component within the multicomponent Incredible Years program.

The parent training component of the Dinosaur School consists of groups of 10–12 parents who meet with a therapist on a weekly basis for approximately 22 sessions for approximately 2 hours. Similar to the child component, parents watch approximately 17 different videotapes containing vignettes modeling appropriate ways for dealing with problematic parent–child interactions. The therapist leads group discussions pertaining to the topics depicted in the videos, and parents are encouraged to ask questions and participate in active discussions of the techniques being presented. The major topics presented during the parent training sessions include effective play techniques, limit setting, ways to handle misbehavior, and communication of emotions (Webster-Stratton, Reid, & Beauchaine, 2013; Webster-Stratton & Hammond, 1997).

Research findings reveal the Dinosaur Schools' effectiveness for decreasing children's aggression and oppositional behaviors (Webster-Stratton et al., 2013); thus the effectiveness of the Dinosaur School and parent training interventions, alone and in combination, appears promising. Findings also reveal that the parent training component has produced significant behavioral gains in comparison to wait-list controls across a number of different studies, even when the parenting videotapes were self-administered without the aid of a therapist (Webster-Stratton, 1984; Webster-Stratton & Hammond, 1997; Webster-Stratton, Kolpacoff, & Hollinsworth, 1988). Overall improvements in parent reports of their children's behavior were still present at 3-year follow-up, with the intervention combining videotaped modeling with therapist-led discussion showing stable improvements (Webster-Stratton, 1990).

A more recent investigation revealed that children who attended the Dinosaur School without parent training experienced a significant reduction in the amount of conduct problems reported in the home and increases in social problem-solving skills in comparison with wait-list controls (Webster-Stratton & Hammond, 1997). Likewise, at 1-year follow-up, nearly two-thirds of children attending this group had parent ratings of behavioral problems in the normal rather than clinically significant range. Although the combination of child and parent training proved superior to each of the component pieces, this finding indicates that cognitive-behavioral treatments directed at young children can be effective in reducing aggressive and disruptive behaviors and could benefit parents who are unwilling or unable to participate in treatment. The Incredible Years program has also been adapted for use as a targeted prevention intervention.

Research findings regarding the effectiveness of Incredible Years across the child, parent, and teacher training interventions have been successfully replicated across several populations. The parent training component has consistently produced significant reductions in child conduct problems at home and school, decreases in negative parenting, and increases in positive parenting in comparison with wait-list control conditions (Webster-Stratton & Hammond, 1997; Webster-Stratton, Reid, & Hammond, 2004). Similarly, the child intervention has produced significant reductions in the amount of conduct problems children exhibit at home and school, as well as producing increases in social problem-solving skills in comparison with wait-list control conditions (Webster-Stratton et al., 2004). Additionally, research findings suggest that overall improvements in children's behavior problems as the result of the parenting intervention can still be seen at 3-year follow-up (Webster-Stratton, 1990). Approximately two-thirds of children who participated in the intervention, at 1-year follow-up, have parent ratings of behavioral problems in the normal rather than clinically significant range (Webster-Stratton & Hammond, 1997). The Incredible Years program is one of the most notable series that provides a rich body of data on children with conduct problems. Several ongoing reviews and empirical studies have been published in recent years (Pidano & Allen, 2015).

Fast Track

The Fast Track program is a multisite comprehensive prevention program targeting high-risk children who display early-onset disruptive behaviors in kindergarten (Conduct Problems Prevention Research Group, 1992). Following a kindergarten screening conducted by teachers, children were randomly assigned to the Fast Track program and received social skills training, tutoring, peer-pairing activities with peers not at risk, and teacher-administered, classroom-wide social competence training in first grade. The parents of the high-risk children participated in parent groups, in parent–child activities, and in home visits. Fast Track is a well-established, developmentally guided intervention that continues with the high-risk children through the elementary school grades.

Research findings reveal significant intervention effects on peer ratings of aggression, on disruptive behavior, and on ratings of classroom atmosphere (Conduct Problems Prevention Research Group, 1999). Likewise, moderate positive social effects on children's social, emotional, and academic skills were observed at the end of the first grade (Conduct Problems Prevention Research Group, 1999). Many of these effects on children's behaviors and social-cognitive processes were maintained at the end of third grade (Conduct Problems Prevention Research Group, 2002) and up to the end of elementary school, through fourth and fifth grades (Conduct Problems Prevention Research Group, 2004). Moreover, among the children with the highest screen scores in kindergarten, children in the Fast Track intervention had lower rates of externalizing diagnoses; once this effect emerged, it continued throughout the high school years (Conduct Problems Prevention Research Group, 2011). Long-term effects on adult criminal behavior at age 25 have been found (Conduct Problems Prevention Research Group, 2015). Indirect effects of the Fast Track intervention indicated that lower parent and youth reports of conduct problems and callous/unemotional behavior were influenced by intervention-produced improvements in children's social-cognitive processes and by parents becoming warmer and less harsh (Dodge et al., 2013; Pasalich, Witkiewitz, McMahon, Pinderhughes, & Conduct Problems Prevention Research Group, 2016).

The Family Check-Up

The Family Check-Up is a brief, three-session intervention based on motivational interviewing techniques that was recently adapted for a preventive intervention for parents of young toddlers (i.e., between 1 and 2 years old) who have socioeconomic, family, and/or child risk factors for future conduct problems (Shaw, Dishion, Supplee, Gardner, & Arnds, 2006). The Family Check-Up includes an initial contact session; a session devoted to assessing child and family functioning and parent–child interactions; and a feedback session focused on supporting existing parenting strengths, exploring parents' willingness to change problematic parenting behaviors, and identifying needed family services (Dishion, Nelson, & Kavanagh, 2003; Shaw et al., 2006). In a randomized trial of the Family Check-Up, families were offered up to six additional follow-up sessions to address parenting practices, other family management issues, and contextual concerns (e.g., marital adjustment, housing, vocational training). At a 2-year follow-up, the intervention group showed significantly greater maternal involvement and reduced child disruptive behavior when compared with families in the control condition.

Recent research documents the process of Family Check-Up effects with young children and has examined whether the program could be disseminated and transferable to community practitioners. In the Early Steps Multisite Trial, high levels of parent–child engagement were associated with less parent–child coercion in the following year for parents of 2- to 5-year-olds, indicating the importance of focusing initially on positive parenting (Sitnick et al., 2015). In addition, families randomly assigned to the Family Check-Up reported increased levels of positive engagement at ages 3 and 5, and the association between positive engagement at age 3 and child problem behavior at age 5 was mediated by reductions in parent–child coercion at ages 3 and 4. Smith, Stormshak, and Kavanagh (2015) reported on feasibility of the Family Check-Up to be disseminated to community partners and found that in three community mental health agencies with 40 therapists working with 71 families with children 5 to 17 years of age, the Family Check-Up condition evidenced significantly reduced youth conduct problems in comparison to youth in usual care.

Intervention in Later Childhood

Universal Prevention Programs

The Seattle Social Development Project

The Seattle Social Development Project (SSDP) is an example of a universal preventive program designed to reduce aggression and problem behaviors in youth by developing a positive school environment. SSDP is a multiyear school-based intervention that includes training for teachers to increase the use of nonpunitive classroom behavioral management techniques, such as positive reinforcement, and includes a parent training component and child problem-solving and social skills training (Berryhill & Prinz, 2003; Hawkins, Catalano, Kosterman, Abbott, & Hill, 1999).

The SSDP has been implemented in Seattle, and research findings reveal that SSDP has produced significant reductions in alcohol use (Hawkins et al., 1999), delinquency, and the frequency of sexual intercourse and number of sexual partners (Hawkins et al., 1999). Students who received SSDP reported more positive feelings and school bonding when compared with control groups. Additionally, adolescents who participated in SSDP were significantly more likely to report condom use when compared with the control group (Lonzak et al., 2002). Furthermore, students who received SSDP had improved academic achievement and less student-reported school misbehavior (Hawkins et al., 1999; Hawkins, Kosterman, Catalano, Hill, & Abbott, 2005).

Positive Behavior Supports

Positive behavior supports (PBS) is a widely used prevention approach designed to promote students' positive social and academic functioning. This strategy has an established record of reducing challenging behaviors in children with developmental and intellectual disabilities (Bradshaw, Waasdorp, & Leaf, 2012; Sugai & Horner, 2006). A review of randomized controlled trials has found PBS to have positive outcomes (Horner, Sugai, & Anderson, 2010). In these controlled studies of school-wide use of the intervention, PBS has led to reduced office referrals (Sherrod, Getch, & Ziomek-Daigle, 2009) and to improved school climate, to children's social-emotional functioning, and to reductions in their suspensions and teacher-rated behavioral problems (Bradshaw et al., 2012; Waasdorp, Bradshaw, & Leaf, 2012). The PBS outcomes have been found to be greatest for at-risk (above the mean for concentration problems and disruptive behaviors) and high-risk (7% of children with the highest levels of concentration and behavioral difficulties) children (Bradshaw, Waasdorp, & Leaf, 2015).

The Child Development Project

The Child Development Project (CDP) is a comprehensive program designed to foster children's social and ethical responsibility and to create a caring school community (Lewis, Watson, & Schaps, 2003). CDP includes cooperative learning, in which students are encouraged to work together (not compete); nonpunitive discipline; reading activities; cross-grade "buddies" activities in which older and younger students are paired together to complete activities; parent activities for home use; and community-building activities that involve all of the students, parents, teachers, and staff in working together within a school (Berryhill & Prinz, 2003; Lewis et al., 2003). Overall, the results indicate that students in schools that had a high fidelity of curriculum implementation showed increases in personal, social, and ethical values and attitudes relative to control schools and to schools that did not implement the curriculum with a high degree of fidelity (Solomon, Battistich, Watson, Schaps, & Lewis, 2000). Additionally, across high change schools, there were significantly positive effects on grade point averages, test scores, and rates of delinquent behaviors (Battistich et al., 2004). Three- and four-year follow-ups of schools with a high degree of program fidelity showed reductions in many measures of substance use and delinquency compared with control schools (Berryhill & Prinz, 2003; Solomon et al., 2000).

Treatment and Targeted Prevention Programs

The Coping Power Program

The Coping Power Program (CPP; Lochman, Wells, & Lenhart, 2008) is a multicomponent intervention for aggressive preadolescents. Grounded in a contextual social-cognitive model of childhood aggression, the CPP includes 34 child group sessions that address additional topics such as emotional awareness, relaxation training, social skills enhancement, positive social and personal goals, and dealing with peer pressure. Other elements of the child component include regular individual sessions that take place every 4–6 weeks and are designed to increase generalization of the program to the children's actual social situations. In addition, periodic consultation is provided to the teachers of children who are making some progress in treatment sessions but who are still having recurrent behavior problems at school.

The CPP has a parent component that consists of 16 parent group sessions that last approximately 2 hours each and are designed to cover the same 15- to 18-month period of time as the CPP child component. The 16 sessions are designed to address issues such as social reinforcement and positive attention, the importance of clear house rules, behavioral expectations and monitoring procedures, the use of appropriate and effective discipline strategies, family communication, positive connection to school, and stress management. Parents are also informed of the skills their children are working on during their sessions, and parents are encouraged to facilitate and reinforce children for using these new skills. The parent component also includes periodic individual contacts with parents through home visits and telephone contacts to promote generalization of skills.

Research data from two separate studies reveal that long-term follow-up effects on youth's externalizing behavior have been found in school settings 3–4 years after the intervention (Lochman, Powell, Boxmeyer, Kelly, & Dillon, 2013; Lochman et al., 2014). In addition, the 1-year follow-up effects on delinquency have found to be mediated by program-induced changes in children's attributional biases, outcome expectations for aggression, internal locus of control, and consistent parental discipline (Lochman & Wells, 2002). In a recent study, children who received the CPP had significant reductions in their parent- and teacher-rated externalizing behavioral problems and in their reported involvement with deviant peers (Lochman et al., 2015). Several randomized trials provide evidence that the CPP provides beneficial effects on children's aggression, academic functioning, and family functioning that continue to be sustained long after treatment (Powell, Lochman, Boxmeyer, Barry, & Pardini, in press).

The CPP has been adapted in several ways. An abbreviated version of the CPP, including 24 child and 10 parent sessions, can be delivered in a single school year with beneficial results (Lochman et al., 2014). A hybrid Internet and in-person implementation has also been developed (Lochman et al., in press), and CPP has been combined with the Family Check-Up to tailor the delivery of the intervention (Herman et al., 2012). CPP is being combined with yoga and mindfulness techniques in a current trial (Boxmeyer et al., 2016). The most recent adaptation includes a developmental adaptation of the CPP for early adolescents during their middle school years. Preliminary data, involving one-third of the intended overall sample, reveal a significant reduction in hyperactivity, aggression, and conduct problems from pre- to postintervention. Furthermore, improvements in impulse control, emotional regulation, and social adjustment were observed among participants (Lochman et al., 2016).

Intervention in Early Adolescence: Universal Prevention Programs

Life Skills Training

The Life Skills Training (LST) program is an example of a universal prevention program designed to prevent substance abuse in adolescents (Botvin

& Griffin, 2004). Rather than solely educating students about the dangers of substance abuse, LST offers an alternative to risky behaviors through designed activities. The program was developed for middle school students. LST has been implemented across 15 class periods during the first year of middle school (11–14 years of age), with supplemental booster sessions during the following 2 years. Specific components of LST include student instruction in personal self-management skills, social skills, and drug resistance skills. The program has been shown to be highly effective in reducing alcohol, tobacco, marijuana, and polydrug use in a series of randomized controlled efficacy trials and in two effectiveness studies. Reductions in smoking and drunkenness were sustained for 5 years after random assignment in both studies (Spoth, Randall, Trudeau, Shin, & Redmond, 2008). Other study results support the long-term effectiveness of the program, as well as its generalizability to diverse geographic, socioeconomic, and racial/ ethnic groups (Botvin, Griffin, & Nichols, 2006). The LST program has produced direct effects on adult substance use; with adolescents, it had demonstrated indirect effects, as intervention reduced adolescent substance use initiation, which, in turn, has predicted reduced substance misuse in young adulthood (Spoth, Trudeau, Redmond, & Shin, 2014). At the time of follow-up at ages 19–22, the effects of LST were similar to the effects of the more comprehensive Strengthening Families Program, in comparison with the control condition (Spoth et al., 2014). The LST program has been adapted for use in international replication and disseminations. Moreover, a German replication found positive program effects on alcohol use and school bonding, with the improved school bonding mediating the reductions in alcohol use (Wenzel, Weichold, & Silbereisen, 2009).

Responding in Peaceful and Positive Ways

Responding in Peaceful and Positive Ways (RIPP) is an example of a school-based violence prevention program designed to develop conflict resolution skills among middle school–age children. RIPP interventionists teach middle school adolescents problem-solving steps, better communication skills, and achievement techniques to aid in the promotion of nonviolence and to reduce aggressive behavior. The original RIPP program was used with sixth-grade students (mean age of 11; Farrell, Meyer, & White, 2001), and a newer version was developed for seventh-grade students (mean age of 12; Farrell, Meyer, Sullivan, & Kung, 2003). This program encourages youth to use critical learning skills and individual management strategies to avoid potential violence. Teens are encouraged to internalize these skills through repetition and mentally rehearsing problem-solving steps, experiential learning, and didactic teaching (Farrell et al., 2001).

Overall results of the RIPP intervention showed that students who were not exposed to RIPP had more than twice the rate of disciplinary code violations related to violence than the RIPP treatment group (Farrell et al., 2003). Additionally, findings reveal that boys who participated in the intervention had significantly more favorable attitudes toward nonviolence at 6-month follow-up. Gender differences were found as boys maintained fewer suspensions compared with the control group 1 year later, whereas girls did not maintain a significantly different number of suspensions compared with controls. RIPP students also reported significantly lower aggression at the 9-month follow-up and significantly lower victimization for boys at the second midpoint in seventh grade. Adolescents in the RIPP program also indicated that they used peer mediation more frequently than did controls. Overall, students who had the highest rates of disruptive behaviors prior to receiving the prevention achieved the greatest benefit from RIPP (Farrell et al., 2001; Farrell et al., 2003).

Case Example

Keith was a 10-year-old boy in the sixth grade at a local middle school. Keith's teacher completed a 6-item scale indicating the frequency of proactive and reactive progressive behaviors on each of her students, and Keith met the criteria to be included in the CPP. Keith's mother, Lisa, was unemployed and overwhelmed by severe financial problems and raising Keith and his brother, Sam, on her own. Lisa described Keith as a well-behaved young man, but, when agitated or picked on, he could become hostile and violent. Lisa said, "He will not bother anyone unless you make him mad, and then you better run for cover."

Keith had trouble staying in school due to fights that resulted in multiple school suspensions. His teacher reported that he was always out of his seat without permission and was violent and disruptive. He not only got into fights with fellow students but also pushed his art teacher and had to attend alternative school for 45 days in the beginning of the school year. The principal met and talked with Keith on several occasions, and Keith had been very defensive and rebellious with him. Once Keith's mother was informed about his eligibility to participate in the CPP, she was relieved and explained that this program might be her only hope. Lisa was very concerned that Keith would continue to get into trouble at school or end up in jail one day.

Lisa recently drove Keith and his younger brother to the local police station and made them spend some time there "to learn the consequences to acting up." She firmly believed that this experience might "scare her boys straight," result in a positive change in their behavior, and, specifically, persuade Keith to behave in school. Lisa went through tremendous effort and invested a lot of time to encourage Keith, and, although many times her actions were unconventional, she demonstrated that she cared a lot about her son's future.

Rachel, the child group leader, worked with Keith to identify a long-term goal that would motivate him to cope with anger and not get into physical fights. Keith said that he would like to play football the following year and pass the sixth grade. Over the next couple of months, during the CPP, Rachel and Keith identified short-term goals that would help Keith stay on track so that he could try out for football and improve his academic grades. Keith decided that he needed to stop getting out of his seat and disrupting class and also that he needed to deal with difficult feelings in other ways than initiating physical fights. Keith also told Rachel that he wasn't keeping up with his homework assignments and had trouble staying organized. Consequently, during the program, Rachel worked with Keith to help him keep his notebooks tidy. Keith was given an organizer and planner to write down his homework assignments. Many sessions were focused on study and organizational skills that would help Keith with his academic goals.

Lisa was very active and responded very positively to the parent component of the program. She said many times during the parent meetings that she would like Keith to be involved in team sports and would like to support him in "doing something positive." Lisa seemed to enjoy the social nature of the parent group and listened keenly to the suggestions of other parents who participated in the group. Lisa specifically bonded and developed a friendship with a grandparent who was raising her granddaughter; she seemed to respect and value her opinion and suggestions to the group. Lisa missed only one out of twelve sessions. She commented that making quality time for Keith had helped her relationship with her son and that she had increased parental monitoring. Lisa also said that being consistent with Keith and establishing clear expectations had strengthened their relationship. She was willing to practice alternative methods to solely physical punishment; she used time-out and privilege removal rather than physical spankings.

During the child component, Keith was introduced to the PICC (problem identification, choices, consequences) model. The PICC model helped Keith to recognize how his actions made others feel. Keith was initially unaware of how his actions and negative comments made his peers feel. During puppet play, Keith practiced coping skills and examined others' perspectives on his actions. Additionally, Keith created a video describing the PICC model and how it could be used in everyday situations. Live role plays tended to be very useful to Keith and other students in the group by allowing the opportunity to practice perspective taking. Specifically, he learned how teasing and picking fights with his peers affected his teachers' feelings about him and his relationships with his classmates. Keith was able to connect with how his actions made teachers and his friends feel. He was very successful in managing his anger by using the anger thermometer, and he made extra efforts outside of the session to understand others' emotions.

Although he was difficult to engage in the beginning, Keith benefited from the positive support and modeling efforts of the CPP group leader. The group leader delivered several of the CPP sessions individually while Keith was in alternative school, which perhaps resulted in meaningful connection and bonding while strengthening engagement.

At the end of the program, Keith demonstrated meaningful gains: decreases in aggressive behaviors, externalizing composite score, and hyperactivity. He also became better at setting goals and demonstrating the emotional knowledge to gauge and control anger. Keith became less impulsive and was able to understand the consequences of his behavior. Rachel praised and rewarded Keith's growth in problem solving and his ability to practice alternative methods to fighting.

Summary

Several empirically supported interventions for children with ODD have been effective for improving deleterious peer relationships, family functioning, academic achievement, and overall health and well-being. The most successful interventions use a multicomponent approach that is applied with parents and children. Unaddressed aggression and delinquency among youth is a serious public health problem. Dissemination and translation of effective programs are critical to improving mental health outcomes.

References

American Psychiatric Association. (2013). *Diagnostic and statistical manual of mental disorders* (5th ed.). Arlington, VA: Author.

Battistich, V., Schaps, E., & Wilson, N. (2004). Effects of an elementary school intervention on students' "connectedness" to school and social adjustment during middle school. *Journal of Primary Prevention, 24*(3), 243–262.

Berryhill, J. C., & Prinz, R. J. (2003). Environmental interventions to enhance student adjustment: Implications for prevention. *Prevention Science, 4*(2), 65–87.

Botvin, G. J., & Griffin, K. W. (2004). Life skills training: Empirical findings and future directions. *Journal of Primary Prevention, 25*(2), 211–232.

Botvin, G. J., Griffin, K. W., & Nichols, T. D. (2006). Preventing youth violence and delinquency through a universal school-based prevention approach. *Prevention Science, 7*(4), 403–408.

Boxmeyer, C., Miller, S., Lochman, J., Powell, N., Romero, D., Jones, S., et al. (2016, April). *Mindful Coping Power: An integrated mindfulness, yoga, and cognitive-behavioral intervention for at-risk aggressive children and their parents.* Poster presented at the 17th Annual Rural Health Conference, Complementary and Integrative Medicine: A Whole Person Approach to Health Care, Tuscaloosa, AL.

Boyle, M. H., & Pickles, A. R. (1998). Strategies to manipulate reliability: Impact on statistical associations. *Journal of the American Academy of Child and Adolescent Psychiatry, 37*(10), 1077–1084.

Bradshaw, C. P., Waasdorp, T. E., & Leaf, P. J. (2012). Effects of school-wide positive behavioral interventions and supports on child behavior problems. *Pediatrics, 130*(5), e1136–e1145.

Bradshaw, C. P., Waasdorp, T. E., & Leaf, P. J. (2015). Examining variation in the impact of school-wide positive behavioral interventions and supports: Findings from a randomized controlled effectiveness trial. *Journal of Educational Psychology, 107*(2), 546–557.

Canino, I. A., & Spurlock, J. (1994). *Culturally diverse children and adolescents: Assessment, diagnosis, and treatment.* New York: Guilford Press.

Cohen, D., & Strayer, J. (1996). Empathy in conduct-disordered and comparison youth. *Developmental Psychology, 32*(6), 988–998.

Conduct Problems Prevention Research Group. (1992). A developmental and clinical model for the prevention of conduct disorder: The Fast Track Program. *Development and Psychopathology, 4*(4), 509–527.

Conduct Problems Prevention Research Group. (1999). Initial impact of the Fast Track prevention trial for conduct problems: I. The high-risk sample. *Journal of Consulting and Clinical Psychology, 67,* 631–647.

Conduct Problems Prevention Research Group. (2002). The implementation of the Fast Track program: An example of a large-scale prevention science efficacy trial. *Journal of Abnormal Child Psychology, 30,* 1–17.

Conduct Problems Prevention Research Group. (2004). The effects of the Fast Track program on serious problem outcomes at the end of elementary school. *Journal of Clinical Child and Adolescent Psychology, 33,* 650–661.

Conduct Problems Prevention Research Group. (2011). The effects of the Fast Track preventive intervention on the development of conduct disorder across childhood. *Child Development, 82,* 331–345.

Conduct Problems Prevention Research Group. (2015). Impact of early intervention on psychopathology, crime, and well-being at age 25. *American Journal of Psychiatry, 172,* 59–70.

de la Osa, N., Granero, R., Domenech, J. M., Shamay-Tsoory, S., & Ezpeleta, L. (2016). Cognitive and affective components of theory of mind in preschoolers with oppositional defiance disorder: Clinical evidence. *Psychiatry Research, 241,* 128–134.

DeGarmo, D. S., Eddy, J. M., Reid, J. B., & Fetrow, R. A. (2009). Evaluating mediators of the impact of the Linking the Interests of Families and Teachers (LIFT) multimodal preventive intervention on substance use initiation and growth across adolescence. *Prevention Science, 10*(3), 208–220.

DeNavas-Walt, C., & Proctor, B. D. (2014). *Income and poverty in the United States: 2013 Current Population Reports.* Washington, DC: U.S. Department of Commerce, U.S. Census Bureau.

Dishion, T. J. (2016). An evolutionary framework for understanding coercion and aggression. In T. J. Dishion & J. Snyder (Eds.), *Oxford handbook of coercive relationship dynamics* (pp. 53–68). New York: Oxford University Press.

Dishion, T. J., Nelson, S. E., & Kavanagh, K. (2003). The family check-up with high-risk young adolescents: Preventing early-onset substance use by parent monitoring. *Behavior Therapy, 34*(4), 553–571.

Dodge, K. A., Godwin, J., & Conduct Problems Prevention Research Group. (2013). Social-information-processing patterns mediate the impact of preventive intervention on adolescent antisocial behavior. *Psychological Science, 24*(4), 456–465.

Dodge, K. A., Pettit, G. S., McClaskey, C. L., Brown, M. M., & Gottman, J. M. (1986). Social competence in children. *Monographs of the Society for Research in Child Development, 51*(2, Serial No. 213).

Domitrovich, C. E., Cortes, R. C., & Greenberg, M. T. (2007). Improving young children's social and emotional competence: A randomized trial of the preschool "PATHS" curriculum. *Journal of Primary Prevention, 28*(2), 67–91.

Eddy, J. M., & Reid, J. B. (2002). Preventive efforts during the elementary school years: Linking the interests of families and teacher projects. In *Antisocial behavior of the adolescent children of incarcerated parents: A developmental perspective* (pp. 219–233). Washington, DC: American Psychological Association.

Ellis, M. L., Weiss, B., & Lochman, J. E. (2009). Executive functions in children: Associations with aggressive behavior and appraisal processing. *Journal of Abnormal Child Psychology, 37*(7), 945–956.

Embry, D. D., & Straatemeier, G. (2001). *The PAX acts game manual: How to apply the good behavior game.* Tucson, AZ: PAXIS Institute.

Farrell, A. D., Meyer, A. L., Sullivan, T. N., & Kung, E. M. (2003). Evaluation of the Responding in Peaceful and Positive Ways (RIPP) seventh grade violence prevention curriculum. *Journal of Child and Family Studies, 12*(1), 101–120.

Farrell, A. D., Meyer, A. L., & White, K. S. (2001). Evaluation of Responding in Peaceful and Positive Ways (RIPP): A school-based prevention program for reducing violence among urban adolescents. *Journal of Clinical Child Psychology, 30*(4), 451–463.

Forgatch, M. S., Snyder, J. J., Patterson, G. R., Pauldine, M. R., Chaw, Y., Elish, K., et al. (2016). Resurrecting the chimera: Progressions in parenting and peer processes. *Development and Psychopathology, 28*(3), 689–706.

Frick, P. J., Lahey, B. B., Loeber, R., Stouthamer-Loeber, M., Christ, M. A. G., & Hanson, K. (1992). Familial risk factors to oppositional defiant disorder and conduct disorder: Parental psychopathology and maternal parenting. *Journal of Consulting and Clinical Psychology, 60*(1), 49–55.

Gibbs, J. T., & Huang, L. N. (1989). *Children of color: Psychological interventions with minority youth.* San Francisco: Jossey-Bass.

Greenberg, M. T. (2006). Promoting resilience in children and youth. *Annals of the New York Academy of Sciences, 1094*(1), 139–150.

Greenberg, M. T., Domitrovich, C., & Bumbarger, B. (2001). The prevention of mental disorders in school-aged children: Current state of the field. *Prevention and Treatment, 4*(1), 1–59.

Greenberg, M. T., & Kusché, C. A. (2006). *Building social and emotional competence: The PATHS curriculum.* Washington, DC: American Psychological Association.

Hawkins, J. D., Catalano, R. F., Kosterman, R., Abbott, R., & Hill, K. G. (1999). Preventing adolescent health-risk behaviors by strengthening protection during childhood. *Archives of Pediatrics and Adolescent Medicine, 153*(3), 226–234.

Hawkins, J. D., Catalano, R. F., & Miller, J. Y. (1992). Risk and protective factors for alcohol and other drug problems in adolescence and early adulthood: Implications for substance abuse prevention. *Psychological Bulletin, 112*(1), 64–105.

Hawkins, J. D., Kosterman, R., Catalano, R. F., Hill, K. G., & Abbott, R. D. (2005). Promoting positive adult functioning through social development intervention in childhood: Long-term effects from the Seattle Social Development Project. *Archives of Pediatrics and Adolescent Medicine, 159*(1), 25–31.

Herman, K. C., Reinke, W. M., Bradshaw, C. P., Lochman, J. E., Boxmeyer, C. L., Powell, N. P., et al. (2012). Integrating the family check-up and the parent coping power program. *Advances in School Mental Health Promotion, 5*(3), 208–219.

Horner, R. H., Sugai, G., & Anderson, C. M. (2010). Examining the evidence base for school-wide positive behavior support. *Focus on Exceptional Children, 42*(8), 1–14.

Lahey, B. B., Applegate, B., McBurnett, K., Biederman, J., Greenhill, L., Hynd, G. W., et al. (1994). DMS-IV field trials for attention deficit hyperactivity disorder in children and adolescents. *American Journal of Psychiatry, 151*(11), 1673–1685.

Lahey, B. B., Loeber, R., Quay, H. C., Frick, P. J., & Grimm, J. (1992). Oppositional defiant and conduct disorders: Issues to be resolved for DSM-IV. *Journal of the American Academy of Child and Adolescent Psychiatry, 31*(3), 539–546.

Langbehn, D. R., Cadoret, R. J., Yates, W. R., Troughton, E. P., & Stewart, M. A. (1998). Distinct contributions of conduct and oppositional defiant symptoms to adult antisocial behavior: Evidence from an adoption study. *Archives of General Psychiatry, 55*(9), 821–829.

Lewis, C., Watson, M., & Schaps, E. (2003). Building community in school: The child development project. In M. Elias, H. Arnold, & C. Steiger Hussey (Eds.), *EQ + IQ = Best leadership practices for caring and successful schools* (pp. 100–108). Thousand Oaks, CA: Corwin Press.

Lochman, J. E., Baden, R. E., Boxmeyer, C. L., Powell, N. P., Qu, L., Salekin, K. L., et al. (2014). Does a booster intervention augment the preventive effects of an abbreviated version of the Coping Power Program for aggressive children? *Journal of Abnormal Child Psychology, 42*(3), 367–381.

Lochman, J. E., Boxmeyer, C. L., Jones, S., Qu, L., Ewoldsen, D., & Nelson, W. M., III. (in press). Testing the feasibility of a briefer school-based preventive intervention with aggressive children: A hybrid intervention with face-to-face and Internet components. *Journal of School Psychology.*

Lochman, J. E., Bradshaw, C. P., Powell, N., Debnam, K., Pas, E., & Ialongo, N. (2016, May). *Can indicated prevention work for conduct problem middle school adolescents?: Preliminary findings for the Early Adolescent Coping Power Program (CP-EA).* Paper presented at the Society for Prevention Research 24th Annual Meeting: Using Prevention Science to Promote Health Equity and Improve Well-Being, San Francisco, CA.

Lochman, J. E., & Craven, S. V. (1993, August). *Family conflict associated with reactive and proactive aggression at two age levels.* Paper presented at the biennial meeting of the Society for Research in Child Development, New Orleans, LA.

Lochman, J. E., Dishion, T. J., Powell, N. P., Boxmeyer, C. L., Qu, L., & Sallee, M. (2015). Evidence-based child preventive interventions for antisocial behavior: A randomized study of the effects of group versus individual delivery. *Journal of Consulting and Clinical Psychology, 83*, 728–735.

Lochman, J. E., & Lenhart, L. A. (1993). Anger coping intervention for aggressive children: Conceptual models and outcome effects. *Clinical Psychology Review, 13*(8), 785–805.

Lochman, J. E., Meyer, B. L., Rabiner, D. L., & White, K. J. (1991). Parameters influencing social problem-solving of aggressive children. *Advances in Behavioral Assessment of Children and Families, 5*, 31–63.

Lochman, J. E., Powell, N. P., Boxmeyer, C. L., Kelly, M., & Dillon, C. (2013). Anger management in schools: The Coping Power program for children and early adolescents. In E. Fernandez (Ed.), *Treatments for anger in special populations: Theory, application, and outcome* (pp. 176–196). New York: Oxford University Press.

Lochman, J., Powell, N., Boxmeyer, C., Young, L., & Baden, R. (2010). Historical conceptions of risk subtyping among children and adolescents. In R. T. Salekin & D. R. Lynam (Eds.), *Handbook of child and adolescent psychopathy* (pp. 49–78). New York: Guilford Press.

Lochman, J. E., Wayland, K. K., & White, K. J. (1993). Social goals: Relationship to adolescent adjustment and to social problem solving. *Journal of Abnormal Child Psychology, 21*(2), 135–151.

Lochman, J. E., & Wells, K. C. (2002). Contextual social-cognitive mediators and child outcome: A test of the theoretical model in the Coping Power Program. *Development and Psychopathology, 14*, 971–993.

Lochman, J. E., Wells, K., & Lenhart, L. A. (2008). *Coping Power: Child group facilitator's guide* (Vol. 2). New York: Oxford University Press.

Lonczak, H. S., Abbott, R. D., Hawkins, J. D., Kosterman, R., & Catalano, R. F. (2002). Effects of the Seattle Social Development Project on sexual behavior, pregnancy, birth, and sexually transmitted disease outcomes by age 21 years. *Archives of Pediatrics and Adolescent Medicine, 156*(5), 438–447.

Lonczak, H. S., Huang, B., Catalano, R. F., Hawkins, J. D., Hill, K. G., Abbott, R. D., et al. (2001). The social predictors of adolescent alcohol misuse: A test of the social development model. *Journal of Studies on Alcohol, 62*(2), 179–189.

Matthys, W., & Lochman, J. E. (2010). *Oppositional defiant disorder and conduct disorder in childhood*. Chichester, UK: Wiley-Blackwell.

Matthys, W., Vanderschuren, L. J. M. J., Schutter, D. J. L. G., & Lochman, J. E. (2012). Impaired neurocognitive functions affect social learning processes in oppositional defiant disorder and conduct disorder: Implications for interventions. *Clinical Child and Family Psychology Review, 15*, 234–246.

McNeil, C. B., Capage, L. C., & Bennett, G. M. (2002). Cultural issues in the treatment of young African American children diagnosed with disruptive behavior disorders. *Journal of Pediatric Psychology, 27*(4), 339–350.

Noordermeer, S. D., Luman, M., & Oosterlaan, J. (2016). A systematic review and meta-analysis of neuroimaging in oppositional defiant disorder (ODD) and conduct disorder (CD) taking attention-deficit hyperactivity disorder (ADHD) into account. *Neuropsychology Review, 26*(1), 44–72.

O'Brien, M., & Chin, C. (1998). The relationship between children's reported exposure to interparental conflict and memory biases in the recognition of aggressive and constructive conflict words. *Personality and Social Psychology Bulletin, 24*(6), 647–656.

Pardini, D. A., Lochman, J. E., & Frick, P. J. (2003). Callous/unemotional traits and social-cognitive processes in adjudicated youths. *Journal of the American Academy of Child and Adolescent Psychiatry, 42*(3), 364–371.

Pardini, D., Lochman, J., & Wells, K. (2004). Negative emotions and alcohol use initiation in high-risk boys: The moderating effect of good inhibitory control. *Journal of Abnormal Child Psychology, 32*, 505–518.

Pasalich, D. S., Witkiewitz, K., McMahon, R. J., Pinderhughes, E. E., & Conduct Problems Prevention Research Group. (2016). Indirect effects of the Fast Track intervention on conduct disorder symptoms and callous-unemotional traits: Distinct pathways involving discipline and warmth. *Journal of Abnormal Child Psychology, 44*(3), 587–597.

Pidano, A. E., & Allen, A. R. (2015). The Incredible Years series: A review of the independent research base. *Journal of Child and Family Studies, 24*(7), 1898–1916.

Powell, N. P., Lochman, J. E., Boxmeyer, C. L., Barry, T. D., & Pardini, D. A. (2017). The Coping Power Program for aggressive behavior in children. In J. R. Weisz & A. E. Kazdin (Eds.), *Evidence based psychotherapies for children and adolescents* (3rd ed., pp. 159–176). New York: Guilford Press.

Reid, J. B., & Eddy, J. M. (2002). Preventive efforts during the elementary school years: The linking the interests of families and teachers project. In J. B. Reid, G. R. Patterson, & J. Snyder (Eds.), *Antisocial behavior in children and adolescents: A developmental analysis and model for intervention* (pp. 219–233). Washington, DC: American Psychological Association.

Reid, J. B., Patterson, G. R., & Snyder, J. (Eds.). (2002). *Antisocial behavior in children and adolescents: A developmental analysis and model for intervention.* Washington, DC: American Psychological Association.

Rey, J. M., & Plapp, J. M. (1990). Quality of perceived parenting in oppositional and conduct disordered adolescents. *Journal of the American Academy of Child and Adolescent Psychiatry, 29*, 157–162.

Schutter, D. J., Van Bokhoven, I., Vanderschuren, L. J., Lochman, J. E., & Matthys, W. (2011). Risky decision making in substance dependent adolescents with a disruptive behavior disorder. *Journal of Abnormal Child Psychology, 39*(3), 333–339.

Shaw, D. S., Dishion, T. J., Supplee, L., Gardner, F., & Arnds, K. (2006). Randomized trial of a family-centered approach to the prevention of early conduct problems: 2-year effects of the family check-up in early childhood. *Journal of Consulting and Clinical Psychology, 74*(1), 1.

Sherrod, M., Getch, Y., & Ziomek-Daigle, J. (2009). The impact of positive behavior support to decrease discipline referrals with elementary students. *Professional School Counseling, 12*(6), 421–427.

Simonoff, E., Pickles, A., Hervas, A., Silberg, J. L., Rutter, M., & Eaves, L. (1998). Genetic influences on childhood hyperactivity: Contrast effects imply parental rating bias, not sibling interaction. *Psychological Medicine, 28*(4), 825–837.

Sitnick, S. L., Shaw, D. S., Gill, A., Dishion, T., Winter, C., Waller, R., et al. (2015). Parenting and the family check-up: Changes in observed parent–child interaction following early childhood intervention. *Journal of Clinical Child and Adolescent Psychology, 44*(6), 970–984.

Smith, J. D., Stormshak, E. A., & Kavanagh, K. (2015). Results of a pragmatic effectiveness-implementation hybrid trial of the family check-up in community mental health agencies. *Administration and Policy in Mental Health and Mental Health Services Research, 42*(3), 265–278.

Solomon, D., Battistich, V., Watson, M., Schaps, E., & Lewis, C. (2000). A six-district study of educational change: Direct and mediated effects of the Child Development Project. *Social Psychology of Education, 4*(1), 3–51.

Speltz, M. L., De Klyen, M., Greenberg, M. T., & Dryden, M. (1995). Clinic referral for oppositional defiant disorder: Relative significance of attachment and behavioral variables. *Journal of Abnormal Child Psychology, 23*(4), 487–507.

Spoth, R. L., Randall, G. K., Trudeau, L., Shin, C., & Redmond, C. (2008). Substance use outcomes 5½ years past baseline for partnership-based, family–school preventive interventions. *Drug and Alcohol Dependence, 96*(1), 57–68.

Spoth, R., Trudeau, L., Redmond, C., & Shin, C. (2014). Replication RCT of early universal prevention effects on young adult substance misuse. *Journal of Consulting and Clinical Psychology, 82*(6), 949–963.

Sugai, G., & Horner, R. R. (2006). A promising approach for expanding and sustaining school-wide positive behavior support. *School Psychology Review, 35*(2), 245–259.

Waasdorp, T. E., Bradshaw, C. P., & Leaf, P. J. (2012). The impact of schoolwide positive behavioral interventions and supports on bullying and peer rejection: A randomized controlled effectiveness trial. *Archives of Pediatrics and Adolescent Medicine, 166*(2), 149–156.

Webster-Stratton, C. (1990). Long-term follow-up of families with young conduct problem children: From preschool to grade school. *Journal of Clinical Child Psychology, 19*(2), 1344–1349.

Webster-Stratton, C. (2005). The Incredible Years: A training series for the prevention and treatment of conduct problems in young children. In E. D. Hibbs & P. S. Jensen (Eds.), *Psychosocial treatments for child and adolescent disorders: Empirically based strategies for clinical practice* (2nd ed., pp. 507–555). Washington, DC: American Psychological Association.

Webster-Stratton, C., & Hammond, M. (1997). Treating children with early-onset conduct problems: A comparison of child and parent training interventions. *Journal of Consulting and Clinical Psychology, 65*(1), 93.

Webster-Stratton, C., & Lindsay, D. W. (1999). Social competence and conduct problems in young children: Issues in assessment. *Journal of Clinical Child Psychology, 28*(1), 25–43.

Webster-Stratton, C., Reid, M. J., & Beauchaine, T. P. (2013). One-year follow-up of combined parent and child intervention for young children with ADHD. *Journal of Clinical Child and Adolescent Psychology, 42*(2), 251–261.

Webster-Stratton, C., Reid, M. J., & Hammond, M. (2004). Treating children with early-onset conduct problems: Intervention outcomes for parent, child, and teacher training. *Journal of Clinical Child and Adolescent Psychology, 33*(1), 105–124.

Wenzel, V., Weichold, K., & Silbereisen, R. K. (2009). The life skills program IPSY: Positive influences on school bonding and prevention of substance misuse. *Journal of Adolescence, 32*(6), 1391–1401.

CHAPTER SEVEN

The Anatomy of Cognitions in Multidimensional Family Therapy

Cynthia L. Rowe
Howard A. Liddle

Decades of research documents that adolescent substance abuse is part of a complex of problem behaviors that has its roots in mutually reinforcing risk and protective factors. As the child develops, risk factors at the individual level interact with parental, familial, and extrafamilial processes to increase vulnerability for substance abuse and related problems during adolescence. Given that substance abuse is multiply determined, it is logical that effective intervention must reduce risk and promote resilience across developmental life domains. In fact, the empirical evidence clearly supports the efficacy of models that are comprehensive, multisystemic, and broad enough to create change not only at the individual level but in other interconnected systems as well (Hawkins, 2009). Family, parenting, and couples approaches are consistently shown to be among the most potent interventions for treating both adolescent and adult substance abuse (Rowe, 2012).

Cognitive processes play an important role in adolescent substance use problems, particularly a teen's positive expectancies about its social and emotional effects, yet these beliefs are largely shaped by parents. Parents' norms against substance use have been shown to have a strong direct link to teens' beliefs about use, as well as an indirect effect on future use

(Sieving, Maruyama, Williams, & Perry, 2000). Children tend to internalize their parents' norms about drinking by early adolescence, which, once internalized, directly influence their own drinking (Brody, Ge, Katz, & Arias, 2000). Thus interventions aimed at changing only the adolescents' cognitions tend not to be powerful enough to reduce their substance use. In fact, in showing the strong effects of parents' drinking on adolescent alcohol expectancies, Martino, Collins, Ellickson, Schell, and McCaffrey (2006, p. 971) concluded: "attempts to alter adolescents' alcohol expectancies are likely to fail unless they address the influence of immediate social models on these beliefs."

We describe a rigorously studied and consistently supported family-based treatment model for addressing adolescent substance abuse, Multidimensional Family Therapy (MDFT; Liddle, 2002, 2010, 2014, 2016). As a companion to our previous publication (Liddle, 1994), this chapter isolates a particular aspect of the approach—cognitions—as a target of change, as well as an instigator of change in other areas. Through the case presentation, MDFT's theory of change, intervention targets, and treatment methods are detailed. Although it is impossible to separate completely the cognitive, emotional, behavioral, and relational changes targeted in a comprehensive approach, it is our intention to show how cognitions are conceptualized and targeted for change in a multisystemic family-based approach.

Theoretical and Empirical Foundations

MDFT is a family-based, comprehensive treatment system for adolescent substance abuse and behavioral and emotional problems (Liddle, 2002, 2010, 2014). It is theory driven, combining aspects of several theoretical frameworks (i.e., family systems theory, developmental psychology, ecological approaches, and risk/protective factors), and incorporating key elements of effective adolescent treatment: comprehensive assessment, integrated interventions, family involvement, developmental specificity, specialized engagement protocols, attention to therapist development, gender and cultural competence, and focus on a range of outcomes. It is a model that effectively and simultaneously reduces adolescent substance abuse, delinquency, and comorbid mental health problems (Hawkins, 2009; Liddle, 2016).

The MDFT Treatment System

MDFT is both a tailored and a flexible treatment delivery system. MDFT teams consist of an MDFT supervisor, two to four certified MDFT therapists, and a therapist assistant (case manager). Treatment duration averages

3–6 months (depending on severity) of one to three weekly sessions, with additional case management services and phone calls. Therapists work simultaneously in four interdependent domains: adolescent, parent, family, and community. Sessions may include one-on-one time with the teen or parent, as well as the family together. Sessions are held in the homes, as well as in clinics, schools, and other community settings.

Tables 7.1 and 7.2 detail the work in MDFT's three stages, as well as the goals for each intervention domain. Briefly, Stage 1 builds a foundation for change, Stage 2 facilitates individual and family change, and Stage 3 solidifies changes. At various points, therapists meet alone with the teen, alone with the parent(s), or conjointly with the adolescent and parent(s), depending on the domain, goals, targeted interventions, and specific problem being addressed.

MDFT through the Lens of a Clinical Case Example

In the case example that follows, we illustrate key cognitive interventions in different domains as the case progresses through the three stages of treatment. Where relevant, we highlight other avenues of change in MDFT

TABLE 7.1. MDFT Stages of Change

Stage	Description
Stage 1: Build a foundation for change	Therapists create an environment in which the youth and parents feel respected and understood. Therapists meet alone with the adolescent, alone with the parents, and with the family, depending on the session's goals. Stage 1 goals are to develop strong therapeutic relationships, to achieve a shared developmental and contextual perspective on problems, to enhance motivation for individual reflection and self-examination, and to begin the change process.
Stage 2: Facilitate individual and family change	Goals for youth, parent, and family functioning (see Table 7.2) are established, evaluated, and revisited throughout. Accomplishments in each individual domain activate and support change in the others.
Stage 3: Solidify changes	The last few weeks of treatment strengthen the accomplishments parents and teens have achieved. The therapist amplifies changes and helps families create concrete plans for responding to future problems, such as substance use relapse, family arguments, or disappointments. The family members reflect on the changes made in treatment, see opportunities for a brighter future, and regain hope.

TABLE 7.2. Goals within the Four MDFT Domains

Domain	Goals
Adolescent domain	• Increase self-awareness and enhance self-worth and confidence • Develop meaningful short-term and long-term life goals • Improve emotional regulation, coping, and problem-solving skills • Improve communication skills • Promote success in school/work • Promote prosocial peer relationships and activities • Reduce substance use, delinquency, and problem behaviors • Reduce and stabilize mental health symptoms
Parent domain	• Strengthen parental teamwork • Improve parenting skills and practices • Enhance parents' individual functioning
Family domain	• Improve family communication and problem-solving skills • Strengthen emotional attachment and connection among family members • Improve everyday functioning and organization of the family unit
Community domain	• Improve family members' relationships with social systems such as school, court, legal system, workplace, and neighborhood • Build families' capacity to access and utilize needed resources

relative to cognitive interventions and how the therapist uses interventions in one domain to prompt change in another area (e.g., individual sessions with a parent or with an adolescent both follow family sessions and set the stage for future family interviews).

Eric was 16 and had been using drugs—mainly marijuana, but also "harder" hallucinogens and stimulants—regularly for 2 years when he was referred to MDFT by his probation officer, Mr. Williams. He lived with his parents, Ron and Sarah, and younger brother, Michael, in a middle-class neighborhood of an urban area in the Northeastern United States. He had been placed on probation for possession of marijuana and was monitored closely by his probation officer for possible placement due to the severity of his substance use and history of self-harm. He had been hospitalized in the months before his treatment referral for a suicide attempt. His probation officer was also very concerned about his pattern of leaving home for days or weeks at a time. He was shy and had few friends growing up, which was partially a function of living in inner-city neighborhoods with limited opportunities to explore independently or socialize with people his age.

At the time of his treatment referral, he was going to an alternative school program and taking medication for attention-deficit/hyperactivity disorder (ADHD), but he stopped both when summer began and he left home for several weeks. His drug use was often triggered by feeling lonely, hurt, and angry; although he found it possible to let all of the harder drugs go after a certain amount of experimentation, "there was something about pot" for him that he could not give up.

Stage 1 Interventions

Entering the Teen's World

In early MDFT sessions, the therapist is primarily focused on engagement and motivation and spends considerable time in individual sessions with teens to "get into their world" and "show them there's something in this for them." Engagement is achieved by showing genuine interest in the adolescent's life, emphasizing that the therapy is for him or her (even if the adolescent was referred by probation or forced to go by parents) and that he or she is the expert on his or her life. The therapist works hard to convey that it truly is up to the teen who he or she wants to be and that the therapy is a collaboration to make his or her dreams possible. Motivation is simultaneously increased by focusing on the things the teen wants for him- or herself (e.g., "getting probation/parents off my back"), drawing discrepancies between the life he or she wants and current circumstances, and amplifying the teen's distress about what isn't working or what he or she seems unhappy about.

In the following account of early sessions with Eric, several cognitive interventions are highlighted as the therapist engages, motivates, and helps the teen build a developmental and contextual sense of himself and his life through self-examination and clarifying what he really wants for himself.

Deepening Engagement and Motivation

THERAPIST: These 2 years have been really bad for you. You think about all that, don't you?

ERIC: Uh huh.

THERAPIST: A lot of things have happened in these 2 years for you.

ERIC: A lot of good, a lot of bad.

THERAPIST: What are the good things?

ERIC: I've learned a lot of lessons. . . . I did a lot of things. Satisfied my curiosity and left it at that.

THERAPIST: That's interesting. I wonder if your mom and dad would be surprised to hear that part. You're saying, "I'm not out of control." If somebody says what you said, they're saying, "I did many things, and part of it was about curiosity and now I've just let it go." You're disagreeing with your parents then . . . seems like you're saying, "I am not out of control." (*Eric nods.*) . . . You said you learned a lot. What kind of lessons?

ERIC: Don't get high and play with guns!

THERAPIST: And to learn *that* you went through hell!

ERIC: I should have known that already, but I'm even more careful now.

THERAPIST: All that scared you. (*Eric nods.*) . . . I would imagine. It would scare anybody. . . .

In this brief exchange, the MDFT therapist pulls out an aspect of Eric's experience that could be a strength. The youth looks back, reflects on what he's been involved in, and says "there were lessons learned," and perhaps that he has decided to leave those activities behind. The therapist highlights the intensity and negativity of his experiences—his cognitive appraisals of those events—underscoring a bottom line that might include assertions about not being out of control, as his parents think he is, and the potential conclusion, worthy of more discussion and reflection, that the curiosity is over, he has learned lessons, what happened was intimidating, and it's not for him.

An important aspect of Stage 1 work with teens is helping them see that there is something "in it for them," which often has to do with getting a better deal with parents or probation. Next, the therapist uses what's right in front of him to motivate the teen concerning the issue of curfew, proposing that they work with the probation officer for something more reasonable. The therapist also elicits distress and the adolescent's fear about losing his freedom to increase motivation and assesses and explores the adolescent's readiness to change.

THERAPIST: So this is a real problem now, I mean, how's this going to get better? How are you going to start feeling like you're connected with others and getting to do things outside the house?

ERIC: Well, I can't do anything because of probation now.

The therapist here focuses on the issue of external pressure from probation. What to do about it is preceded by attempts to get acknowledgment from Eric, an appraisal of it as an issue of worry and importance, and, of course, something that, in addition to his thinking about it and drawing certain conclusions, has emotional aspects. Here we see how Eric's cognitive appraisal of his circumstances, as well as, of course, his emotional reactions to those circumstances, are brought into focus in a certain way (note the steps to this process). The circumstance is pinpointed and framed in a certain way. Confirmation is sought from Eric—not for insight but as a foundation for taking action—for acting in relation to that circumstance in a way that raises self-efficacy and reflection, challenges cynicism and passivity, and begins a new process for Eric. This effort is something that will hopefully have concrete behavioral outcomes, but also outcomes concerning how Eric experiences himself and how others (parents and those outside the family) see him, which is not unimportant. Outcomes are approached in small, pinpointed, and collaborative ways, and focal areas must be something of interest to Eric.

Therapists' cognitions are always at play as well. The clinician is capable of having big-picture systems and intersystem (subsystems) interactions in mind, as well as individual-level dynamic processes. Knowledge about the importance of different aspects of functioning, cognitive appraisals, emotions, and behavior in different social environments and situations is key to changing human behavior. In this approach, practical, change-oriented thinking that organizes this knowledge within developmental and dynamic systems is a fundamental cognitive process that therapists use to decide what to focus on and what to do in sessions.

THERAPIST: What do you mean?

ERIC: I can only hang out until 7, and then I have to be home.

THERAPIST: Well, we have to talk about that. You have to feel like there's a way to work your way out of that, no? If you don't feel that, you're going to get really pissed off and do something stupid.

ERIC: I think it's true though, all that pressure from probation, you know?

This interaction shows an intervention, stemming from a therapeutic principle, being formed in the usual way in a session: The therapist's idea comes from something said by the client. It could be something related to the client's thinking, but it does not need to have cognition-related or schema-related content. The content triggers a cognitive process in the therapist about the client's actual situation and an aspect of it and the client's participation in it (or response to it or response to others in it, for example). Here the cognitive process in the therapist seems to be about change; it appears that it was something that relates to a change principle or even the potential application of a change principle. The therapist realizes that this circumstance (Eric's frustration with probation restrictions) might be used to channel motivation and change, or at least be used as a context to shape competent problem solving on Eric's part. The sequence starts to show the gradual and systematic honing in on details of personal circumstances and the meaning or the interpretation Eric gives to them. The therapist is not simply reflecting at this point as much as shaping, or sharpening a point—a point about Eric's interpretation of the probation strictures. A rationale is also connected to the sharpening: "If you don't feel that there's a way to work your way out of all this, you'll be angry and may do something stupid." Eric agrees that pressure is felt, which is a good thing, as the external pressure is used within the therapy and as one element of motivation.

THERAPIST: Agree. But it doesn't have to last forever. Can I invite your probation officer here for a meeting—to really talk about your probation, curfew, the whole thing?

ERIC: Oh, I want to do that. Definitely. I want to do that.

THERAPIST: OK. 'Cause I don't think it's good for you to be moaning every day, week in and week out, "I got a seven o'clock curfew. . . . " You've got to have something you can look at down the road.

ERIC: Right, even if I could work something out like . . . staying out late one night a week. Then if I manage to stay out of trouble, make it two, and then three . . . you know, if I'm still coming up clean, after like 2 months? I don't see why he wouldn't let me go.

The therapist's actions focus on agency, problem solving, collaboration, and partnering with Eric on something important to him. Eric's receptivity to the problem-solving session is taken as an alignment of different dimensions of his possible response, and, as such, he is responsive to the therapist's suggestion and participating in moving it ahead and planning for the meeting.

> "Good, you're thinking ahead and being practical about it. You're starting to deal directly and work out something with probation. That's also dealing with your parents by doing that—you should be able to get something good back from them if you keep going down that road, right?"

Cognitive interventions include naming aspects of Eric's response—his initiative, its problem-solving orientation, and its capacity to influence the negative mindset his parents have developed after many previous attempts in and out of therapies to help their son. Identifying small movements or areas of progress is important, as they allow the therapist to use these steps forward as stepping stones toward broader change and also as touchstones to come back to in discussions about related topics or as positive markers of change when relapses occur.

THERAPIST: I would just hate to see you lose your freedom. You're in a situation where the very thing that you hate the most, having people run

your life . . . well, that's happening, isn't it? I think it's really scary, you
know? Are you scared about what's happening? Sometimes it's good
to be a little scared . . . not too scared, a little bit. You can see things
differently. What do you think?

ERIC: (*Quietly, looking down, almost to himself.*) I'm scared. If I wasn't
scared, I wouldn't care. . . .

The therapist's stance as an advocate is seen within an intervention
that seeks to establish, and then in the next sequence use, the reality of a
difficult situation—a situation that is going to be "bad for me," and, moreover, an intimidating situation that arouses fear.

THERAPIST: Do you ever think about how you're gonna feel if you really
start to change things? I mean, do you ever think, like, "Geez, wouldn't
that be great? Wouldn't I feel good? Wouldn't I just feel better day-to-
day? I'm working, I have a certain kind of life, relationships, friends,
less hassles with Mom and Dad. . . . " Do you ever envision that? We're
talking about this probation thing now. We've got to get Mr. Williams
over here to talk about something that's good for you. Do you ever
think about your life like that—working towards those things that are
down the road?

ERIC: I think about it every day.

THERAPIST: How do you envision it? Like "It's there," "I can see it . . . "
—like that?

The previous exchange is a foundation or a springboard for an exploration of what changes are needed, or what change might be like. This
is not done in a problem-solving intervention mode just yet. The journey
to finding and shaping alternatives that can be developmentally beneficial
and, importantly, thought of as useful and interesting to the client occurs
through conversation—interchanges that help Eric's exploration and reflection.

ERIC: I'm scared to think what my life would be like if I stopped doing this
or started doing that . . .

THERAPIST: How come?

ERIC: It's new. I don't know what's gonna happen. In my usual routine I
know what'll happen.

THERAPIST: So you're saying "no, I can't visualize it."

ERIC: Right, I can only see a little.

THERAPIST: OK, so what is the little that you *do* see? I was just using my
words before. I don't know if it's those things you see or want to see.

Those things that I said—is that what you're trying to see out there? What do you see when you look out there, down the road for yourself?

ERIC: Sometimes I try . . . I wonder what would happen if I stopped this or started doing that. . . .

THERAPIST: You get scared? (*Eric nods and looks down.*) So all right. Track it down. What comes up?

ERIC: Just fear. . . .

THERAPIST: Of the unknown? Or of failure or getting hurt or . . .

ERIC: If I try it, am I gonna succeed? And if I don't, what's that gonna be like? What was the point in trying? What if I do it? What's it gonna be like?

THERAPIST: Uh huh . . . and what is it about the alternative, the sliding back or staying in a bad spot? It's what, familiar, comfortable or something?

ERIC: Yeah, there I just know what's gonna happen.

THERAPIST: So, when you say that, what do you mean? I have an image of that, but what do you mean?

ERIC: Like I know if I fight with my parents, and I get high, it's not gonna bother me that much. But what happens if I fight with them and I don't get high? That's just something little, but . . .

THERAPIST: Mmm hmm . . . getting high is like medication. But the house and all the bad feelings there. . . . Do you ever think about the option that says, "I don't have to fight with them so much"?

ERIC: Not usually.

THERAPIST: You're not optimistic about them changing . . . ? (*Eric shakes his head "no."*) Eric, I think the main thing is for you to be thinking clearly right now. I think that's the most critical thing. What are you thinking about day-to-day? Are you able to look at yourself over there and visualize a future for yourself? I think that's where it's at. We've got to talk about this more . . . about what happens when you visualize it and you get afraid. OK? So, good luck with your work and things at home. I'll call you about the meeting with Mr. Williams.

Fear of change, the unknown, and failure prevail but are expressed in somewhat nonconcrete terms. The therapist converses with goals of increasing the specificity and helps to craft a workable aspect of Eric's situation. A common clinical construction, supported by research, is the "adaptiveness" or "helpfulness" of getting high. Eric's example has to do with the atmosphere in his home, his relationship with his parents, and their responses to him. A critical cognitive aspect of this segment concerns Eric's progression toward clarity about his conflict with his parents. Here he is clear about what usually happens and how he copes with the day-to-day conflict.

Getting high is understood as something that relates to those environmental and relationship circumstances, and the prospect of changing drug-taking behaviors presents the possible loss of a means of coping. Again, cognitive aspects of the therapist's formulation are present, but, as usual, they are complimented by the multidimensional focus that includes emotion and behavior (planning/anticipating) aspects that address individual *and* familial (interpersonal) dimensions. Sorting through and naming different aspects of the individual and relationship aspects takes time, and not too many aspects of complex conflicts like this can be addressed in useful ways all at once. The work proceeds systematically in stages.

Stage 2 Interventions

The Journey of Self-Examination

As the therapy enters Stage 2, deeper self-examination and behavioral change are sought. Here, more direct attention is placed on the substance use and problem behaviors in order to initiate Eric's own reflection about what the substance use/problem behavior is about, the meaning it holds for him, what it does for him, and ultimately the costs relative to the gains.

ERIC: I didn't get high yesterday, and I didn't get high today.

THERAPIST: Nice. What do you think goes into it for you?

ERIC: Working has been good for me. 'Cause when I got nothing to do I get high. And I don't get high at work.

THERAPIST: So let's trace through a day like that, when you're not doing anything.

ERIC: Well, if I'm not doing nothing, I probably worked the day before, which means I was high that night. So I wake up, and maybe in an hour and a half or two hours I get high.

THERAPIST: So when you don't have work you're feeling worse about yourself? (*Eric nods.*) On those days, what do you think about? What's going on with you?

ERIC: I don't know . . . just nothing to do, so I get high. It's like, "There's nothing to do today." I'm up early, nobody else is up. Nowhere to go. Either everybody I know is working or out or something. I don't have anybody to hang around with.

THERAPIST: How does it help you to get high?

ERIC: It relaxes me. I say, "screw it, I don't have anything going on right now."

THERAPIST: You're less likely to think about problems or bad stuff then.

ERIC: Yeah, like, "Nothing to do," feeling bad. When I get in a fight with my parents, I'll get high.

THERAPIST: Eric, let me ask, do you ever think about, sort of look at yourself from outside? Like now, make believe you're over there in that chair (*points at empty chair*), and you look back at where you are now, and you say, "What's going on with this guy? Who is this person?"

ERIC: Yeah, every once in a while I do. Like, I don't know, for some reason I just have to stop and think and say, "What the f—k are you doin'?"(*Therapist nods, encouraging Eric, and pauses.*) I say to myself, "You gotta slow down."

THERAPIST: Yeah, see, I think the way to think about using is, what's going on in your life? For you to have more moments or more days when you're able to do what you said you sometimes do. Like you were thinking the other day, "Who is this kid?" 'Cause it's unlikely for you to be thinking about yourself when you're using. You can't do those two things at the same time. It's more unlikely for you to be using when you're in a spot of thinking about yourself. (*Eric nods.*) The other thing is, what has to be in your life, or what's not in your life? Usually if a kid is using a lot, then there are other things that are not in your life. If those things were there, you probably wouldn't be using so much, or even using at all. So what's missing?

ERIC: Well, I thought about this a lot . . . that I think has to do a lot with the way I was brought up. . . .

Crisis as Opportunity

About 2 months into treatment, Eric hit a crisis point when his drug use escalated, the conflict with his parents worsened, and he left home to live with an adult family friend. In MDFT, these kinds of crisis points are seen as opportunities to increase focus, attention, and motivation for change. In the sessions during this crisis, the therapist increased the intensity of the treatment, maintained close contact with the probation officer, and used the phone between sessions to create continuity and maintain focus with Eric and his parents. Eric was willing to meet with the therapist, probation officer, and his parents, so the therapist used this crisis to deepen Eric's self-examination about himself and in relationship to his parents.

THERAPIST: So where you're living, I think it becomes a problem if it goes on too long, if you're out of touch with Mr. Williams . . . certainly if you get in trouble. I want to talk about the living situation. I mean, there are some things we just can't clarify now, but it seems we ought to have a plan. You and me ought to have a plan that we start talking about today about at least in your mind, how long you want to stay over there and when you want to make a move back home.

ERIC: I think that depends on how things go in here.

THERAPIST: With your parents in here? (*Eric nods yes.*) . . . So say more about that.

ERIC: I don't know. I was just thinking yesterday, that I noticed I keep getting into a pattern. Like I get into a fight and things just keep going with it and I do something to make a change, like a drastic change, like moving out and trying to kill myself or something like that. Which tells me I want to change, but no changes are happening.

THERAPIST: That's interesting, because actually that's what I wanted us to talk about most of all today—how you make sense of these things. You know, you try and kill yourself, you try and hurt yourself, you mess yourself up in various ways 'cause you're feeling so bad. This time you leave home, and I'm trying to understand and have you understand before you start dealing with them. . . . I think it's important for you to have decent clarity about what those things mean to you.

The therapist aims to deepen Eric's understanding of himself to be in a better position to talk to his parents. Here we see more clearly that self-examination is not sought only as a target in and of itself but also as a means for healing the relationship with his parents. The therapist defines "moving out" as making a drastic change but mentions the suicide attempt as well in order to increase urgency, focus, and clarity and to stimulate Eric to look at himself.

THERAPIST: For sure—you tried to hurt yourself, you could have fallen off the edge there. You could be dead. You had this thing with the gun. You got shot. You've been involved in very extreme stuff. Being out of the house is extreme and potentially dangerous, so here you go again. You're in another situation where you felt like you had to do something.

ERIC: Something had to change. It just ain't working. . . .

THERAPIST: Right, but what are you telling them about who you are and how you are? If a baby cries in the middle of the night, it's saying something to the world and whoever's there to hear, right? What are the things that it says? "I'm wet, I'm hungry, I can't sleep through the night." You're 16 years old. You do certain things in your life and you're telling everybody what's going on with you. So what are the things that you tell the world with all these things? (*Eric shrugs.*)

The extreme behaviors have an attempted solution aspect, and it is that side of the situation (Eric's experience at this time with his parents) that the therapist is attempting to expand first with Eric alone, and then in conversation with Eric and his parents.

THERAPIST: I'm interested to see what you think of this, but I think it's important to do two things with all of this. First, we'll talk about what those things mean to you. Then, you can speak to your parents about it, and I can help them listen to you and respond to you and so on. What do you think?

ERIC: That makes sense to me, but what will change?

THERAPIST: Let's not jump right into practicalities and problem solving about you and your brother fighting and other day-to-day things. I think there are things that are more basic—things in your soul, things inside of you. You don't feel good. Day to day, you don't feel good. Right or wrong?

ERIC: Right.

THERAPIST: Right. And you think, sometimes when things really go bad, you feel that you have to do something. This is an extreme step. You know, leaving, taking money . . . what's that gonna yield? I'm not talking good or bad behavior now, and I know a lot of the discussion with your parents goes to good boy/bad boy. This time, we'll start with what's going on with you. There are some hurtful things you're feeling. You've been on the edge for a while. So let's talk about this. You've been thinking about this, what this means to you. In a way you're telling them something every time something like this happens. What kinds of things are you telling them?

ERIC: Something's got to change?

THERAPIST: But what are you telling. . . .

ERIC: That there was no way to solve anything between me and them, and I felt lousy so I left.

THERAPIST: What kinds of things are you talking about?

ERIC: Just getting along with my parents, all of us together. . . . (*Therapist nods, encouraging him.*) Favoritism between me and my brother and privacy . . . is probably the biggest . . . respect.

THERAPIST: Did you ever succeed with them around any of these things? (*Eric shakes his head no.*) . . . Did you ever influence them? Did you ever win an argument?

ERIC: Yeah, I have but. . . . Not about the big things, no.

THERAPIST: These are big things. I feel it's important for your parents to understand what's going on with you. But that's hard to talk with them about, huh? (*Pauses. Eric looks down.*)

ERIC: I get upset if I think about all that.

THERAPIST: You're just not there now, are you?

ERIC: I don't know. I think it's just how I am.

THERAPIST: See, I'm trying to present this from a point of view of what's going to reach them. You want them to change, right? (*Eric nods.*)

Here the therapist shifts and slows down his response. He is distinguishing a few issues here: Eric's readiness, his clarity with himself, and his capacity to speak to his parents.

THERAPIST: You want them to change because you're not happy over there. You're not happy in general. I would imagine it's hard for you just in terms of who you are and how you do things, I guess, but it's also hard 'cause you're worried about how they'll react?

ERIC: I know I have to stay with it but I don't know if I can do it.

THERAPIST: OK, stay with it, talk about whatever is there. The thing about leaving home, that would be a good thing to talk about. Let's say you go back home and things get bad again. You start thinking about leaving again or worse. . . . I think that's what we ought to be talking about, no?

Here the therapist starts troubleshooting possible negative outcomes with Eric.

ERIC: Yeah, then I think about it before I talk about it.

THERAPIST: Yeah, but I mean *really* think about it. I mean like go back and forth about it, struggle with it. . . . Everybody worries about kids lying to other people. Sure, but I also worry if people lie to themselves. You've heard me say, "What's going on with this guy?" OK, fine, you took your stand with them. You got their attention . . . your parents. You said, "Things are not good there." You have their attention now, and that's what we're going to try to do—get something done. So tell me what you think about what I'm telling you here. Talk to me about this.

He repeats attempts to help Eric focus on his core experiences of day-to-day living.

ERIC: I've gotta stop using.

THERAPIST: OK, fine, but what are the basics here? Remember we talked about thinking clearly. "What's bothering me? What's wrong? I left home. Why?" You did that the other day. You said something like, "There's a cycle. There's this thing. I do these really extreme things to try and change things. Nothing changes." That's what I mean about being clear. That was fantastic!

Here the therapist is not only positive but also connecting substance use with psychological processes and feeling states, as well as conclusions about Eric's life at present.

THERAPIST: Eric, do you realize how good that was when you say something like that or no?

ERIC: No.

THERAPIST: OK, well, I'll tell you. That was fantastic. That's what I mean by thinking clearly.

ERIC: I don't know . . . but I think you're right. I gotta stop doing it.

THERAPIST: Are you thinking about yourself lately? Are you coming back to earth with stuff? (*Eric nods.*) So tell me about your using these days. Is it an automatic thing?

ERIC: Yeah, I just do it.

THERAPIST: OK, then that means you don't think you have a grip on yourself. Do you know what that expression means? (*Eric nods his head yes.*) "Get a grip on yourself." What does it mean to you?

ERIC: Get control of yourself.

THERAPIST: Yeah, like here, let's do this. Go and sit over there in that chair. Take a look at who's here, look at yourself. Nobody can do this for you, Eric. A therapist can't do this. Your parents can't do this. Nobody can do this, Eric. I'm not talking about "straightening out." I'm not talking about "being good" or "being bad." I'm talking about something more basic than that. How you're thinking . . . and I think using gets in the way right now of getting a grip on yourself, no?

ERIC: Obviously!

This intervention is a simple method to dramatize the questions: "Who am I? What is going on in my life? Do I know? Can I specify the issues in useful ways?"

THERAPIST: What's the way that you're gonna re-enter that home? What's the way that you're going to go back? If that's where it's going, sooner rather than later, it seems like you have to use your time and start thinking about things. It's like we were talking about the other day about focus, right?

The therapist is helping Eric by doing several things in this segment: thinking ahead, moving beyond impulsiveness, using rehearsal, and troubleshooting potential challenges.

THERAPIST: I said to you the other day, "Are you ready to start talking to them?" You said, "There's some big things between me and talking to them." So it seems to me we gotta get to these things.

ERIC: I don't know. I just know I gotta do it. I just got to do it.

THERAPIST: But what goes into it? (*Pauses, thinking, and looks down.*) What's a recipe?

ERIC: A whole bunch of ingredients.

THERAPIST: Any old ingredients? (*Eric shakes his head no.*) Right, specific things. What are the ingredients here—from your point of view?

ERIC: I don't know. We just gotta work it out.

THERAPIST: Come on, that's too vague. Think ingredients. Think: What's on my mind? The starting place is talking to yourself first and then eventually with them about when you left—what that's about for you and what that means to you. We will get to the practical things about going back, but first we've got to get clear. So let's practice some of this. Moving out—what's it about?

The therapist here is breaking down the elements of attacking and improving on a distressing interpersonal situation in Eric's relationship with his parents.

ERIC: About running away?

THERAPIST: Wait, is that what it was? I don't think it was "running away." I don't think that's the phrase to use with your parents, right? It's what they said, but what was it for you?

ERIC: I guess I took a stand.

THERAPIST: OK, I think that's closer. Better to start talking about what's wrong and what you think.

ERIC: Yeah, what's wrong . . . what's wrong with me?!?!

This line of exploration is a simple reframing on one level; but, more than that, it is a frame or interpretation that the therapist feels is more hopeful and positive in terms of Eric's agency. The therapist aims to develop more complexity for Eric concerning the parents' interpretation of his leaving the house as troublemaking and impulsiveness by an "out-of-control son."

THERAPIST: What's wrong in that house for you? That's what we gotta talk about. You left to give them a message. You left to try some stuff out. You left because you were angry, because you're hurt about the way things go there. That's the stuff we've got to get on the table with them.

ERIC: I think trust is one thing that has to change. They've never trusted me! (*The therapist nods, encouraging Eric to continue.*) . . . I can't explain it. It just pisses me off. I get so mad.

THERAPIST: Right, it pisses you off. Say more. This is what we were talking about—staying with things.

ERIC: Right . . . they don't respect me, they don't treat me my age, they're unfair about my brother.

THERAPIST: And that makes you think what? See, there's even a more basic level. You worry about what? Whether they love him more than you? Care about him more than you? (*Eric nods.*)

The therapist is very persistent to promote active thinking and expression by Eric.

THERAPIST: Yeah. What's more basic than that in life? Not much. See, that's basic. That hurts to think that, doesn't it? That hurts. See, now why can't they deal with that with you? They have to deal with that. They have to. They do. It's not easy for them to deal with that. You left that house and you pushed them. You pushed on them in a certain way. But you didn't push on them to deal with that. They have a lot of reactions to you, but they don't deal with this. This is one thing, and it comes up a lot, and it hurts you a lot. So you leave, you hurt yourself, you try and kill yourself, and they have to deal with you. They have to deal with you in some way, but they don't deal with you around this thing that hurts you a lot. See what I'm saying? They have to deal with you about that and other things. How are we going to help you push them to deal with you about this?

ERIC: I don't know. I guess just keep talking about it.

THERAPIST: I would imagine it hurts to talk about this. It's upsetting. I mean, if we started talking about this now, wouldn't it be easier to put the headphones on? It's impossible if you had the headphones on and you turned it on, even softly, and I said, "Let's talk about this, let's talk about how you feel," it would be hard to do. Yeah? (*Eric nods his head yes.*) Right now, when you use, you can't think about that, can you? You can't deal with yourself or with them when you're high.

ERIC: Right, I think that's one of the points of doing it.

THERAPIST: Sure. When you're out of that house, when you leave, when you try and hurt yourself, you also are not dealing with that. I mean you are in a real indirect way, but the basics of it, "Hey, this is how I feel, this really hurts me, this is what I think about things," you aren't dealing with. Do you believe this, really? Are we focused in on something now that's really important? Is this very important, or is it not so important? I want to make sure. . . .

This segment illustrates more expansion of what the issues are from Eric's point of view. The therapist is attempting to help him clarify and express, and then become ready to discuss, these issues with his parents in a new way—a more competent and more readily receivable way.

ERIC: I think it's very important.

THERAPIST: But even to say it's very important is hard, isn't it? (*Eric nods his head yes.*) Yeah. See, that's why this is all going to be hard. I hope you can push them. I hope we can find a way to start to help you deal with this with them. You can't talk to them about things because . . . why?

ERIC: I did talk to them. Nothing ever happened.

THERAPIST: But do you think you talk in a good way?

ERIC: Sometimes.

THERAPIST: If you were to get better in the way that you talk about these particular things . . . how would you get better? How would we know you're getting better? What would you do differently?

ERIC: I don't know. I guess just stop getting so angry.

THERAPIST: Maybe, but I'm not convinced that the getting angry is the culprit here. Tell me if I'm wrong. You say something, your mom or your father might say something, it goes back and forth, and somebody gets mad, and then it sort of ends. I think the thing about getting mad is it doesn't continue. Like, "Oh, OK, screw you." Is it possible for you to be mad in any situation and to keep the thing going? (*Eric shakes his head no.*) No? I think it is. You don't think it is?

Again, the therapist attempts to help Eric unpack the multidimensionality of the intrapersonal, interpersonal, historical, and current family conflicts—to change his cognitive processing of these conflicts.

THERAPIST: They're gonna come over here in the morning. Getting back home is very, very important for them, for you. Do you think this is important? I think there's a lot at stake this time around. Do you agree with me? I think we have to meet with them tomorrow. What do you think?

ERIC: All right.

THERAPIST: I'd like you to think about starting to talk to them about this stuff. I'm gonna say, "Look, this coming back home thing, it can't be like before. Everybody's got to feel like we're entering into this with reasonable spirits." You have to feel that they're going to be reasonable with you, and they have to feel that you're gonna be reasonable with them. You want them to change something, and I think the medicine to help them start to deal with you is these things.

ERIC: Me talking?

THERAPIST: You talking about those sorts of things: "Well, let me tell you why I left. Let me tell you what was going on. Let me tell you how I feel about it. Let me tell you how I feel in that house. Let me tell you how I feel about myself. Let me tell you how I feel about my life. . . . " That's gonna get their attention, I mean *really* get their attention. That's gonna move them. It is. I'm talking about doing this for you. I'm talking about doing this for you, for your life, not for them. I mean it will affect them, but I think mainly this is for you. This is the medicine for you to get a grip on what's going on with you. Tell me what you think about what I'm saying.

ERIC: In order for things to get better, I have to deal with them.

THERAPIST: Do you know that it's also dealing with you?

ERIC: I gotta do it for myself, not for them.

THERAPIST: Yeah, and do it for yourself, but see it's *dealing* with yourself, see. . . . It's . . . if you have the headphones on, it's hard to think clearly about yourself. You're distracted. If you're using, you're distracted. You go through a lot of your life miserable right now, very unhappy. That's no good. You hear me talk about taking care of yourself. I think you doing this is taking care of yourself. You left that house for valid reasons. I think things are not at all in a good spot for you and I'm saying, "What are you going to do, Eric? What are you going to do?" Use this to do something. Use this thing to get a grip on yourself—for you. OK, see you in the morning.

The next morning, Eric and his parents meet for a family session. When the parents bring up an episode regarding Eric leaving school after being dropped off, the therapist keeps the focus on the theme of creating a "road back home" and avoids haggling over details and parents voicing their doubt and lack of trust in Eric. The therapist shapes them to communicate their love to Eric.

THERAPIST: I mean, some of these things are not winnable . . . are not resolvable. In the grand scheme of things, in the bigger picture of things, this would be one. This would be one, OK, you see something, you bring it up, it looks fishy, you think it is reasonable to ask for an answer about something. But how is it ever going to get through to him in a way that's acceptable to him? There's something there that is inevitably going to lead to a stalemate and more bad feelings. That's what I was trying to say to Sarah in a way, that too much focus on the negatives. . . . I'm not saying to sweep things under the rug, but I am saying that too much focus, taking that road too far to the exclusion of other things, won't help. There's one thing that you want to say to him over and over and over, and it's about wanting him home with you. It wouldn't be about things like where did you go after being dropped off at school, or we can't trust you or we doubt you. . . .

MOTHER: But there's a real safety issue. I'm sure it doesn't look to him like a safety issue, but a couple years ago, a female teacher was stopped by a policeman because she parked over where he wandered off, in the same area. She heard this car coming along and slowing down—it was the police. And they said, "It's not safe to walk here. Don't walk over here by yourself." So I might be a worrisome parent, you know, but seeing him going over into that area, alone. . . .

THERAPIST: Uh huh, well, OK, that's a different discussion now. But that's not, "We don't trust you," or "We think you're doing bad stuff." That's about, "We're worried sick about you and we want you to be safe because we love you so much. We have to keep you safe." That's a different message. Eric, does that sound different to you? Does that sound more reasonable?

ERIC: A little bit. . . .

FATHER: We're not saying you're in danger, but. . . .

THERAPIST: Right, a little bit more reasonable, right? Well, let's leave that for now, because I don't see a resolution to exactly what happened, and I don't think that's where things are right now. What I want to say again, Ron and Sarah. . . . When he first left and you were frantic about him being gone, I kept saying to you over and over, there is one thing that you have to tell him, that you have to get through to him, and that's that you want him in that house. I said, above everything else you say to him, you want him home. You don't want to pick on him about how he looks or about how he doesn't do chores, or you can't trust him. . . . If a more basic message does not get through to him . . . my own feeling is that that's a problem. Eric, is that right? Is that what you were saying the other day when we talked about what's in the way of creating this road home?

ERIC: Yeah, it's a problem for me. I get to where it's too much. . . .

THERAPIST: 'Cause I think what you need to hear from them loud and clear over and over is that it is important to them, that your parents want you home now. That you can live there, not where Mr. Williams fills out a piece of paper in Pittsburgh or wherever it's going to be if you can't make it back home. I was on their back about saying to you in very clear terms, regardless of what else goes on day to day, "We want you to live in our house." Do you get that from them?

ERIC: Sometimes. . . .

THERAPIST: And if there's anything that you can do to help them. . . . See, sometimes people need encouragement to say things, too. I happen to think that that's very important for you to hear that from them, but *you* have to let them know that. Am I wrong? (*Eric shakes his head no.*) I mean I just think this. . . . I feel really strongly about this, knowing you to the degree that I do. So I kept saying to your mom and dad, you must communicate this to him. That's the first thing, and everything else comes after that. We've gotta be talking about what's gonna keep you in some sort of stabilized spot so that you can make it back home and you don't feel like you have to do extreme things. We've talked about this many times. When you start to feel too pressured and too panicked, you start to think about extreme solutions, don't you? We just talked about this. You start hanging around with really funky people, you try and kill yourself, and you start messing up at school and you leave the house, right? When you get very upset and pushed against the wall, you can take matters into your own hands and do things like we talked about in terms of impulsive things and extreme things. So I kept saying to them that they have to find it in their hearts to tell you this, OK? But they might need your encouragement.

THERAPIST: (*To the parents.*) So you heard it here from the horse's mouth. If there's one thing that I'm really standing behind, you know, it's that one: that you want him home, period. I think that's gonna stabilize him now. I think that's gonna make him available to deal with the stuff that he's gotta deal with in his life now. I want him to feel solid about that. Are you with me?

FATHER: Yes. Eric, we love you, and we want you home. We'll work things out. We'll work it out.

MOTHER: Yes, of course, that's what we want. That's all we want, Eric. . . . (*Wipes away tears.*)

Of course there are many aspects of the situation, and different members of the family interpret events differently. The therapist brings the concern, worry, commitment, and love for their son to the forefront with the parents, making the case that those matters can and should be discussed and, moreover, that those aspects are central to helping Eric stabilize, come back home, and begin to express his concerns more directly. Problem-solving aspects of their day-to-day lives, matters of curfew, what seems fair or unfair, and the negotiations around those important topics are all vital, of course. However, this approach first centers on relationship topics as a way of reestablishing an atmosphere of trust in which family members make good-faith efforts and promote compassion and empathy and family love and connection—all of which create motivation that sponsors reasonable give-and-take even after very conflictual and hurtful events have occurred.

Stage 3 Interventions: Sealing the Changes

The last phase of therapy seals the changes that have been made during therapy, anticipates "bumps in the road" (healthy expectations), and helps parents and teens be as optimistic as possible about launching their next life chapter. For Eric and his parents, day-to-day life had become more stable, less conflicted, and Eric had a period of clean time in which he was back home and going to school. Probation was still monitoring him but had eased up on his restrictions, given his good progress. In a family session at the end of treatment, the therapist helped Eric and parents address remaining issues. After the family negotiated some new rules that gave Eric more freedom, the therapist highlighted their changes and new ways of relating.

THERAPIST: You've come in here more than most kids come here. You've done a lot, you know. You've done a lot. Your parents have done a lot. You should get a lot of credit for that. You know, I said to your parents last week how good they were doing, and I think of how good you're doing with this, too, you know, as I said. You're doing your best and that's really good. So all right, so let's do this. Ron and Sarah, I'll trust you to relay all this to Mr. Williams.

FATHER: OK, I think that's a good plan.

THERAPIST: It is. You've come a long way, all of you. And my mode with you and I've told you this a hundred times. . . . I think, Eric, you've got to get the message by now that regardless of everything that's happened in the past and regardless of the stuff you do not like day to day, that there's one thing that comes in front of all that, and that's that they want you, they want you home, they want you to live with them. I think that's what's going to keep you reasonable with them, on the beam, not moving to any extremes. So my mode is that things had to improve between you and them before we could start talking about anything else, or working out anything else.

Discussion

This chapter has attempted to detail the ways MDFT, an empirically supported treatment for adolescent substance abuse and delinquency, works with the adolescent's and parents' cognitions as a target of change, as well as an avenue for prompting change in other areas. Through the case of Eric and his parents, we illustrated intrapersonal and interpersonal aspects of the change process through the exploration of beliefs and attributions about oneself and others. We have also attempted to illustrate the inextricable links and the ongoing interplay between cognitions, emotions, and behaviors in a multisystemic therapeutic approach.

Designed with adolescent development and developmental psychopathology research on adolescent problems at its core, MDFT was developed specifically to target multiple, mutually reinforcing risk and protective factors. This approach has changed the lives of countless youth and families in both research and clinical applications. Specifically, MDFT has been evaluated and found to have significant effects in randomized controlled trials (RCTs) using active treatment comparisons with a range of clinical populations (Dennis et al., 2004; Hogue, Liddle, Becker, & Johnson-Leckrone, 2002; Liddle et al., 2001; Liddle, Dakof, Turner, Henderson, & Greenbaum, 2008; Liddle, Rowe, Dakof, Henderson, & Greenbaum, 2009; Rigter et al., 2012). These RCTs have adhered to methodological criteria, including randomization, fidelity to manuals, sound measures, and high data capture rates at follow-ups (Austin, Macgowan, & Wagner, 2005; Becker & Curry, 2008).

The results of RCTs evaluating MDFT have shown positive effects in comparison with individual cognitive-behavioral therapy, peer group therapy, and multifamily group therapy in reducing adolescent substance use, delinquency, and emotional and behavioral problems and improving school performance and parent/family functioning (Liddle et al., 2001; Liddle et al., 2008; Liddle et al., 2009; Rigter et al., 2012). The data suggest that MDFT treatment gains hold up over time, showing durable effects on substance use at 1-year follow-up (Brannigan, Schackman, Falco, & Millman, 2004) and may even strengthen further after treatment completion (Vaughn & Howard, 2004). MDFT is less expensive than standard outpatient and residential treatments across the United States (French et al., 2003; Zavala et al., 2005) and has been applied with African American, Hispanic, and white non-Hispanic youth and families (Huey & Polo, 2008). Based on the empirical support, the model is recognized as an exemplary best practice for adolescent substance use disorders and delinquency (e.g., National Institute on Drug Abuse, 1999; National Registry of Evidence-Based Programs and Practices, 2008) and is widely disseminated in community-based organizations.

Identifying MDFT's effective ingredients, such as the focus on cognitive interventions, has been a primary focus in process research on adolescent and parent interventions. Current directions include the refinement and testing of the approach for other challenging issues and populations (e.g., transitional age drug abusers).

References

Austin, A. M., Macgowan, M. J., & Wagner, E. F. (2005). Effective family-based interventions for adolescents with substance use problems: A systematic review. *Research on Social Work Practice, 15*, 67–83.

Becker, S., & Curry, J. (2008). Outpatient interventions for adolescent substance abuse: A quality of evidence review. *Journal of Consulting and Clinical Psychology, 76*(4), 531–543.

Brannigan, R., Schackman, B. R., Falco, M., & Millman, R. B. (2004). The quality of highly regarded adolescent substance abuse treatment programs. *Archives of Pediatrics and Adolescent Medicine, 158*, 904–909.

Brody, G. H., Ge, X., Katz, J., & Arias, I. (2000). A longitudinal analysis of internalization of parental alcohol-use norms and adolescent alcohol use. *Applied Developmental Science, 4*, 71–79.

Dennis, M., Godley, S. H., Diamond, G., Tims, F. M., Babor, T., Donaldson, J., et al. (2004). Main findings of the Cannabis Youth Treatment (CYT) randomized field experiment. *Journal of Substance Abuse Treatment, 27*(3), 197–213.

French, M. T., Roebuck, C., Dennis, M. L., Godley, S. M., Liddle, H. A., & Tims, F. M. (2003). Outpatient marijuana treatment for adolescents: Economic evaluation of a multisite field experiment. *Evaluation Review, 27*, 421–459.

Hawkins, E. H. (2009). A tale of two systems: Co-occurring mental health and substance abuse disorders treatment for adolescents. *Annual Review of Psychology, 37*, 262–301.

Hogue, A., Liddle, H. A., Becker, D., & Johnson-Leckrone, J. (2002). Family-based prevention counseling for high-risk young adolescents: Immediate outcomes. *Journal of Community Psychology, 30*, 1–22.

Huey, S. J., & Polo, A. J. (2008). Evidence-based psychosocial treatments for ethnic minority youth. *Journal of Clinical Child and Adolescent Psychology, 37*, 262–301.

Liddle, H. A. (1994). The anatomy of emotions in family therapy with adolescents. *Journal of Adolescent Research, 9*(1), 120–157.

Liddle, H. A. (2002). Multidimensional family therapy for adolescent cannabis users (Cannabis Youth Treatment [CYT] Series, Vol. 5). Rockville, MD: U.S. Department of Health and Human Services, Substance Abuse and Mental Health Services Administration, Center for Substance Abuse Treatment. Available at *http://adaiclearinghouse.org/downloads/Multidimensional-Family-Therapy-for-Adolescent-Cannabis-Users-207.pdf*.

Liddle, H. A. (2010). Treating adolescent substance abuse using multidimensional family therapy. In J. R. Weisz & A. E. Kazdin (Eds.), *Evidence-based psychotherapies for children and adolescents* (3rd ed., pp. 416–432). New York: Guilford Press.

Liddle, H. A. (2014). Adapting and implementing an evidence-based treatment with justice-involved adolescents: The example of multidimensional family therapy. *Family Process, 53*(3), 516–528.

Liddle, H. A. (2016). Multidimensional family therapy: Evidence base for transdiagnostic treatment outcomes, change mechanisms, and implementation in community settings. *Family Process, 55*(3), 558–576.

Liddle, H. A., Dakof, G. A., Parker, K., Diamond, G. S., Barrett, K., & Tejeda, M.

(2001). Multidimensional family therapy for adolescent drug abuse: Results of a randomized clinical trial. *American Journal of Drug and Alcohol Abuse, 27*(4), 651–688.

Liddle, H. A., Dakof, G. A., Turner, R. M., Henderson, C. E., & Greenbaum, P. E. (2008). Treating adolescent drug abuse: A randomized trial comparing multidimensional family therapy and cognitive behavior therapy. *Addiction, 103*, 1660–1670.

Liddle, H. A., Rowe, C. L., Dakof, G. A., Henderson, C. E., & Greenbaum, P. E. (2009). Multidimensional family therapy for young adolescent substance abuse: Twelve-month outcomes of a randomized controlled trial. *Journal of Consulting and Clinical Psychology, 77*, 12–25.

Martino, S. C., Collins, R. L., Ellickson, P. L., Schell, T. L., & McCaffrey, D. (2006). Socio-environmental influences on adolescents' alcohol outcome expectancies: A prospective analysis. *Addiction, 101*(7), 971–983.

National Institute on Drug Abuse. (1999). Scientifically based approaches to drug addiction treatment. In *Principles of drug addiction treatment: A research-based guide* (NIH Publication No. 99-4180, pp. 35–47). Rockville, MD: National Institutes of Health, National Institute on Drug Abuse.

National Registry of Evidence-Based Programs and Practices. (2008). *Multidimensional family therapy: Intervention summary.* Available at *http://legacy.nrep-padmin.net/ViewIntervention.aspx?id=16.*

Rigter, H., Henderson, C., Pelc, I., Tossmann, P., Phan, O., Hendriks, V., Schaub, M., & Rowe, C. L. (2013). Multidimensional family therapy lowers the rate of cannabis dependence in adolescents: A randomized controlled trial in Western European outpatient settings. *Drug and Alcohol Dependence, 130*(1–3), 85–93.

Rowe, C. L. (2012). Family therapy for drug abuse: Review and updates 2003–2010. *Journal of Marital and Family Therapy, 38*(1), 59–81.

Sieving, R. E., Maruyama, G., Williams, C. L., & Perry, C. L. (2000). Pathways to adolescent alcohol use: Potential mechanisms of parent influence. *Journal of Research on Adolescence, 10*(4), 489–514.

Vaughn, M. G., & Howard, M. O. (2004). Adolescent substance abuse treatment: A synthesis of controlled evaluations. *Research on Social Work Practice, 14*, 325–335.

Zavala, S. K., French, M. T., Henderson, C. E., Alberga, L., Rowe, C., & Liddle, H. A. (2005). Guidelines and challenges for estimating the economic costs and benefits of adolescent substance abuse treatments. *Journal of Substance Abuse Treatment, 29*, 191–205.

CHAPTER EIGHT

Treatment of Cognitively Able Youth with Autism Spectrum Disorder

Rogelio J. Mercado
Hillary E. Kratz
Hannah E. Frank
Megan Wolensky
Connor M. Kerns

Autism spectrum disorder (ASD) is a complex neurodevelopmental disorder characterized by impairments in social communication and the presence of restricted, repetitive behaviors, interests, or activities (American Psychiatric Association, 2013). Recent estimates from the Centers for Disease Control and Prevention (CDC; U. S. Department of Health & Human Services, Centers for Disease Control & Prevention, 2014) indicate a prevalence rate of 1 in 68 children, representing approximately 1 in 42 boys and 1 in 189 girls. This rate reflects a rapid increase in prevalence and highlights the importance of identifying evidence-based interventions for ASD.

A challenge in developing and implementing ASD interventions is the heterogeneity observed in individuals with ASD. Individuals with ASD vary dramatically in their cognitive functioning, communication, reciprocal social interaction, and types and presence of restricted behaviors, interests, and activities, and they often present with diverse symptoms above and beyond the core symptoms of autism (e.g., intellectual impairment, comorbidity; Lam, Bodfish, & Piven, 2008; Matson & Nebel-Schwalm, 2007). This heterogeneity manifests in treatment response as well. Individuals with ASD respond differently to the same intervention, and no single intervention has been identified to meet the needs of all individuals with ASD (Warren et al., 2011).

Interventions for ASD fall into two broad categories: (1) comprehensive intervention models, which are designed to address multiple domains of learning and development, and (2) focused intervention practices, which are designed to address a single skill or goal (Wong et al., 2015). Rogers and Vismara (2008) note that comprehensive intervention models are often "branded" interventions in that each consists of a set of intervention strategies that is commonly known by a brand name, often requiring a set training program and proprietary materials to administer. In contrast, focused intervention practices are designed to address a more specific skill deficit or symptoms, such as social and communication skills, vocational skills, or a comorbid condition such as anxiety. Across both of these categories, interventions that use applied behavior analysis (ABA) strategies have the strongest evidence base in addressing the core and associated symptoms of ASD (Smith, 2008). ABA-based interventions involve applying principles of operant conditioning to provide specialized instruction for promoting skill development (National Research Council, 2001). Studies using ABA teaching strategies have shown improvements in social skills, communication, behavior regulation, adaptive behavior, cognitive development, academics, and vocational tasks (Warren et al., 2011; Wong et al., 2015).

Despite this long history of behavioral interventions for ASD, the study of cognitive-behavioral therapy (CBT) for ASD is relatively new. Thus far, CBT has been used primarily as a focused intervention to address comorbid conditions often associated with ASD, particularly anxiety. Although promising, using CBT for youth with ASD often necessitates both adaptation and augmentation of standard CBT approaches. In addition, a challenge that is not unique to CBT but that is particularly salient given its short-term focus is the issue of limited generalization and stability of treatment effects (e.g., Hwang & Hughes, 2000). Last, although CBT is typically time-limited and aimed at symptom remission, individuals with ASD often require support across the life span, and complete amelioration of ASD symptoms is rare (Howlin, 2000). These issues and others expanded on throughout this chapter.

CBT Approaches for Youth with ASD

Anxiety

Because the majority of research on CBT in youth with ASD has focused on addressing anxiety, CBT for anxiety is the focus of this chapter. Anxiety disorders are among the most common presenting concerns in children and adolescents with ASD, with anxiety disorders affecting 11–84% of the sampled children in multiple studies (Kerns & Kendall, 2012; White, Ollendick, Scahill, Oswald, & Albano, 2009). A meta-analysis of 31 existing studies had similar findings, with 39.6% of children with ASD meeting criteria for an anxiety disorder (van Steensel, Bögels, & Perrin, 2011). Children with ASD and anxiety experience more self-injurious behavior, symptoms of depression, family stress, gastrointestinal difficulties, and health care needs than children with ASD alone (Bellini, 2004, 2006; Chang, Quan, & Wood, 2012; Kerns et al., 2015; Mazurek et al., 2013). These findings have brought additional attention to how CBT can be used to address anxiety among youth with ASD.

Given this substantial evidence demonstrating the efficacy of CBT for treating anxiety disorders in youth without ASD (e.g., Compton, Burns, Egger, & Robertson, 2002), numerous researchers have sought to determine whether CBT is appropriate and efficacious for youth with ASD. A recent systematic review of randomized controlled trials (RCTs) and open trials using CBT to treat anxiety in youth with ASD identified 14 studies, with a total of 511 participants (Ung, Selles, Small, & Storch, 2015). They found that CBT was superior to control conditions (i.e., wait list or treatment as usual) with a moderate effect size (Hedges's $g = -.76$), similar to effect sizes for treatment of anxious youth in general (Reynolds, Wilson, Austin, & Hooper, 2012). Studies in the meta-analysis of Ung and colleagues (2015) showed important heterogeneity in method of delivery: modular treatments, group approaches, varying levels of parental involvement. Although none of these were found to be treatment moderators (likely due to low sample size), they highlight the multiple ways that CBT can be delivered.

Group treatments have many potential advantages, including the normalization of anxiety through peers, increasing social contact, and the delivery of services in a timely and affordable manner. Research into group approaches with youth with ASD show that they can be effective when they include a substantial parental component. Indeed, some approaches without parental involvement have not shown efficacy above treatment-as-usual-conditions (e.g., Ooi et al., 2008). In contrast, group approaches with varied forms of parental involvement have shown promising results. One treatment, Cool Kids, contains parent sessions that mirror topics presented to children, in addition to including specific modules on parental stress and relapse prevention (Chalfant, Rapee, & Carroll, 2007). Other approaches include training parents to support their child at home and explaining the link between autism and anxiety (Coping Group: Fighting Worry and Facing Fears; Reaven, Blakeley-Smith, Culhane-Shelburne, & Hepburn, 2012) or training parents to be "cotherapists" in all stages of the intervention (Sofronoff, Attwood, & Hinton, 2005). The content of group treatment also varies. Some are brief interventions that do not include exposures in session, though exposures are completed at home by families (Sofronoff et al., 2005). Others include exposures both in sessions and as part of homework (e.g., Chalfant et al., 2007; Reaven et al., 2012). Despite the differences, research suggests that group interventions that include a parental component did better than wait-list and treatment-as-usual conditions (Chalfant et al., 2007; Reaven et al., 2012), as well as individual CBT sessions that did not include parental involvement (Sofronoff et al., 2005)

Other treatment approaches include individual CBT, with varying degrees of parental involvement. Coping Cat, an individual CBT program for anxious youth (e.g., Kendall, Hudson, Gosch, Flannery-Schroeder, & Suveg, 2008), has been adapted for use with anxious youth with ASD. McNally Keehn, Lincoln, Brown, and Chavira (2013) adapted Coping Cat to make the treatment friendlier to youth with ASD by increasing the length of the session to 90 minutes, integrating the youth's specific interests and preoccupations, using more concrete and visual materials, and making other changes to accommodate the child's language skills and attention difficulties. They also added in additional dedicated time to review the session content with the parents every week. Their approach has been found to be superior to a wait-list condition in one RCT (McNally Keehn et al., 2013) across multiple outcome measures. A second RCT examining the efficacy of Coping Cat in youth with anxiety and ASD is currently under way (Kerns, Wood, et al., 2016).

Researchers have developed modular approaches out of the belief that core ASD deficits, such as social problems and restricted and repetitive behaviors, contribute to the development of anxiety and must be addressed within the context of a behavioral treatment program. These modular treatments provide modules that focus on addressing each core issue in a CBT framework. One such program, Behavioral Interventions for Anxiety in Children with Autism (BIACA), provides anxiety-focused treatment with a modular approach. Specific modules are used to treat both anxiety and core ASD deficits, including social skills training, peer relationship development, difficulties with adaptive tasks, creating a more flexible range of interests, and minimizing repetitive behaviors. BIACA, however, typically also includes a substantial parent component, with each session having time roughly split between individual therapy and parent training. Across a variety of trials, BIACA has been found to be superior to wait-list and treatment-as-usual conditions (Storch et al., 2013; Storch et al., 2015; Wood et al., 2015).

Another program, Multimodal Anxiety and Social Skills Intervention (MASSI; White et al., 2013), includes social skills training and enhances CBT with principles from ABA. Designed to include group, individual, and parent sessions, MASSI has been found to be effective in improving social skills in youth with ASD, with promising results in the treatment of anxiety (White et al., 2013).

Core ASD Symptoms

More recently, there has been an emerging focus on the use of CBT to address core ASD deficits, rather than focusing on associated symptoms such as anxiety, with the goal of more broadly improving functioning. For example, Unstuck and On Target (UOT; Kenworthy et al., 2014) is a cognitive-behavioral, school-based intervention that targets specific executive functions related to flexibility, big-picture thinking, and planning that have been found to be impaired in ASD. It is designed to teach new skills and accommodate impairments by teaching what flexibility, goal setting, and planning are; why they are important; and how to use self-regulatory scripts that guide flexible, goal-directed, and playful behavior. Although interventions such as UOT are relatively new, early results are promising. In a randomized controlled effectiveness trial of 67 third through fifth graders comparing UOT to a social skills intervention (both delivered by school staff), children in the UOT group showed greater improvements in problem solving, flexibility, planning/organizing, and classroom behavior (Kenworthy et al., 2014). These findings suggest that CBT has the potential to address the core symptoms of ASD, in addition to comorbid conditions such as anxiety (for a review, see Danial & Wood, 2013).

Assessment

In order to gauge whether CBT is appropriate for a given child or adolescent with ASD and to develop a plan for treatment, careful assessment is critical. As the most researched comorbidity with ASD, anxiety is a particularly relevant focus. Clinically distressing anxiety is common in individuals with ASD, and it continues to muddy the diagnostic waters for clinicians. Considerable overlap, wide-ranging and ambiguous behavioral manifestations of anxiety (e.g., avoidant behavior, fears of change and social unpredictability, unusual phobias), and the restrictions of self-report are just a few of the complications inherent in accurately assessing co-occurring anxiety among youth with ASD (Kerns, Rump, et al., 2016). In general, CBT interventions are most indicated for those youth who are conceptualized to have traditional anxiety symptoms (i.e., rather than ASD-related or ambiguous anxiety manifestations) and who have an intellectual capacity appropriate for participation. To determine whether CBT is appropriate, a multimodal assessment is conducted.

Diagnostic overshadowing happens when co-occurring clinical phenomena are minimized as being part of the chief complaint or diagnoses

(Kerns, Rump, et al., 2016; Mason & Scior, 2004). This frequently occurs in ASD, where anxiety is often conceptualized as a consequence of the developmental disability, rather than being identified and treated distinctly. If certain symptoms are ignored or marginalized in favor of an ASD-only conceptualization, treatment planning may become distorted, and the chances of running into obstacles during the treatment phase are increased. Fortunately, anxiety disorders in individuals with ASD are frequently recognizable and separately diagnosable according to DSM-5 (American Psychiatric Association, 2013). Studies suggest that anxiety and ASD symptoms are separate phenomena that can be reliably distinguished (Kerns, Rump, et al., 2016; Renno & Wood, 2013). Nevertheless, anxiety presentation can both influence and be influenced by the unique manifestation of ASD, as would be the case with any comorbid disorder. Wood and Gadow (2010) describe three roles that anxiety may play in ASD: (1) a downstream consequence of ASD symptoms, (2) a moderator of ASD symptom severity, and (3) a proxy of core ASD symptoms. Vague, anxiety-like symptoms are frequently inherent in ASD. For example, research estimates that almost half of children with ASD experience varied and diffuse fears and worries that cannot be accounted for by traditional diagnoses (Kerns et al., 2014; Mayes et al., 2013). Common anxieties that appear to be related to the cardinal features of ASD, such as fears of novelty/routine change, social avoidance, or compulsive behavior, further compound the diagnostic picture (Kerns, Rump, et al., 2016; Kerns & Kendall, 2012). Differential diagnosis rests on the assessor's knowledge and ability to distinguish vague anxieties common to ASD manifestations from those that are identifiable as anxiety beyond what one would expect, given the case conceptualization. We recommend that ASD and anxiety be seen not as discrete but as related phenomena. The importance of appropriately identifying and conceptualizing anxiety among youth with ASD is paramount in order to address symptom presentation and enhance treatment outcome.

Kerns, Rump, et al. (2016) recently delineated a four-step framework for differentiating anxiety and ASD symptoms. The first step is to determine whether any anxiety symptoms are disproportionate to the child's developmental level. The second step is to determine whether there is a specific impairment that is caused by the anxiety symptoms themselves. The third step is to distinguish between anxiety-related symptoms (e.g., fears, worries, and avoidance behaviors due to anticipatory anxiety) and ASD-related symptoms (e.g., problems with emotional regulation or sensory sensitivities following an event or stimulus). Lastly, a determination is made as to whether the anxiety symptoms exceed what is considered characteristic of ASD. An in-depth explanation of the four-step framework is beyond the scope of this chapter, and readers are encouraged to see Kerns, Rump, et al. (2016) for a description. The framework is also used in the case example below.

Measures

Recent studies have introduced increasingly valid diagnostic methods and instruments, which have aided in further distinguishing ASD from other mental health disorders in children (Chakrabarti & Fombonne, 2005; White et al., 2010). For present purposes, a few of the most recommended and current measures are reviewed. All of these measures are relatively new and will benefit from continued investigation, and the issues related to measures to assess anxiety in youth with ASD have been discussed (Kerns & Kendall, 2012; Kerns, Rump, et al., 2016). Rather than relying on single measures, caution is encouraged, and diagnoses should be interpreted only in situations in which other supportive data have been gathered.

Semistructured behavioral interviews conducted with individuals with ASD are best done when they are sensitive to considerations of cognitive and language capabilities (Blakeley-Smith, Reaven, Ridge, & Hepburn, 2012). Many children with ASD have some difficulty identifying and labeling cognitions and emotions, making assessment through self-report challenging (Baron-Cohen, 2002). As a result, it is recommended that assessors heavily rely on the reports of other informants (typically parents) for this information. As suggested by Davis, White, and Ollendick (2014), information regarding the anxiety response, collateral and other problem behaviors, and antecedents and consequences of the behavior should be collected through the interview process. Information gathered is best when descriptive in nature and not biased by caregivers' attempts at interpreting the function of children's behavior.

The *Anxiety Disorders Interview Schedule Child and Parent Version* (ADIS-C/P; Silverman & Albano, 1996) is a psychometrically sound tool to assess for the presence of anxiety disorders in youth in general. Kerns et al. (2014) introduced the *Autism Spectrum Addendum* (ASA) to expand and adapt the ADIS for use with individuals with ASD. The ASA allows clinicians to gather other relevant data (e.g., sensitivity concerns, notable disabilities) during the assessment that could be useful when making a differential diagnosis, and it also inquires about the presence of ambiguous manifestations of anxiety in youth with ASD. Although new, the ASA has been shown to have favorable psychometric properties and interrater reliability (Kerns et al., 2014; Kerns, Renno, Kendall, Wood, & Storch, 2017).

Another instrument, the *Children's Interview for Psychiatric Syndromes* (ChIPS), assesses 20 disorders, including phobias, social anxiety, separation anxiety, generalized anxiety, and obsessive–compulsive disorder (OCD). It is administered in about an hour, it is appropriate for use with children ages 6–17, and it has been found to be appropriate for use in youth with ASD (Witwer, Lecavalier, & Norris, 2012). The psychometrics are generally sound, but the instrument becomes less reliable in detecting the presence of additional disorders for youth with IQs less than 70 or for youth with generalized anxiety disorder (GAD), OCD, attention-deficit/hyperactivity disorder (ADHD), and mood disorders.

The *Autism Comorbidities Interview—Present and Lifetime Version* (ACI-PL; Leyfer et al., 2006) is a semistructured interview based on the *Kiddie Schedule for Affective Disorders and Schizophrenia for School-Age Children* (K-SADS; Ambrosini, 2000). It was modified for use in children and adolescents by developing additional screening questions and coding options that more accurately reflect comorbid psychopathology seen in ASD. The ACI-PL takes 1–3 hours to administer and is appropriate for youth ages 5–17 years. Reliability has been established for OCD, ADHD, and major depression in the ASD population, but its psychometric properties for anxiety disorders remains to be explored.

Factors to Consider
when Using CBT with Youth with ASD

There are several important issues that are necessary to consider when beginning CBT with youth on the autism spectrum; for example, being aware of the difficulties with which children with ASD often present and how these difficulties can affect treatment. We highlight several of these issues and then discuss ways in which they can be addressed throughout therapy: reduced verbal, abstract, and executive functioning abilities; the presence of special interests; parental factors; and the impact of core ASD symptoms.

Reduced Verbal, Abstract, and Executive Functioning Abilities

Youth with ASD often present with difficulties in cognitive and verbal abilities, including restricted speaking abilities, reduced abstract thinking, and reduced executive functioning. For example, youth with ASD have been shown to be impaired on tasks that measure cognitive flexibility or the ability to shift the manner in which they approach problems (e.g., Hill, 2004). They also have difficulties in aspects of attention, including filtering out distracting information and disengaging attention from one stimulus to another (Keehn, Lincoln, Müller, & Townsend, 2010). These difficulties can exist in addition to the deficits in verbal and social communication described as typical of ASD (American Psychiatric Association, 2013), including a propensity for rigidity in language and thought.

There are ways in which treatment can be adapted to accommodate the cognitive styles of youth with ASD. For example, programs have advocated for the use of concrete, visual materials. Reaven et al. (2012) provide youth with ASD with worksheets to go along with each new concept taught and provide multiple-choice quizzes to help youth with ASD learn key concepts. Other programs emphasize the use of drawings and cartoons to teach new concepts. In BIACA (e.g., Wood et al., 2015), cartoons are used to teach identification of somatic feelings of anxiety and to aid in the process of cognitive restructuring. The MASSI protocol (White et al., 2010) encourages the therapist to work with the client to develop specific cues or images, such as a character, that is then used to teach various strategies.

This approach can also be used when developing the fear hierarchies. For example, typical CBT approaches for child anxiety call for therapists to work with youth to develop a fear hierarchy that is described as a ranking, from easiest to hardest, of situations that the child fears. In working with youth with ASD, however, it is preferable to create fear hierarchies not only for an individual disorder but also for other areas that require special treatment. These fear hierarchies can be visual (e.g., pictures, flowcharts, tables) or physical representations (e.g., clay sculptures, puzzles, or board games) of the tasks of therapy. They can ready children for the road ahead and provide structure to upcoming sessions.

Although multiple manual-based treatments for youth in general include visual supports in the form of a manual or a workbook for the child, treatments for youth with ASD incorporate this as a more essential part of the treatment. In addition to their traditional goal of keeping the child engaged, these concrete, visual techniques are important because of the concrete thinking patterns seen in those with ASD and the visual or multimodal learning style that can be preferable for youth with ASD. Increasing the length of sessions may give the therapist more time to explore these ideas and accommodate the difficulties in task switching and learning that youth with ASD often have.

Special Interests

Youth with ASD often present with restricted or repetitive interests. Although these interests may be targets of treatment in themselves, they can also help in increasing participation in therapy. Clinicians are encouraged to explore the child's special interests and to use these as a tool in developing rapport and for teaching specific skills. Indeed, youth with ASD often present with circumscribed interests that can be incorporated in a variety of ways. BIACA, for example, encourages therapists to work with parents to find out what the child's special interest is and have the child bring something related to this interest to the first session. A client who is interested in *Star Wars* can be encouraged to bring in his or her favorite *Star Wars* toy, and discussions of his or her favorite character can be used throughout treatment. A character can be used to model coping skills (e.g., "How would a Jedi handle being afraid?") and social skills, or it can be used in cartoon scenarios or role plays. These strong or special interests can also be used as rewards or incentives for participation in treatment both in session (e.g., "We can talk about *Star Wars* for 5 minutes after we finish our exposure") or at home (e.g., earning points for a new toy). Of course, the therapist remains cognizant of keeping a balance between using special interests to motivate and build rapport and being careful not to allow these special interests to take over the therapy or to reinforce discussion of special interests at inappropriate times. If the child becomes too interested in the special toy or activity, a visual chart or agenda can be used to delineate specific periods in which the special interest can be discussed or used.

Parental Factors

It is important to focus on the both the stress that parents may face in their daily lives and how their actions help to shape their child's environment and problem behaviors. For example, parents of youth with ASD experience high levels of burden and stress as a result of caring for a child with a developmental disability (Drahota, Wood, Sze, & Van Dyke, 2011; Hayes & Watson, 2013; Lai, Goh, Oei, & Sung, 2015; Reaven, 2011). As a way of managing this stress, parents of children with ASD may adopt a protective parenting style, which may involve taking over social interactions for the child, helping the child manage personal hygiene, and allowing the child to avoid anxiety-provoking situations (Reaven & Hepburn, 2006). These actions are consistent with the notion of parental accommodation, defined as parents' efforts to reduce or alleviate the child's anxiety symptoms by changing activities, behaviors, or expectations. Another important factor to consider is parents' interaction styles. These are often considered on a continuum from responsive through directive styles, with a dynamic course as children's initiations change with development (Bornstein, Tamis-LeMonda, Hahn, & Haynes, 2008). For children with ASD, who may have poor "readability," parents may have more difficulty appropriately scaffolding a child's behaviors (Adamson et al., 2012). Thus sometimes parents of children with ASD are *under*responsive, which decreases opportunities for language development and social behavior (Kasari, Paparella, Freeman, & Jahromi, 2008).

Let us consider how the two factors just discussed may affect CBT treatment. Accommodation, while effectively reducing anxiety in the short term, maintains anxiety in the long term. Moreover, studies have shown that reduced parental accommodation is associated with better treatment outcomes (e.g., Merlo, Lehmkuhl, Geffken, & Storch, 2009). Thus one aim of CBT is to reduce parental accommodation (e.g., particularly with self-help skills that the child is capable of doing). Although removing parental accommodations may come with an increase in parental burden in the short term (i.e., dealing with distress that comes with the removal of accommodations), it ultimately allows the child to operate more independently. Involving parents and helping them to reduce accommodation also improves child engagement and understanding of treatment and allows the child to approach feared stimuli more frequently outside of session (e.g., Drahota et al., 2011).

A second point of intervention may be a parent intervention that focuses on increasing social communication and language in families. Shire, Gulsrud, and Kasari (2016) found a significant increase in parent responsive behavior and joint engagement when using such an intervention. Thus, when employing CBT for youth with ASD, it is important to find an appropriate balance between parental responsiveness to the child's needs and decreasing accommodation that may interfere with treating anxiety symptoms.

Indeed, the therapist strives to involve the parent as much as possible. For example, one study found that individual CBT without a parent component was less effective than individual CBT with a parent component (Sofronoff et al., 2005). RCTs evaluating CBT for youth anxiety have reported that parental involvement was significantly better for those youth with elevated ASD symptoms (Puleo & Kendall, 2011).

In addition to the two points of intervention described, there are multiple other areas of CBT that can be used as a point of discussion with parents. For example, group treatments often have a concurrent parent group that provides an opportunity for teaching important parenting skills and reviewing what the child is learning in his or her sessions (Chalfant et al., 2007). In the context of individual therapy, parents can be included in every stage of treatment (as in Coping Cat). In one approach, each 90-minute therapy session is divided into separate parent and child portions (e.g., BIACA; Wood et al., 2015). Parents have a chance to be involved and learn about the content of their child's therapy sessions, as well as to have their own, parent-specific modules. Specifically, modules can include (1) psychoeducation about ASD and anxiety, (2) explorations of independence and adaptive functioning, and (3) opportunities to work with their child's therapist to review weekly homework and address any difficulties the family is having in implementation.

Impact of Core ASD Symptoms

Another consideration in using CBT with youth with ASD is the interaction of the ASD symptoms and the anxiety symptoms. For example, youth with ASD may present with social anxiety and *also* have social deficits. Youth who have comorbid ASD and social anxiety have been found to have more social functioning deficits (e.g., lack of assertiveness, limited awareness of social rules) than youth without social anxiety (Chang et al., 2012). More specifically, there appears to be a reciprocal relationship between assertion skills and social anxiety, such that youth report of poorer assertion skills is related to higher social anxiety (Bellini, 2004). Given that this relationship was significant only for youth (rather than parent) report of social skill functioning, it suggests that youths' *perception* of more social skills deficits may lead to higher anxiety and greater avoidance and/or distress in social situations. Similarly, increased anxiety may lead to inaccurate interpretation of social cues, more avoidance of social interactions, and fewer opportunities to practice implementing newly learned social skills (White et al., 2014; Wood et al., 2009).

At various times within the context of treatment, it is worthwhile to pay attention to the impact of core ASD symptoms. For example, a child with ASD may have social anxiety. Rather than beginning with traditional exposures for social anxiety, it may be prudent to first begin with some social skills training. Multiple modular programs mentioned herein have modules for teaching social skills. BIACA, for example, includes a module in which the therapist works with the youth to teach him or her social skills in an easy and controllable situation. The therapist role-plays the situation with the child and creates specific expectations for the exposure task. When the exposure takes place, the therapist can press "pause" and intervene in real time to provide further teaching. The therapist then shares the information with (teaches this same skill to) the parents so the child can be encouraged to practice at home. Once there is a foundation of social skills, other social anxiety exposures can be conducted. In this way, the chance of success for a higher-level social exposure is maximized because the underlying social deficit has begun to be addressed.

Multicultural Issues in Assessment and Treatment

ASD occurs across cultures, and initial research has identified some important cultural differences with regard to its prevalence, assessment, diagnosis, and treatment. Within the United States, there are differential prevalence rates of ASD across ethnic and racial groups. Kogan and colleagues (2009) found that the odds of having ASD were significantly lower for African American, non-Hispanic multiracial, and non-Hispanic other race (not African American or European American) children than for non-Hispanic European American children. These differences may reflect differential rates of parental reporting and access to services for ASD (i.e., ethnic/racial minorities may have less access) rather than a true racial or ethnic difference in prevalence.

There are also cultural considerations with regard to etiology, assessment, and treatment, and it is important to note that many studies have not sufficiently addressed issues of race. This insufficiency makes it less easy to assume the transportability of established treatments to more diverse groups. Although this problem is, of course, an issue that the entire field struggles with broadly, we can highlight the ways in which the presence of ASD can provide extra layers of difficulty. Differences in beliefs about etiology may be particularly important, especially if the family adheres to theories outside of those presented by mainstream Western medicine. Such a situation would require increased communication with the family and work in the service of building rapport. Differing cultural norms may also complicate the assessment or treatment of youth with ASD. For example, youth with ASD are often taught to look at people in the eyes when they engage with them socially, but this would not be preferred in cultures in which children are taught not to have eye contact with adults.

Case Example

History and Initial Evaluation

We use the fictitious case of Madelyn, a hybrid of multiple real cases, to illustrate a CBT approach to treating anxiety and disruptive behavior in a child diagnosed with ASD. Madelyn was a 10-year-old female with ASD who was referred for outpatient treatment by her teacher and school counselor. Madelyn's teachers reported that she was disruptive and disrespectful at school. They were concerned that her disruptive behavior was becoming worse throughout the year and beginning to affect her education and the classroom environment. Although Madelyn had a history of being uncooperative, her behavior became worse in her current grade as school demands increased. For example, her current teacher would have students work in pairs on classroom assignments and often called on the students without warning. Madelyn's teacher allowed her aide to help her with assignments, but Madelyn was less cooperative with both the teacher and the aide, and she often threw tantrums in the classroom when she was asked to participate. She seemed unaware of how her behavior affected her peers and unmoved by their reactions. Because of her difficulties in calming herself, Madelyn was allowed to leave to visit the counselor during these moments. Her teachers believed she was being intentionally disruptive and recommended she get treatment.

At the initial visit, the therapist met with Madelyn's parents, followed by another meeting with Madelyn. In addition to reporting on her disruptive behavior at school, her parents also reported that Madelyn was very "needy" throughout the day. For example, they reported that Madelyn was unable to shower in the bathroom without someone else present and often got angry when she was encouraged to be in the bathroom by herself. They also noted that Madelyn often forgot to wash her hair and did not do a good job of cleaning her body. The parents also said that she slept in their bed every night; however, they could not remember when this started, and the family had largely become comfortable in this routine.

In the past, they had tried to get Madelyn to sleep in her own bed, but she refused and became angry to the point that her parents stopped trying. Madelyn's parents noted that she had difficulty getting ready in the morning and getting onto her school bus. They reported their belief that Madelyn lacked the organization and skills necessary to get started on her own, and they stated that having Madelyn sleep in their room made it easier for them to get Madelyn to school. In addition to the difficult morning and night routines, Madelyn's parents stated that she would often cling to them (especially her mother). For example, her parents tried to have her stay with a babysitter so they could go out to dinner, but Madelyn began screaming and throwing objects when they tried to leave, so they stayed home. They reported that Madelyn began to become distressed about their dinner plans once she found out, a week ahead of time. Madelyn frequently asked them questions about where they were going, what would happen to them, and if they would return home safe. Madelyn had similar reactions when her parents planned to go somewhere without her. However, if she was allowed to come, she instantly became happy and was no longer concerned for their well-being.

Madelyn's parents noted social skill deficits. She did not know how to start conversations with her peers, nor did she have any close friends that she saw outside of school. Madelyn denied wanting any friends or feeling like she was missing out on social interactions. Nevertheless, Madelyn began to avoid numerous social situations in which she had been previously engaged. She did not go to birthday parties, interact with members of the community, or give presentations to the entire class. If asked to engage socially, she would either have a tantrum or become clingy with her mother. On days when she had to give presentations, she resisted going to school. Madelyn consistently became upset in social situations but was not able to identify why; she did not indicate being anxious or afraid of being judged or rejected. Her interest in other children was limited to younger kids in her neighborhood.

During the separate interview with Madelyn, she was initially able to separate from her parents and go to the room next door with minimal difficulty. However, approximately 30 minutes into the interview, Madelyn became visibly upset and refused to answer more questions. With some probing by the interviewer, it became apparent that Madelyn wanted to see her parents. Madelyn was given a short break, during which she hugged her parents and then returned to the interview room. Throughout the interview, Madelyn had difficulty making eye contact, looked down toward the ground, and spoke quietly. She denied anxiety in most situations. She reported that she needed to be near her mother as much as possible because she loved her mom and said that she did not want to interact with her peers because she "doesn't enjoy it" and "doesn't need to." Madelyn also reported that she did not like it when her "parents make her do things."

Madelyn spoke willingly and eagerly during the interview only when the topic focused on Minecraft, her special interest.

Diagnostics in the case of Madelyn were hampered by multiple factors. Supporting a diagnosis of social anxiety disorder, Madelyn was found to be avoidant of multiple social situations, such as presenting in class, working with other people, and interacting with members of her community. However, Madelyn also had limited social skills and a lack of interest in her peers and other people, a presentation consistent with ASD. Further, Madelyn herself did not report fears of being judged or feeling embarrassed around other people. When considering a diagnosis of social anxiety disorder, the focus was on Madelyn's reaction during social situations. Beyond avoidance, Madelyn also had strong emotional reactions during social situations. She would cling to her mother when possible or throw a tantrum at school when she had to interact with peers or present to her class. A diagnosis of Other Specified Anxiety Disorder was considered most appropriate given (1) Madelyn's clear discomfort and anxiety in social situations and (2) the lack of reporting of social or evaluative concerns. This diagnosis is also consistent with the framework offered by Kerns et al. (2014). Specifically, Madelyn's anxiety was disproportionate to her developmental level (Step 1) and was causing her substantial impairment (e.g., having tantrums, avoiding important academic and social situations; Step 2). Further, Madelyn had clear anticipatory anxiety, as evidenced by her behavior on days when she had to give presentations, and was clearly distraught when forced to interact with peers and others (Step 3). Finally, her anxiety was excessive in comparison with that of other children with ASD (Step 4).

Madelyn showed many symptoms of separation anxiety disorder, such as the inability to sleep alone, difficulty transitioning to school, avoidance of being with a babysitter, and constantly being near her parents. As with her social difficulties, Madelyn struggled to put words to her fears. Despite the lack of direct verbal reporting of fears of something bad happening to her parents, a diagnosis of separation anxiety disorder was given because there was clear evidence of anticipatory worry about being separated from her parents. Although she did not identify them directly, she often asked questions that betrayed an extreme concern for her parents' well-being. It is also worth noting that there was nothing to suggest that her anxiety was due to an ASD-related concern. For example, Madelyn was not adherent to any strict routine that a babysitter might mess up, nor was she overly distraught by changes in her daily routine. There was no particular routine the family had at night, either, and no observable "rules" that Madelyn had about sleeping with her parents. Because the behaviors were excessive for her developmental level and caused meaningful impairment for the family, separation anxiety disorder was an appropriate diagnosis. Use of the framework provided by Kerns et al. (2014) also supports a diagnosis of separation anxiety. As with her previous diagnosis, Madelyn's separation anxiety was disproportionate to her developmental level (Step 1) and was causing substantial impairment (Step 2). Madelyn also had clear anticipatory worry (Step 3), and her worries were not explained by her ASD (Step 4). Thus use of the four-step framework further supports a diagnosis of separation anxiety.

Treatment

Treatment focused on Madelyn's anxiety in social situations and her difficulty in separating from her parents. It was decided that an adapted CBT approach would be taken, with the addition of a large parental component, as is often the case for youth with ASD. It was recommended to the family that therapy begin with weekly sessions, starting with psychoeducation about anxiety for both the parents and Madelyn, followed by the teaching of coping strategies and then an emphasis on exposure-based treatment.

Child

Madelyn was initially resistant to engaging in treatment and had difficulty separating from her parents during early sessions. She was provided with rewards for increasingly longer periods of time, during which her parents sat outside of the room rather than in the room. By the third session, Madelyn was able to spend the majority of the session in the room with just the therapist. Establishing a therapeutic alliance with Madelyn was somewhat difficult. Due to her anxiety about being separated from her parents and her anxiety about social interactions, Madelyn was unhappy about being "forced to be there" and appeared to struggle with much of the session content. The therapist integrated Madelyn's special interest (Minecraft) into the therapy sessions to increase her engagement. Rather than having Madelyn learn material in larger "chunks," she was given smaller amount of information (i.e., 2–3 minutes at a time) and then rewarded with an equal amount of time playing Minecraft. In addition, only the core information (i.e., regarding psychoeducation and coping strategies) was shared with Madelyn with minimal elaboration. Furthermore, more time was spent with her parents to ensure that they understood the content and could incorporate it at home.

Although Madelyn became increasingly engaged with the use of Minecraft as a topic of discussion throughout the session, she appeared to have low comprehension of the content that was being taught. The therapist tried to explain "thinking traps" to Madelyn, but she quickly became frustrated because she did not understand what the therapist meant by "thoughts." Instead of explaining all of the details of thinking traps, the therapist instead incorporated language and examples from Minecraft when explaining content. For example, "catastrophizing" was explained as assuming that your "hearts" in Minecraft would go down right away if you ever left your shelter in survival mode, a variation of the world-building game in which the main character can die due to physical accidents (e.g., fire) or by attacks from enemies. Madelyn was able to identify that always expecting the worst to happen would not ever let her enjoy playing the game. The therapist also encouraged Madelyn to think of her own ways to explain what she had to do when she was faced with a "challenge" (i.e., an exposure). Madelyn became increasingly engaged when the session content was tied to her special interest and when explanations were shortened. Madelyn even suggested calling exposures chances to "be brave" and described situations in which she was brave when playing Minecraft. The idea of the "Worry Monster" was introduced to Madelyn as a way of externalizing her worries, and, to increase engagement with this idea, it was relabeled as the "Creeper," a foe in the Minecraft game. She was told that she, her family, and her therapist were all on the same team fighting against the Creeper.

Despite her increased engagement during the psychoeducation phase of treatment, when Madelyn was told that she would begin "being brave" in real-life situations, she screamed at the therapist, threw a number of magazines on the floor, and hid underneath the table, refusing to participate. The therapist made it clear that the expectation was for Madelyn to use a "calm" voice and keep a safe body and that she would wait until Madelyn was ready to discuss what would be an appropriate challenge. She also reminded Madelyn that she had the opportunity to earn a reward for completing a challenge. Every time that Madelyn stopped yelling, the therapist praised her for being quieter and reminded her of the expectations and potential opportunity to earn a reward. Eventually, Madelyn began to engage in a conversation in a calmer voice from underneath the table. The therapist reminded Madelyn of how practicing "being brave" could help her earn more Minecraft time at the end of the session. Madelyn remained upset but reluctantly agreed to participate. To reengage Madelyn in the session, she and the therapist drew a picture of the Creeper, who was to blame for the quick increase in anxiety. Then Madelyn and the therapist talked about how they could fight the Creeper and earn more Minecraft time in the process. With this approach in mind, Madelyn agreed to engage in her first exposure, which was to say "hi" to a new person at the clinic. Treatment with Madelyn continued with multiple exposures designed to target her areas of anxiety, with an initial emphasis on other social exposures, such as making eye contact when talking with someone, conducting a survey, asking for directions, and ordering food at a restaurant.

Parents

Concurrent with the initial psychoeducation provided to Madelyn, the therapist worked with her parents to provide psychoeducation about anxiety and autism. In the early sessions, her parents identified Madelyn's tantrums as the priority for treatment. For the family, they represented a new, problematic behavior that had begun in school and was beginning to spill into their home life as well. Her parents described being flustered and being unable to identify a trigger for her tantrums, either at home or at school. Over the course of several sessions, her parents were asked to record specific instances of tantrums using a worksheet designed to help the family track the behavior in question. The therapist provided and modeled the use of the ABC analysis approach, in which families tracked behaviors that fell under the umbrella of "tantrums." They tracked the antecedent, the activity that immediately preceded the problem behavior; the behavior itself (e.g., throwing chairs, leaving the classroom, yelling at parents); and the consequence of the behavior (i.e., what happened immediately after). Afterward, the therapist worked with the family to determine what could be the possible function of each behavior. Across situations, it became apparent to the therapist that Madelyn often threw tantrums when she was about to, or perceived she was about to, separate from her parents and/or face challenging social situations. For example, Madelyn would be asked to get ready in the morning and to put on her outfit, and she would throw a tantrum when she could not find her bag. At school, it became apparent that Madelyn had tantrums when she had to work with other people or began assignments that had to be presented to the class. Several consequences were maintaining these behaviors, including getting to avoid anxiety-provoking situations and receiving attention from her parents. At home, her parents often immediately tried to help her to calm down and worked hard to make her feel better. When she had a tantrum at home in the morning, she was sometimes allowed to stay home from school that day or to go in later in the day to give her time to calm down. When she had a tantrum when her parents planned to go somewhere without her, her parents often allowed her to come along with them. Through discussion with her parents, it also became clear that they often avoided difficult situations by planning to take Madelyn with them; if they perceived any anger or negative attitude from Madelyn, they offered her the chance to go with them. They were taught how these behaviors, though well intended, could reinforce anxiety and other problematic behaviors (e.g., tantrums, avoidance).

The parents were taught behavioral strategies to change their response to Madelyn in these moments. For example, they were taught planned ignoring, and the therapist role-played with the parents how to ignore her negative and aggressive behaviors. They were also instructed to reward her for positive behaviors once she had calmed down, thereby reinforcing behavior that was desired and not providing reinforcement for her negative outbursts.

This discussion of how to manage her behavior when she became upset and angry was used at the framework to set up a reward-based system for participating in exposures. Madelyn's parents worked with her therapist to create a hierarchy of separation- and social-related exposures of increasing difficulty that Madelyn could work on during therapy sessions and at home. Her parents were taught how to use a detailed reward chart, which included both traditional exposures (i.e., opportunities to "be brave") and specific behavioral goals to help Madelyn with her anxiety and outbursts. The therapist worked with the parents to discuss what exposure task and behavioral goals would be the focus at home each week, as well as how the parents could address noncompliance. Exposure tasks included on the reward chart varied each week and addressed separation (e.g., sleeping alone, staying at home alone for a brief time) and social anxiety (e.g., giving a presentation to a few classmates, inviting a friend over). Examples of behavioral goals included "keeping my cool when I go to school in the morning" and "being respectful when mom and dad ask me to do something." Parents were instructed to provide daily rewards to Madelyn when she completed all of her therapy goals for the day. They also kept track of each goal by placing a small sticker on her reward chart when each individual goal was accomplished. This served as a tool to increase motivation; if a certain number of stickers were attained each week, an extra reward was provided. The use of a daily and a weekly reward allowed for continued motivation to engage in all of the day's goals, even if one was not met.

Over the course of therapy, Madelyn's parents had varying degrees of success in adhering to the reward chart. The therapist reviewed the reward chart every week with both Madelyn and her parents. Several times throughout treatment, the rationale behind the need for consistency was explained, and every attempt was made to make the reward chart accessible to the parents. For example, it was decided early in treatment that a strong daily reward for Madelyn would be extra time every day to play Minecraft. However, her parents had difficulty in monitoring her daily allotment of Minecraft time. When Madelyn began to refuse to do her exposures, it was revealed that she had been playing a version of the game on a readily accessible iPad. The therapist worked with the parents to come up with strategies to limit access to electronics and eventually worked with the family to make all Minecraft time contingent on completion of the daily goals.

Conclusion

We reviewed the challenges and the promise that CBT offers for youth with ASD. Indeed, there exists an emerging body of research that suggests that CBT can be effectively used to address certain difficulties in youth with ASD. In particular, multiple RCTs have shown that CBT for youth with anxiety and ASD can be comparably effective to CBT for youth with anxiety in general. We reviewed special factors that clinicians should consider when implementing CBT with this population and provided strategies to address these factors. It is prudent that clinicians adapt their CBT approach to account for the unique ways in which youth with ASD learn: Concrete examples and multimodal presentation of materials are two examples. Youth with ASD may be more motivated to participate in the therapy process if they can engage with their special interests or activities, and outcomes may be better when families are an integral part of the process.

The case example of Madelyn is one way in which CBT can be used with youth with ASD. In this example, we highlighted some of the difficulties in making differential diagnoses and provided suggestions for how to engage youth with ASD in therapy. As we continue to pursue such matters, we encourage the field to study optimal ways to tailor CBT for youth with ASD. Indeed, youth with ASD are extremely heterogeneous in presentation, often presenting with other behavioral or medical difficulties, requiring researchers and clinicians to explore the best ways to integrate care for ASD.

References

Adamson, L. B., Bakeman, R., Deckner, D. F., & Nelson, P. B. (2012). Rating parent–child interactions: Joint engagement, communication dynamic, and shared topics in autism, Down syndrome, and typical development. *Journal of Autism and Developmental Disorders, 42*, 2622–2635.

Ambrosini, P. J. (2000). Historical development and present status of the Schedule for Affective Disorders and Schizophrenia for School-Age Children (K-SADS). *Journal of the American Academy of Child and Adolescent Psychiatry, 39*(1), 49–58.

American Psychiatric Association. (2013). *Diagnostic and statistical manual of mental disorders* (5th ed.). Arlington, VA: Author.

Baron-Cohen, S. (2002). The extreme male brain theory of autism. *Trends in Cognitive Sciences, 6*(6), 248–254.

Bellini, S. (2004). Social skill deficits and anxiety in high-functioning adolescents with autism spectrum disorders. *Focus on Autism and Other Developmental Disabilities, 19*(2), 78–86.

Bellini, S. (2006). The development of social anxiety in adolescents with autism spectrum disorders. *Focus on Autism and Other Developmental Disabilities, 21*(3), 138–145.

Blakeley-Smith, A., Reaven, J., Ridge, K., & Hepburn, S. (2012). Parent–child agreement of anxiety symptoms in youth with autism spectrum disorders. *Research in Autism Spectrum Disorders, 6*(2), 707–716.

Bornstein, M. H., Tamis-LeMonda, C. S., Hahn, C. S., & Haynes, O. M. (2008). Maternal responsiveness to young children at three ages: Longitudinal analysis of a multidimensional, modular, and specific parenting construct. *Developmental Psychology, 44*(3), 867–874.

Chakrabarti, S., & Fombonne, E. (2005). Pervasive developmental disorders in preschool children: Confirmation of high prevalence. *American Journal of Psychiatry, 162*(6), 1133–1141.

Chalfant, A. M., Rapee, R., & Carroll, L. (2007). Treating anxiety disorders in children with high functioning autism spectrum disorders: A controlled trial. *Journal of Autism and Developmental Disorders, 37*(10), 1842–1857.

Chang, Y.-C., Quan, J., & Wood, J. J. (2012). Effects of anxiety disorder severity on social functioning in children with autism spectrum disorders. *Journal of Developmental and Physical Disabilities, 24*(3), 235–245.

Compton, S. N., Burns, B. J., Egger, H. L., & Robertson, E. (2002). Review of the evidence base for treatment of childhood psychopathology: Internalizing disorders. *Journal of Consulting and Clinical Psychology, 70*(6), 1240–1266.

Danial, J. T., & Wood, J. J. (2013). Cognitive behavioral therapy for children with autism: Review and considerations for future research. *Journal of Developmental and Behavioral Pediatrics, 34*(9), 702–715.

Davis, T. E., White, S. W., & Ollendick, T. H. (2014). *Handbook of autism and anxiety*. Cham, Switzerland: Springer.

Drahota, A., Wood, J. J., Sze, K. M., & Van Dyke, M. (2011). Effects of cognitive behavioral therapy on daily living skills in children with high-functioning autism and concurrent anxiety disorders. *Journal of Autism and Developmental Disorders, 41*(3), 257–265.

Hayes, S. A, & Watson, S. L. (2013). The impact of parenting stress: A meta-analysis of studies comparing the experience of parenting stress in parents of children with and without autism spectrum disorder. *Journal of Autism and Developmental Disorders, 43*(3), 629–642.

Hill, E. L. (2004). Evaluating the theory of executive dysfunction in autism. *Developmental Review, 24*(2), 189–233.

Howlin, P. (2000). Outcome in adult life for more able individuals with autism or Asperger syndrome. *Autism, 4*(1), 63–83.

Hwang, B., & Hughes, C. (2000). The effects of social interactive training on early social communicative skills of children with autism. *Journal of Autism and Developmental Disorders, 30*(4), 331–343.

Kasari, C., Paparella, T., Freeman, S., & Jahromi, L. B. (2008). Language outcome in autism: Randomized comparison of joint attention and play interventions. *Journal of Consulting and Clinical Psychology, 76*(1), 125–137.

Keehn, B., Lincoln, A. J., Müller, R. A., & Townsend, J. (2010). Attentional networks in children and adolescents with autism spectrum disorder. *Journal of Child Psychology and Psychiatry, 51*(11), 1251–1259.

Kendall, P. C., Hudson, J. L., Gosch, E., Flannery-Schroeder, E., & Suveg, C. (2008). Cognitive-behavioral therapy for anxiety-disordered youth: A randomized clinical trial evaluating child and family modalities. *Journal of Consulting and Clinical Psychology, 76*(2), 282–297.

Kenworthy, L., Anthony, L. G., Naiman, D. Q., Cannon, L., Wills, M. C., Luong-Tran, C., et al. (2014). Randomized controlled effectiveness trial of executive function intervention for children on the autism spectrum. *Journal of Child Psychology and Psychiatry, 55*(4), 374–383.

Kerns, C. M., & Kendall, P. C. (2012). The presentation and classification of anxiety in autism spectrum disorder. *Clinical Psychology: Science and Practice, 19*(4), 323–347.

Kerns, C. M., Kendall, P. C., Berry, L., Souders, M. C., Franklin, M. E., Schultz, R. T., et al. (2014). Traditional and atypical presentations of anxiety in youth with autism spectrum disorder. *Journal of Autism and Developmental Disorders, 44*(11), 2851–2861.

Kerns, C. M., Kendall, P. C., Zickgraf, H., Franklin, M. E., Miller, J., & Herrington, J. (2015). Not to be overshadowed or overlooked: Functional impairments associated with comorbid anxiety disorders in youth with ASD. *Behavior Therapy, 46*(1), 29–39.

Kerns, C. M., Renno, P., Kendall, P. C., Wood J. J., & Storch, E. (2017). Anxiety Disorders Interview Schedule—Autism Addendum: Reliability and validity in children with autism spectrum disorder. *Journal of Clinical Child and Adolescent Psychology, 46*(1), 88–100.

Kerns, C. M., Rump, K., Worley, J., Kratz, H., McVey, A., Herrington, J., et al. (2016). The differential diagnosis of anxiety disorders in cognitively-able youth with autism. *Cognitive and Behavioral Practice, 23*(4), 530–547.

Kerns, C. M., Wood, J. J., Kendall, P. C., Renno, P., Crawford, E. A., Mercado, R. J., et al. (2016). The Treatment of Anxiety in Autism Spectrum Disorder (TAASD) Study: Rationale, design and methods. *Journal of Child and Family Studies, 25*(6), 1889–1902.

Kogan, M. D., Blumberg, S. J., Schieve, L. A., Boyle, C. A., Perrin, J. M., Ghandour, R. M., et al. (2009). Prevalence of parent-reported diagnosis of autism spectrum disorder among children in the US, 2007. *Pediatrics, 124*(5), 1395–403.

Lai, W. W., Goh, T. J., Oei, T. P. S., & Sung, M. (2015). Coping and well-being in parents of children with autism spectrum disorders (ASD). *Journal of Autism and Developmental Disorders, 45*(8), 2582–2593.

Lam, K. S. L., Bodfish, J. W., & Piven, J. (2008). Evidence for three subtypes of repetitive behavior in autism that differ in familiality and association with other symptoms. *Journal of Child Psychology and Psychiatry and Allied Disciplines, 49*(11), 1193–1200.

Leyfer, O. T., Folstein, S. E., Bacalman, S., Davis, N. O., Dinh, E., Morgan, J., et al. (2006). Comorbid psychiatric disorders in children with autism: Interview development and rates of disorders. *Journal of Autism and Developmental Disorders, 36*(7), 849–861.

Mason, J., & Scior, K. (2004). "Diagnostic overshadowing" amongst clinicians working with people with intellectual disabilities in the UK. *Journal of Applied Research in Intellectual Disabilities, 17*(2), 85–90.

Matson, J. L., & Nebel-Schwalm, M. S. (2007). Comorbid psychopathology with autism spectrum disorder in children: An overview. *Research in Developmental Disabilities, 28*(4), 341–352.

Mayes, S. D., Calhoun, S. L., Aggarwal, R., Baker, C., Mathapati, S., Molitoris, S., et al. (2013). Unusual fears in children with autism. *Research in Autism Spectrum Disorders, 7*(1), 151–158.

Mazurek, M. O., Vasa, R. A., Kalb, L. G., Kanne, S. M., Rosenberg, D., Keefer, A., et al. (2013). Anxiety, sensory over-responsivity, and gastrointestinal problems in children with autism spectrum disorders. *Journal of Abnormal Child Psychology, 41*(1), 165–176.

McNally Keehn, R. H., Lincoln, A. J., Brown, M. Z., & Chavira, D. A. (2013). The Coping Cat program for children with anxiety and autism spectrum disorder: A pilot randomized controlled trial. *Journal of Autism and Developmental Disorders, 43*(1), 57–67.

Merlo, L. J., Lehmkuhl, H. D., Geffken, G. R., & Storch, E. A. (2009). Decreased family accommodation associated with improved therapy outcome in pediatric obsessive–compulsive disorder. *Journal of Consulting and Clinical Psychology, 77*(2), 355–360.

National Research Council. (2001). *Educating children with autism.* Washington, DC: National Academies Press.

Ooi, Y. P., Lam, C. M., Sung, M., Tan, W. T., Goh, T. J., Fung, D. S., et al. (2008). Effects of cognitive-behavioural therapy on anxiety for children with high-functioning autistic spectrum disorders. *Singapore Medical Journal, 49*(3), 215–220.

Puleo, C. M., & Kendall, P. C. (2011). Anxiety disorders in typically developing youth: Autism spectrum symptoms as a predictor of cognitive-behavioral treatment. *Journal of Autism and Developmental Disorders, 41*(3), 275–286.

Reaven, J. (2011). The treatment of anxiety symptoms in youth with high-functioning autism spectrum disorders: Developmental considerations for parents. *Brain Research, 1380,* 255–263.

Reaven, J., Blakeley-Smith, A., Culhane-Shelburne, K., & Hepburn, S. (2012). Group cognitive behavior therapy for children with high-functioning autism spectrum disorders and anxiety: A randomized trial. *Journal of Child Psychology and Psychiatry and Allied Disciplines, 53*(4), 410–419.

Reaven, J., & Hepburn, S. (2006). The parent's role in the treatment of anxiety symptoms in children with high-functioning autism spectrum disorders. *Mental Health Aspects of Developmental Disabilities, 3*(9), 73–80.

Renno, P., & Wood, J. J. (2013). Discriminant and convergent validity of the anxiety construct in children with autism spectrum disorders. *Journal of Autism and Developmental Disorders, 43*(9), 2135–2146.

Reynolds, S., Wilson, C., Austin, J., & Hooper, L. (2012). Effects of psychotherapy for anxiety in children and adolescents: A meta-analytic review. *Clinical Psychology Review, 32*(4), 251–262.

Rogers, S. J., & Vismara, L. A. (2008). Evidence-based comprehensive treatments for early autism. *Journal of Clinical Child and Adolescent Psychology, 37*(1), 8–38.

Shire, S. Y., Gulsrud, A., & Kasari, C. (2016). Increasing responsive parent–child interactions and joint engagement: Comparing the influence of parent-mediated intervention and parent psychoeducation. *Journal of Autism and Developmental Disorders, 46*(5), 1737–1747.

Silverman, W. K., & Albano, A. M. (1996). *The Anxiety Disorders Interview Schedule for DSM-IV—Child and Parent Versions.* San Antonio, TX: Graywind.

Smith, T. (2008). Empirically supported and unsupported treatments for autism spectrum disorders. *Scientific Review of Mental Health Practice, 6,* 3–20.

Sofronoff, K., Attwood, T., & Hinton, S. (2005). A randomised controlled trial of a CBT intervention for anxiety in children with Asperger syndrome. *Journal of Child Psychology and Psychiatry and Allied Disciplines, 46*(11), 1152–1160.

Storch, E. A., Arnold, E. B., Lewin, A. B., Nadeau, J. M., Jones, A. M., De Nadai, A. S., et al. (2013). The effect of cognitive-behavioral therapy versus treatment as usual for anxiety in children with autism spectrum disorders: A randomized, controlled trial. *Journal of the American Academy of Child and Adolescent Psychiatry, 52*(2), 132–142.

Storch, E. A., Lewin, A. B., Collier, A. B., Arnold, E., De Nadai, A. S., Dane, B. F., et al. (2015). A randomized controlled trial of cognitive-behavioral therapy versus treatment as usual for adolescents with autism spectrum disorders and comorbid anxiety. *Depression and Anxiety, 32*(3), 174–181.

Ung, D., Selles, R., Small, B. J., & Storch, E. A. (2015). A systematic review and meta-analysis of cognitive-behavioral therapy for anxiety in youth with high-functioning autism spectrum disorders. *Child Psychiatry and Human Development, 46*(4), 533–547.

U.S. Department of Health & Human Services, Centers for Disease Control & Prevention. (2014). Prevalence of autism spectrum disorder among children aged 8 years—Autism and Developmental Disabilities Monitoring Network, 11 sites, United States, 2010. *Morbidity and Mortality Weekly Report Surveillance Summaries, 63*, 1–21.

van Steensel, F. J. A., Bögels, S. M., & Perrin, S. (2011). Anxiety disorders in children and adolescents with autistic spectrum disorders: A meta-analysis. *Clinical Child and Family Psychology Review, 14*(3), 302–317.

Warren, Z., McPheeters, M. L., Sathe, N., Foss-Feig, J. H., Glasser, A., & Veenstra-VanderWeele, J. (2011). A systematic review of early intensive intervention for autism spectrum disorders. *Pediatrics, 127*(5), e1303–e1311.

White, S. W., Albano, A. M., Johnson, C. R., Kasari, C., Ollendick, T., Klin, A., et al. (2010). Development of a cognitive-behavioral intervention program to treat anxiety and social deficits in teens with high-functioning autism. *Clinical Child and Family Psychology Review, 13*(1), 77–90.

White, S. W., Mazefsky, C. A., Dichter, G. S., Chiu, P. H., Richey, J. A., & Ollendick, T. H. (2014). Social-cognitive, physiological, and neural mechanisms underlying emotion regulation impairments: Understanding anxiety in autism spectrum disorder. *International Journal of Developmental Neuroscience, 39*, 22–36.

White, S. W., Ollendick, T., Albano, A. M., Oswald, D., Johnson, C., Southam-Gerow, M. A., et al. (2013). Randomized controlled trial: Multimodal anxiety and social skill intervention for adolescents with autism spectrum disorder. *Journal of Autism and Developmental Disorders, 43*(2), 382–394.

White, S. W., Ollendick, T., Scahill, L., Oswald, D., & Albano, A. M. (2009). Preliminary efficacy of a cognitive-behavioral treatment program for anxious youth with autism spectrum disorders. *Journal of Autism and Developmental Disorders, 39*(12), 1652–1662.

Witwer, A. N., Lecavalier, L., & Norris, M. (2012). Reliability and validity of the Children's Interview for Psychiatric Syndromes—Parent Version in autism spectrum disorders. *Journal of Autism and Developmental Disorders, 42*(9), 1949–1958.

Wong, C., Odom, S. L., Hume, K. A., Cox, A. W., Fettig, A., Kucharczyk, S., et al. (2015). Evidence-based practices for children, youth, and young adults with autism spectrum disorder: A comprehensive review. *Journal of Autism and Developmental Disorders, 45*(7), 1951–1966.

Wood, J. J., Drahota, A., Sze, K., Har, K., Chiu, A., & Langer, D. A. (2009). Cognitive behavioral therapy for anxiety in children with autism spectrum disorders: A randomized, controlled trial. *Journal of Child Psychology and Psychiatry and Allied Disciplines, 50*(3), 224–234.

Wood, J. J., Ehrenreich-May, J., Alessandri, M., Fujii, C., Renno, P., Laugeson, E., et al. (2015). Cognitive behavioral therapy for early adolescents with autism spectrum disorders and clinical anxiety: A randomized, controlled trial. *Behavior Therapy, 46*(1), 7–19.

Wood, J. J., & Gadow, K. D. (2010). Exploring the nature and function of anxiety in youth with autism spectrum disorders. *Clinical Psychology: Science and Practice, 17*(4), 281–292.

CHAPTER NINE

Facilitating Understanding and Management of Attention–Deficit/ Hyperactivity Disorder

Arthur D. Anastopoulos
Sarah R. O'Rourke
Allison C. Bray

At face value, the idea of using cognitive therapy as a tool in the clinical management of attention-deficit/hyperactivity disorder (ADHD; American Psychiatric Association, 2013) may seem counterintuitive. After all, ADHD is commonly conceptualized as a behavioral condition, characterized by developmentally deviant levels of inattention and/ or hyperactivity–impulsivity, whose etiology stems primarily from genetics and other biological factors (Barkley, 2015). Thus ADHD would not seem to be amenable to cognitive therapy, given its emphasis on the identification and amelioration of faulty thinking patterns that presumably underlie the development and maintenance of maladaptive emotions and behaviors. In support of this contention are the results of early cognitive therapy efforts, which typically failed to bring about clinically meaningful improvements in primary ADHD symptoms (Abikoff, 1985).

Although cognitive therapy may not be the first-line approach for treating primary ADHD symptoms, it would be premature for practitioners to cast cognitive therapy aside when providing clinical services to children and adolescents with ADHD. Many possibilities exist for using cognitive therapy with these youth, and this chapter brings many of these to light. First, however, it is valuable to have an understanding of what ADHD is and how it presents itself clinically in child and adolescent samples. Against this background, two case examples will highlight some of the many ways in which cognitive therapy strategies can be employed.

Overview of ADHD

Although a comprehensive depiction of ADHD is beyond the scope of this chapter, readers interested in learning more are encouraged to consult other sources (e.g., Barkley, 2015). What follows is a summary of the major issues that have direct bearing on the use of cognitive therapy with children and adolescents displaying ADHD.

Diagnostic Criteria

As outlined in the fifth edition of the *Diagnostic and Statistical Manual of Mental Disorders* (DSM-5; American Psychiatric Association, 2013), the five major criteria needed to diagnose ADHD are: (1) a high frequency of primary ADHD symptoms, (2) an onset of these symptoms prior to 12 years of age, (3) evidence that these symptoms occur in two or more settings, (4) evidence that these symptoms cause clinically significant impairment in daily functioning, and (5) clear evidence that these symptoms and impairment are not better accounted for by the presence of some other mental health or medical condition. Depending on the relative distribution of primary symptoms, the clinical presentation of ADHD can be further subclassified as combined, predominantly inattentive, or predominantly hyperactive–impulsive.

Situational Variability

In practice, one of the most confusing aspects of ADHD is that its primary symptoms often present inconsistently. At times, this inconsistency in performance can lead to characterizations of children as being "lazy"; at other times, it may even cause some individuals to question the accuracy of the diagnosis. In anticipation of these possibilities, it is critically important for practitioners to understand that ADHD symptoms do not present in an all-or-none, always present–never present fashion. Instead, ADHD symptoms are subject to situational variability, and their presence or absence depends on contextual factors, such as novelty, interest level, and the immediacy and frequency of feedback. In this way, ADHD can be thought of as a disorder of performance *variability* rather than inability. Armed with such knowledge, practitioners are well positioned to cognitively reframe parental and teacher misperceptions of how ADHD may present itself.

Comorbidity

ADHD is often accompanied by co-occurring or comorbid conditions. Up to 60% of youth with ADHD have at least one co-occurring condition (Pliszka, 2015). Oppositional defiant disorder (ODD) is the most prevalent comorbid condition, with roughly 40% of children and adolescents with ADHD meeting full diagnostic criteria for ODD; of these, another 25% may develop more serious antisocial behavior in the form of conduct disorder (CD). Around 25–35% of children and adolescents with ADHD may meet criteria for an anxiety disorder, the most common of which is generalized anxiety disorder (GAD; Elia, Ambrosini, & Berrettini, 2008). Rates of depression in children and adolescents with ADHD have consistently been reported to be higher than in community samples, falling between 25 and 30% (Angold, Costello, & Erkanli, 1999; Pliszka, 2015). Similarly, high rates of diagnosable depression and anxiety have been reported among college students with ADHD (Anastopoulos et al., 2016). Together, such findings highlight the need to take various comorbid conditions into account in the routine assessment and treatment of children and adolescents with ADHD. Specifically, this increased risk for depression and anxiety speaks to the need for including cognitive therapy and other evidence-based strategies in the clinical management of these comorbid conditions.

Impairment

The combined impact of ADHD and its comorbid features increases the risk for a myriad of psychosocial difficulties across the life span (Barkley, Murphy, & Fischer, 2008). In terms of educational functioning, most clinic-referred children with ADHD exhibit academic underachievement relative to their aptitude, including lower test scores, higher rates of course failure, more suspensions and expulsions, greater use of special education services, and lower grade-point averages (DuPaul & Stoner, 2015). As a direct consequence of academic impairment experienced by the majority of youth with ADHD, up to 80% of individuals with ADHD do not initially enroll in a 4-year college (Barkley et al., 2008). The subset of individuals with ADHD who do pursue postsecondary education tend to have lower grade-point averages (GPA), poorer organization and study skills, and time-management difficulties, and they are less likely to graduate than college students without ADHD (Barkley et al., 2008; DuPaul, Weyandt, O'Dell, & Varejao, 2009; Norwalk, Norvilitis, & MacLean, 2009).

Children and adolescents with ADHD may experience impairment at home, particularly in terms of relationships with family members. Families of children and teens with ADHD are characterized by greater intrafamily conflict, negativity, and parenting stress than control families (Barkley, Anastopoulos, Guevremont, & Fletcher, 1992; Johnston & Mash, 2001). Compounding difficulties between parents and their children with ADHD is the finding that biological mothers and fathers of children with ADHD may also have ADHD themselves and that they are also more likely to experience other psychological conditions, including depression, anxiety, learning disabilities, and conduct problems and antisocial behavior (Barkley, 2015).

In terms of social functioning, children and teens with ADHD may experience a pattern of rejection in social situations, as they tend to exhibit poor social and communication skills and have fewer close friendships (Bagwell, Molina, Pelham, & Hoza, 2001; Klimkeit et al., 2006). Adolescents with ADHD are also at risk for impairment in terms of driving behavior; use and abuse of alcohol, nicotine, and drugs; and risky sexual behavior (Barkley, Guevremont, Anastopoulos, DuPaul, & Shelton, 1993; Flory, Molina, Pelham, Gnagy, & Smith, 2006; Molina, Marshal, Pelham, & Wirth, 2005). Research on ADHD in college students suggests that both male and female students with ADHD exhibit social skills deficits and more problems accessing social support compared with their counterparts without ADHD (Kern, Rasmussen, Byrd, & Wittschen, 1999; Shaw-Zirt, Popali-Lehane, Chaplin, & Bergman, 2005).

Assessment

Comprehensive assessment of ADHD is essential to ensure that all DSM-5 criteria for ADHD are met. Comprehensive assessment also allows practitioners to assess for any comorbid conditions and sets the stage for comprehensive treatment planning. A multimethod, multi-informant approach to the assessment of ADHD is recommended (Anastopoulos & Shelton, 2001). Key features of this approach include the use of clinical interviews and behavior rating scales completed by parents and teachers and by self-report when older adolescents are involved. In some cases, medical evaluations, psychoeducational assessment, continuous performance tests, or direct observation of the child may also be useful (see Anastopoulos & Shelton, 2001, for further discussion).

Clinical interviews are useful in gathering relevant historical information, as well as assessing whether the child meets diagnostic criteria for ADHD and other disorders. An unstructured interview with parents may be conducted to gather background data, including the presenting concerns, developmental and health history, educational history, family history, and social history. An unstructured interview with the child can also shed light on the child's perceptions of the presenting concerns and history. To ensure diagnostic accuracy, it is recommended that a structured or semistructured interview be given to assess whether the child meets diagnostic criteria for ADHD and/or other specific conditions. Commonly used structured and semistructured interviews include the Child and Adolescent Psychiatric Assessment (CAPA; Angold, Prendergast, Cox, Harrington, Simonoff, & Rutter, 1995), the Diagnostic Interview for Children and Adolescents–IV (DICA-IV; Reich, Welner, Herjanic, & MHS Staff, 1996), the Diagnostic Interview Schedule for Children–IV (DISC-IV; Shaffer, Fisher, Lucas, Dulcan, & Schwab-Stone, 2000), and the Kiddie Schedule for Affective Disorders and Schizophrenia for School-Age Children (K-SADS; Kaufman et al., 1997). None of these interviews has yet been updated for DSM-5. Given that there were few changes in the diagnostic criteria for ADHD from DSM-IV to DSM-5, these interviews are likely still appropriate for assessing ADHD. However, DSM-5 contains more substantial changes to the diagnostic criteria for common co-occurring conditions and also added new diagnoses, such as disruptive mood dysregulation disorder (DMDD), that are not covered at all in these existing structured interviews. Practitioners may therefore need to supplement these older structured and semistructured interviews with additional questions to ensure that DSM-5 diagnostic criteria are applied. Practitioners are also encouraged to rapidly adopt updated versions of these interviews as they become available.

Narrow band rating scales focus specifically on ADHD symptoms and are useful in establishing frequency counts and whether symptoms of inattention and hyperactivity–impulsivity are developmentally deviant. Narrow band ADHD measures include the ADHD Rating Scale–5 (DuPaul, Power, Anastopoulos, & Reid, 2016), the Conners 3rd Edition (Conners 3; Conners, 2008a), the SNAP-IV (Swanson, 1992), and the Vanderbilt ADHD Rating Scales (Wolraich, Feurer, Hannah, Pinnock, & Baumgaertel, 1998). Of these, both the ADHD Rating Scale–5 and the Conners 3 are updated for DSM-5. The ADHD Rating Scale–5 was written and normed based on DSM-5 criteria for ADHD. Parent and teacher versions are available, and both versions include the 18 symptoms of ADHD, along with six items that directly address impairment stemming from these symptoms. The Conners 3 was published before the release of the DSM-5, but a scoring update has since been released for DSM-5. The Conners 3 assesses symptoms of ADHD, ODD, and CD and has parent, teacher, and self-report versions.

Broadband rating scales assess a wide range of child behaviors. In the context of ADHD assessment, they may be particularly useful in screening for conditions that co-occur with ADHD or that provide a better explanation for the presenting concerns. Commonly used broadband scales include the Achenbach System of Empirically Based Assessment (AESBA; Achenbach, 2009), the Behavior Assessment System for Children—Third Edition (BASC-3; Reynolds & Kamphaus, 2015), and the Conners Comprehensive Behavior Rating Scales (Conners CBRS; Conners, 2008b) and Conners Early Childhood (Conners EC; Conners, 2009). Each of these measures has been released or updated since the release of DSM-5, include parent-, teacher-, and self-rated versions (with the exception of the Conners EC, which includes only parent- and teacher-rated versions), and provide adequate coverage of internalizing, externalizing, and social-developmental domains. In addition, DSM-5 includes a "DSM-5 Parent–Guardian-Rated Level 1 Cross-Cutting Symptom Measure—Child Age 6–17" and "DSM-5 Self-Rated Level 1 Cross-Cutting Symptom Measure, Child Age 11 to 17." These cross-cutting measures screen for a range of emotional and behavioral concerns and guide users to areas in which further inquiry is indicated.

Overview of Treatment

The earliest cognitive-behavioral treatments for young children characterized as "impulsive" were cognitive self-instructional training procedures in which children were trained to provide themselves with verbal commands, at first spoken aloud and later spoken to themselves, to enhance their self-control (e.g., Meichenbaum & Goodman, 1971). Although this approach received some support in studies of impulsive children (Kendall & Braswell, 1982), therapeutic benefits were far more limited for children with more severe ADHD-type problems (Abikoff, 1985). Thus the field began shifting its attention toward behavior modification and other treatments for ADHD.

A series of reviews of psychosocial treatments for children and adolescents with ADHD have been published over the last two decades (Evans, Owens, & Bunford, 2014; Pelham & Fabiano, 2008; Pelham, Wheeler, & Chronis, 1998). These reviews have used the Chambless and Hollon (1998) criteria, outlined in the opening chapter of this volume, to evaluate the empirical evidence for these psychosocial treatments. In the most recent review, Evans, Owen, and Bunford (2014) classified psychosocial treatments thus:

Level I: Well Established

- Behavioral parent training (BPT)
- Behavioral classroom management (BCM)
- Behavioral peer intervention (BPI)
- Combined behavior management interventions (e.g., elements of both BPT and BCM)
- Organization training

Level II: Probably Efficacious

- Combined interventions (i.e., Challenging Horizons Program; Evans, Schultz, DeMars, & Davis, 2011; Molina et al., 2008)

Level III: Possibly Efficacious

- Neurofeedback

Level IV: Experimental

- Cognitive training

Level V: Not Effective

- Social skills training

In this chapter, we highlight two well-established treatments for younger children and two promising treatments that can be used with younger and older adolescents. For younger children, we cover BPT and organization training, which are commonly employed and most practicably implemented by practitioners working in office settings. We then describe the problem-solving communication training (PSCT) approach for younger adolescents and a newly developed cognitive-behavioral treatment for older adolescents with ADHD attending college.

Treatments for Children

Behavioral Parent Training

In general, BPT for school-age children with ADHD involves teaching parents to implement behavioral techniques in the home setting. Behavioral techniques typically include use of "special time" to enhance the warmth of the parent–child relationship; positive attending to desired behaviors; providing effective directions; implementation of a home contingency management system to improve compliance with parental requests; response cost; and time-out. As part of BPT, practitioners may also facilitate the implementation of a daily report card system, used by the child's classroom teacher, to improve the child's classroom behavior. There are many manualized variations on BPT for ADHD, such as the Defiant Child program (Barkley, 2013) and the Community-Oriented Parenting Education (COPE) program (Cunningham, Bremner, & Secord-Gilbert, 1998). BPT is usually delivered in 8–12 sessions and may be delivered to parents in individual and/or group formats. Importantly, despite many years of extensive research establishing the efficacy of BPT, little is known about what child or parent characteristics moderate the effectiveness of this treatment (Evans et al., 2014).

As the name suggests, BPT is primarily behavioral in nature. However, we also routinely incorporate cognitive strategies when addressing parental cognitions about their child, their child's behavior, and the treatment itself in order to enhance parental acceptance and compliance with BPT (Anastopoulos, Rhoads, & Farley, 2006). For instance, parents may enter BPT with misperceptions about the causes of ADHD or the extent to which their child's symptoms are within the child's own control. Here, psychoeducation about ADHD at the start of BPT can help parents gain a clearer understanding of their child's behavior. Other parents may respond to initial therapist attempts to describe behavioral strategies that will be included in BPT, with cognitions such as "I've tried all these strategies before and they didn't work." In this instance, practitioners can help parents to understand that the behavioral strategies contained in the treatment package are *specialized* variations on these strategies that they have not likely used before. Yet other parents present with concerns about how their mere engagement in BPT reflects on their own parenting or about using behavioral strategies in public settings; for example, some parents report thoughts that "I must be a bad parent if I need parenting advice" or "Other parents would think my child was out of control if they saw me making my child serve a time-out in a public setting." Traditional cognitive restructuring strategies are often useful, including Socratic questioning and helping the parent arrive at a more adaptive and realistic appraisal of the situation. For example, more useful, balanced cognitions could include "I am showing love for my child by learning ways to enhance our relationship and decrease arguing" or "I can't be sure what other parents think when they see me discipline my child in public, and what other parents think about me doesn't matter much anyway."

Organizational Training

Organizational training is based on the observation that many children with ADHD have skills deficits in the areas of organization, time management, and planning (Abikoff et al., 2013). In organizational training, practitioners work directly with children to teach specific organization, time-management, and planning skills. In the particular organizational training treatment developed by Abikoff and colleagues (2013), the therapist uses an analogy to encourage the child to maximize his or her executive functioning skills (or the "Mastermind") and to successfully navigate executive functioning deficits (e.g., "glitches"). The clinician teaches the child skills that include recording assignments and due dates, organizing school materials into binders, monitoring their own organization and supplies using checklists, accurately estimating and tracking the time needed to complete tasks, and breaking larger tasks down into smaller tasks. Parents typically join the final few minutes of the session to learn how to support and reward the use of these new skills. One manualized version of organizational training for elementary-age students is the *Organizational Skills Training for ADHD* manual (Gallagher, Abikoff, & Spira, 2014).

Treatments for Younger Adolescents

Despite Evans and colleagues' (2014) characterization of BPT as a well-established treatment in their review of psychosocial treatments for ADHD, they acknowledge that behavior management interventions (including BPT, BCM, and BPI) can really only be considered well-established for children between ages 4 and 12. Both Evans and colleagues' (2014) review and Pelham and Fabiano's (2008) review noted the need for additional study of psychosocial treatment approaches for teens with ADHD. The Challenging Horizons Program (CHP; Evans et al., 2011; Molina et al., 2008) is a probably efficacious treatment that was developed for adolescents with ADHD. CHP is delivered as an after-school program for middle and high school students that involves organization training, academic skills training, and social skills training. An organizational skills program for middle school students that is delivered by school mental health personnel is also promising (homework, organization, and planning skills [HOPS] program; Langberg et al., 2012).

Problem–Solving Communication Training

Problem-solving communication training (PSCT) has been named a promising approach for this age group (Pelham & Fabiano, 2008) but has not been classified according to task force criteria in the two most recent reviews due to a dearth of related studies. In the absence of other treatments for teens with ADHD that are designed to be implemented in an office setting, we describe PSCT here. The evidence base for PSCT is reviewed first (as it has not been extensively reviewed elsewhere), followed by a description and case illustration of this treatment.

Two studies have compared PSCT to BPT in adolescent samples (Barkley, Guevremont, Anastopoulos, & Fletcher, 1992; Barkley, Edwards, Laneri, Fletcher, & Metevia, 2001). In the earlier study, families of 12- to 17-year-olds with ADHD were assigned to one of three treatment conditions: BPT involving parents only, PSCT involving both teens and their parents, or structural family therapy (SFT), also involving both teens and their parents. All three of the treatment approaches resulted in improvements in externalizing and internalizing symptoms, parent–teen communication, number of conflicts, anger intensity during conflicts, and maternal depression, and participants in the three treatments reported similar levels of satisfaction with the treatments. There were no changes, however, in raters' observations of the families' communications. In the second study (Barkley et al., 2001), families were assigned to one of two treatment conditions: 18 sessions of PSCT involving teens and their parents or 9 sessions of BMT involving parents only followed by 9 sessions of PSCT. As in the earlier study, these two groups produced similar improvements in parent ratings of teen behavior, teen ratings of parent behavior, and observer ratings of mothers' behavior, and no changes in raters' observations of the families' communications. The dropout rate in the PSCT-only condition was, however, significantly greater than the dropout rate in the BMT + PSCT condition.

As noted in Barkley and colleagues' (1992) study, PSCT and other family-based approaches to treating teens with ADHD have the potential not only to manage the core symptoms of ADHD but also to alleviate distress in the family system that may be related to the challenges of parenting a teen with ADHD. PSCT is based on treatment principles and procedures outlined by Robin and Foster (1989) and generally involves three major components: problem solving, communication training, and cognitive restructuring. Families, including teens and parents, are trained in a five-step problem-solving method that involves defining the problem, brainstorming possible solutions, evaluating solutions and negotiating, making a decision about a solution, and implementing and evaluating the solution. A written behavior contract, which outlines specific behaviors expected on the part of the teen and the parents, as well as specific contingencies, is typically generated as part of the problem-solving approach. The therapist also helps parents and teens to develop more effective communication skills for discussing conflicts, including using active listening skills, attending to one's own tone of voice and volume, using "I" statements, and avoiding insults and ultimatums. In contrast to BPT, cognitive restructuring is included as one of the formal components of PSCT. The therapist helps parents and teens identify and examine extreme or inflexible beliefs about other family members' behaviors. It is common for teens and parents alike to endorse misattributions for the others' behaviors (e.g., "My child is purposely trying to get under my skin" or "My parents never let me do fun things with my friends because they're completely out of touch"). Parents and teens also commonly hold unreasonable beliefs on themes of ruination, obedience, perfectionism, self-blame, autonomy, or malicious intent (Robin & Foster, 1989). These misattributions and unreasonable beliefs may inflame family conflict and distress. After these misattributions and unreasonable beliefs have been identified and examined, the therapist guides the parents and teens to develop more accurate and useful cognitions that are less likely to contribute to conflict. This approach is described further in the *Defiant Teens* manual (Barkley & Robin, 2014).

Case Example: A Younger Adolescent

To protect privacy, identifying data have been removed from the following case.

Background

At the time these services were provided, Taylor was a 14-year-old Caucasian male who attended approximately 6 months of weekly psychotherapy along with his mother. Taylor had been previously evaluated and diagnosed with ADHD and ODD at an ADHD clinic, using a multimethod, multi-informant assessment (Anastopoulos & Shelton, 2001).

Taylor and his mother, Mrs. S., presented to therapy with concerns regarding his functioning in several domains. At home, Taylor was frequently oppositional and forgetful with requests from parents (e.g., arguing with requests, not following through on chores, respectively). Taylor lived with his mother, father, and younger sister. His mother worked full time at a school, and his father traveled often for his job. When his father was home, Taylor demonstrated notably significantly more compliance with requests than when his father was away. Taylor acknowledged that he did not view his mother as an authority figure, and his mother admitted that she struggled to follow through with rewards and consequences for Taylor's behavior.

Taylor also had consistent difficulty remembering school supplies, which often necessitated his parents' retrieving his belongings and bringing them to school. Mrs. S. also left for work very early in the morning, requiring Taylor to get himself ready most mornings. Mrs. S. expressed concern that Taylor regularly forgot to close the front door (let alone lock it) on his way out in the morning. Taylor was also intermittently compliant with his stimulant medication, and, a few weeks after starting therapy, he decided that he was not going to take medication at all.

Taylor began attending therapy in the fall of his ninth-grade year. At school, Taylor had trouble concentrating in class and was easily distracted, particularly later in the day. This difficulty was exacerbated when Taylor stopped taking his stimulant medication. He also had trouble keeping track of homework and assignments. Despite an IQ in the high average range and doing relatively well on exams, Taylor's grades were mostly C's and D's, primarily as a result of incomplete work. Taylor had an individualized education plan (IEP) on the basis of his ADHD diagnosis, which allowed him to arrange his class schedule such that he took two academic classes with two electives per quarter to spread out his academic load. His IEP also afforded him extra time on exams, as well as testing in a private room. Taylor expressed self-consciousness about utilizing these accommodations, as he did not want to "stand out" from his peers. Taylor was also a talented athlete and was at risk of being removed from his sports teams for poor academic performance.

Treatment Plan

A multimodal treatment plan was created to address the multiple targets for therapy. This treatment plan included a combination of intervention approaches, encompassing home management strategies and communication skills training as guided by the PSCT framework, periodic individual counseling for Mrs. S., strategies for classroom and homework success, and consideration of reinstituting stimulant medication therapy.

Regarding pharmacotherapy, Taylor had previously taken stimulant medication with notable improvement observed by parents and teachers, as well as by Taylor himself, particularly in terms of his ability to focus and complete tasks. However, Taylor became self-conscious about taking medication and did not really understand why it was needed. Taylor also experienced some side effects, including appetite suppression, which had led his teachers to be concerned that he was not eating his lunch at school. Mrs. S. suspected that her husband had undiagnosed ADHD as well and was initially opposed to medication, which may have influenced Taylor's thinking. Given Taylor's reluctance to take medication, it was agreed that he could conditionally go without it for the time being. If his academic performance did not improve and specific goals were not met (e.g., having teachers sign his planner) by the second quarter of the academic year, medication would be reinstituted. Taylor, Mrs. S., and the therapist agreed to this plan.

Problem-Solving Communication Training

Given Taylor's ADHD and ODD diagnoses, and to address the conflicts between Taylor and his mother, PSCT was selected as a treatment modality. PSCT is a family-based approach that relies on both parent and teen involvement, with components including problem solving between family members, effective communication skills, and cognitive therapy strategies (see Table 9.1).

First, positive communication skills were reviewed and rehearsed in session. For Taylor and his mother, "I" statements, making eye contact, and using a calm tone of voice were specific targets for practice. Next, the therapist introduced problem-solving skills, first by teaching Taylor and his mother how to define their areas of conflict. For example, problems were defined in specific, descriptive terms, such as "cleaning his room when asked," and "identifying a weekend curfew." Taylor and his mother then alternated suggesting potential solutions, with occasional help from the therapist, which were written on a whiteboard in the therapy room.

TABLE 9.1. Summary of Problem-Solving Communication Training

Five-step behavioral problem solving	Communication skills	Cognitive therapy skills	Structural family therapy
The goal is to compromise rather than insist on "my way or the highway":	*The goal is to avoid communication patterns that fan the flames of conflict, including:*	*The goal is to avoid misperceptions that fan the flames of conflict, such as:*	*The goal is to make adjustments to family structure that contribute to conflict, such as:*
• Define problem in concise, neutral terms. • Creatively brainstorm multiple solutions. • Evaluate each solution. • Select solution most agreeable to all. • Implement and then evaluate the effectiveness of the agreed-upon solution.	• Parental lecturing, bringing up the past, yelling, labeling • Teen sarcasm, silent treatment, insults	• Mind reading ("I know you hate me.") • Negative fortune telling ("You won't be able to get a job looking like that.") • All-or-none thinking ("You never let me do things with my friends.")	• A parent–parent alliance weakened by marital issues or disagreements over parenting • Improper parent–teen boundaries (parent complaining to teen about the other parent)

Solutions were not evaluated until the list was compiled, which aimed to include at least two suggestions from each party. Next, each solution was rated by both Taylor and his mother as either acceptable or unacceptable with a simple plus sign (+) or minus sign (–), respectively. A solution was then identified that was rated as acceptable by both parties. Typically, neither party got his or her most highly preferred solution, but both were encouraged to compromise. Taylor and his mother would then employ the chosen solution over the following week and discuss its efficacy at the next session, at which time the therapist would help to troubleshoot any obstacles or revisit the solutions list to identify an alternative solution.

As another goal of PSCT, the therapist helped create a behavioral system that allowed Taylor to earn privileges based on compliance with specific behavioral expectations. This behavior system was formalized in a written and signed behavior contract (see Figure 9.1). Specific behavioral targets for Taylor included asking teachers to sign his planner at the end of each class period; using a polite tone of voice; completing his homework before 8 P.M.;

Behavior Contract

I, Taylor S., agree to do the following on a daily basis:
- Close and lock the front door after leaving for school.
- Take ADHD medication.
- Have all of my teachers sign my planner.
- Complete my homework each night before 8:00 P.M.

I, Mrs. S., agree to provide the following privileges if Taylor completes the above:
- Daily: up to 1 hour of television and/or computer time after completion of homework.
- Weekly: an outing with friends, if Taylor earns daily privileges on 4/5 weekdays.
- Taylor may also earn 1 point per day for completing the above; when he earns 30 points, he may have use of a cell phone.

I, Mrs. S., also agree to remove the following privileges if Taylor does not complete the above:
- Loss of television and/or computer time that day.

This contract may be renegotiated at any time by mutual agreement between Taylor and Mrs. S.

Signed,

_____

Taylor S.

_____

Mrs. S.

FIGURE 9.1. Sample parent–teen behavior contract.

taking his medication; closing and locking the front door each morning; remembering to bring all school materials and sports equipment to school; and complying with one- or two-step requests immediately when asked. Typically, only four to five behaviors were included on the behavior chart at any one time, including behaviors with high, medium, and low probability of success. The notion of earning privileges was explained to Taylor as a means of "getting credit" for complying with expectations. Privileges to be earned included daily rewards, such as computer and TV time, as well as weekly rewards (e.g., a weekend outing with friends) and longer term rewards (e.g., a cell phone). Together with the therapist, Taylor and his mother identified rewards that his mother (and father, when he was home) would be able to realistically and consistently implement.

Also incorporated into PSCT is an emphasis on using cognitive therapy principles to create reasonable expectations for Taylor's behavior and reasonable rewards and consequences that his mother could realistically implement. The therapist also used cognitive restructuring in regard to how both Mrs. S. and Taylor thought about his behavior, as well as negativistic thoughts about each other (e.g., "He's defying me on purpose" and "She's so unfair"), with the goal of reducing conflict between them. Approximately once a month, Mr. S. attended therapy as well in order to provide input on the behavior plan and learn to consistently implement these strategies when he was home and to support the system even when he was away from home.

Parent Counseling

Cognitive therapy principles were employed with Mrs. S. to address negative views of herself as a parent. For example, she expressed a lack of confidence in her parenting abilities in thoughts such as "He'll never listen to me," "I won't be able to follow through," and "I should've started making changes a long time ago." Identifying these negative thoughts about herself helped the therapist and Mrs. S. to identify a negative core belief: "I'm a weak parent." The therapist used Socratic questioning to challenge her negative automatic thoughts. For example, negative expectations about the outcome of her parenting efforts, such as "He'll never listen to me" were challenged with questions such as "Do I know for sure that he won't listen?" "Where is the evidence that he won't listen, and where's the evidence that he will listen?" and "What would you suggest to a friend who was having trouble getting her child to listen to her?" Ultimately, the therapist and Mrs. S. were able to challenge the core belief that she is a weak parent and to think about herself and her parenting in a more realistic way (e.g., "I am working to improve my parenting of a child who requires specialized parenting").

School

A variety of problem-solving and cognitive-behavioral strategies were employed to target the specific goal of improving Taylor's academic performance. One of Taylor's biggest areas of difficulty was that he frequently did not earn credit on his homework assignments, either because he didn't do them or because he forgot to turn them in. Taylor frequently told his mother that he did not have homework, but she did not know whether Taylor was being deliberately untruthful, whether he did not remember, or whether he was correct. This caused nightly arguments between Taylor and his mother about whether or not he had homework to do. Through the problem-solving method, Taylor and his mother decided that having teachers sign his planner at the end of each class period would help with the goal of completing homework. Behavioral strategies included using a timer to complete a homework assignment within a certain time frame, and "finishing homework assignments" was added to the behavior plan for which Taylor earned access to privileges. Mrs. S. also began corresponding with teachers via email on a weekly basis to facilitate better communication, rather than waiting to receive a progress report to learn of Taylor's performance.

Medication

Despite a good effort on Taylor's part to implement the strategies learned in therapy, his academic performance had not substantially improved by the end of the second quarter. Although all parties had agreed to resume medication under such circumstances, Taylor balked at this. To address his concerns about medication, a sports-related analogy was discussed via Socratic questioning to explain the deficits inherent in ADHD and to cognitively reframe the purpose of taking medication:

THERAPIST: So, are you a fast runner, Taylor?

TAYLOR: Yup.

THERAPIST: If you and your best friend ran a race, who would win?

TAYLOR: I would.

THERAPIST: OK. But who would win if you had 10-pound weights around your ankles?

TAYLOR: I guess my friend would.

THERAPIST: Is that because he is faster than you?

TAYLOR: No, it's because I have weights around my ankles that slow me down.

THERAPIST: Exactly. And having ADHD is like running a race with weights tied to your legs. You may be a fast runner but because of the ADHD "weight," you will not be able to run as fast as you can. Taking medication removes some of the ADHD "weight," which then allows you to run up to your ability.

Psychoeducation on the effects of medication on the brain, as well as cognitive restructuring, were also employed to address Taylor's (and, during a family session, his father's) perspective on medication. For example, cognitive restructuring was used to address his negative thoughts about himself as a person who takes medication (e.g., "I'm weird"): "Everybody has different areas of strength and difficulty, and many areas of difficulty, like ADHD, are invisible." Taylor and the therapist also generated a list of celebrities who have publicly disclosed their ADHD diagnoses, in order to demonstrate that ADHD is a common disorder and that many successful people struggle with it. Through such efforts, Taylor was receptive to another medication trial. Under the care of his pediatrician, he resumed taking a stimulant medication that had previously worked for him. The medication was closely monitored for the appetite-suppression side effect that he had experienced before. "Taking medication daily" was added to the behavior contingency chart. Over time, Taylor observed numerous medication benefits and therefore became more accepting of this form of treatment.

Outcome

After 6 months of weekly therapy, Taylor had improved his academic performance, and both Taylor and Mrs. S. reported that they were getting along much better at home. Both parents demonstrated an ability to implement the behavior plan and make adjustments as needed, and Taylor was consistently earning most privileges. They also repeatedly provided examples in session of successfully using problem-solving and positive communication skills to address conflicts at home. A booster session was offered about a month later, at which time Taylor and Mrs. S. reported ongoing success, and all parties agreed to end therapy.

Treatments for Older Adolescents in College

Over the past few years there has been a surge of interest in the impact that psychosocial interventions may have on college students with ADHD (He & Antshel, 2016). Initial research efforts examined this issue from a diverse array of therapeutic perspectives, including cognitive-behavioral therapy (CBT; Anastopoulos & King, 2015; Eddy, Canu, Broman-Fulks, & Michael, 2015; LaCount, Hartung, Shelton, Clapp, & Clapp, 2015), dialectical behavior therapy (DBT; Fleming, McMahon, Moran, Peterson, & Dreessen, 2015), coaching (Prevatt & Yelland, 2015), self-monitoring (Scheithauer & Kelley, 2014), and organization, time-management, and planning (OTMP) skills training (LaCount, Hartung, Shelton, & Stevens, 2015).

Generally speaking, findings from these initial investigations have revealed significant improvements in primary ADHD symptoms (Anastopoulos & King, 2015; Eddy et al., 2015; Fleming et al., 2015; LaCount, Hartung, Shelton, Clapp, & Clapp, 2015) and self-reported executive functioning (Anastopoulos & King, 2015; Fleming et al., 2015). Results have been mixed with respect to reductions in comorbid depression and anxiety symptoms (Anastopoulos & King, 2015; Fleming et al., 2015). Although there have been reports of improvements in self-reported learning strategies (LaCount, Hartung, Shelton, & Stevens, 2015; Prevatt & Yelland, 2015) and increased use of disability services and other campus resources (Anastopoulos & King,

2015), corresponding changes in GPA have thus far not been reliably demonstrated (Anastopoulos & King, 2015; Fleming et al., 2015).

Taken together, results from this emerging literature offer much promise for the role that psychosocial interventions may ultimately play in the overall clinical management of college students with ADHD. To give readers a better understanding of how treatment might be delivered to an older adolescent with ADHD in college, we present the following case study, describing a college student who participated in ACCESS (Accessing Campus Connections and Empowering Student Success), a psychosocial intervention that we developed, pilot tested (Anastopoulos & King, 2015), and are now in the process of examining in the context of a large-scale, multisite randomized controlled trial.

Case Example: An Older Adolescent in College

Background

At the time she underwent treatment, Nicole was an 18-year-old student enrolled in her first year of college. Nicole had initially been diagnosed with ADHD at 9 years of age by her family physician. From that time through her enrollment in college, she had taken stimulant medication for her ADHD. In addition, she received Section 504 Plan accommodations to address her ADHD during her elementary and middle school years, and intermittently participated in individual counseling to address self-esteem issues as well. Despite her having access to treatment resources, Nicole's parents and teachers frequently complained that she was not working up to her capabilities, especially when she received D grades in two of her required classes. Nicole's friends also complained that she was "rude" and inconsiderate because she regularly interrupted them and did not follow through on social commitments. Additional difficulties occurred in her job as a server in a restaurant, where her supervisor would often reprimand her for being inattentive to customers, forgetting their orders, and at times misplacing their bills or payments.

Nicole learned about the availability of treatment for her ADHD in college during a summer freshman orientation session. Prior to her receiving treatment, however, it was first necessary for her to undergo a screening evaluation, the main purpose of which was to confirm her ADHD diagnosis, to screen for co-occurring mental health conditions, and to determine that the available treatment was a good fit for her needs. The screening evaluation, which followed the format of the multimethod, multi-informant assessment approach described earlier, did indeed confirm that Nicole met DSM-5 criteria for ADHD, Combined presentation. At the same time, however, this evaluation also revealed that Nicole was dealing with anxiety symptoms that met criteria for GAD. Although she had never been formally diagnosed with GAD, Nicole was not surprised to receive this diagnostic feedback, because she acknowledged that for the past few years she had been worrying several hours each day over a multitude of things, including her grades, her friends, her family, money matters, losing things, and being fired from her job.

Based upon the results of this screening evaluation, it was clear that Nicole was a good candidate to receive the cognitive-behavioral treatment that was available to her on campus. She began this program in the fall semester of her first year in college.

Accessing Campus Connections and Empowering Student Success

Nicole received cognitive-behavioral treatment in the context of ACCESS. A detailed description of the rationale, nature, and development of this program may be found elsewhere (Anastopoulos & King, 2015). Briefly, ACCESS is delivered via group therapy and individual mentoring across two consecutive semesters, the first of which is an 8-week active phase, followed by a maintenance phase. The goals of ACCESS are to (1) increase knowledge of ADHD and awareness of campus resources, (2) improve organization, time-management, and other behavioral skills, and (3) increase adaptive thinking via restructuring and other cognitive therapy techniques. To the extent these goals are achieved, improvements in ADHD symptoms and other domains of functioning are expected to occur. Within ACCESS, therefore, knowledge of ADHD, behavioral strategies, and adaptive thinking are conceptualized as the mechanisms of clinical change responsible for improvements in functioning.

Nicole participated actively in the CBT group sessions, attending all but one of the eight planned 90-minute sessions (see Table 9.2). In discussions covering knowledge of ADHD, she openly shared personal life experiences and expressed great appreciation for gaining a new understanding of ADHD that allowed her to view her past, as well as her future, in a less critical and more optimistic light. Hearing similar stories from others in the group in particular allowed her to realize that she was not "weird" and that she was not alone in her daily efforts to deal with ADHD. Moreover, she came to realize that treatments other than stimulant medication needed to be in place to address not only her ADHD but also the generalized anxiety she had been experiencing. Although Nicole was open to trying some of the new behavioral strategies for improving her organization and planning, there were times when she voiced resistance to trying new behavioral techniques. For example, when discussing time-management strategies for completing papers, she noted that procrastination had "worked" for her in the past. Using Socratic questioning, this belief was challenged and ultimately reconceptualized ("The data do not support this belief, and so I need to consider an alternative approach"), leading her to use a more effective approach to completing papers. During the CBT portion of the group, Nicole easily and freely provided examples of maladaptive thinking related to her constant worrying. With input from the group leader, as well as from other group members, she generally was able to develop alternative, more realistic thoughts that served to reduce her worrying.

Concurrent with the eight weekly group CBT sessions, Nicole received one-on-one mentoring sessions and attended all of her scheduled mentoring appointments. She benefited greatly from using her mentoring sessions as a vehicle for reviewing and refining what she had learned in the CBT group. Consistent with another objective of the mentoring process, Nicole enjoyed receiving guidance on setting short- and long-term goals pertaining not only to school-related objectives but also to various personal goals. In consultation with her supportive mentor, she also learned about various

TABLE 9.2. Session-by-Session Outline of the ACCESS Program

Session	ADHD knowledge	Behavioral strategies	Cognitive therapy
1	• Introduction to ACCESS What is ADHD?	• Assessing campus resources	• What is cognitive therapy?
2	• What causes ADHD?	• Choosing tools: using a planner and notebook	• Recognizing maladaptive thinking (MAT)
3	• Assessment of ADHD	• Getting organized	• Replacing MAT with adaptive thinking (AT)
4	• How does ADHD affect school? • Does ADHD only affect school?	• Getting the most from classes	• How can AT help manage ADHD and improve schoolwork?
5	• Depression, anxiety, and other things that may go with ADHD • Sex, drugs, and ADHD	• Studying effectively	• Dealing with emotions and resisting harmful temptations
6	• What medications are used to treat ADHD?	• Taking exams • Managing papers and long-term projects	• Sticking with treatment
7	• Is medication the only way to treat ADHD?	• Healthy lifestyle • Handling relationships	• Improving relations with friends and family
8	• A look into the future	• Setting long-term goals • Maintaining your skills	• An (AT) look into the future • Relapse prevention

resources on campus that might benefit her and ultimately agreed (1) to register with the disability service office in order to receive accommodations in some of her courses and (2) to begin receiving regular, individually delivered CBT services from the counseling center on campus to address her excessive worrying.

By the end of the active phase of ACCESS, Nicole had learned a great deal more about ADHD, developed more effective study strategies, learned to stick to a study schedule, and learned better note-taking procedures and test-taking strategies. In addition, she developed better time awareness with respect to both her schoolwork and her social life and improved in her use of "to do" lists and in setting reminder alarms. She also developed better awareness of how her thought patterns were related to her worrying tendencies, which in turn allowed her to begin the process of bringing her anxiety under better control. Additional work on her anxiety was in progress through her participation in individual CBT sessions at the campus counseling center. Nicole was also registered with and utilizing academic accommodations through the disability services office and participated in campus tutoring as well. Together, such changes very likely were at least partially responsible for her receiving fall semester grades that represented a definite improvement over grades she had been receiving in high school.

During the following maintenance phase semester, Nicole attended a required group CBT booster session, as well as five mentoring sessions. She continued to have a strong relationship with her mentor and was eager to meet with her. She stated that her transition to the new semester was easier than she had anticipated because, for the most part, she was continuing to use the knowledge and strategies she had learned from the active phase of the ACCESS program. Overall, Nicole was extremely pleased with the considerable progress she had made and expressed much gratitude for the valuable support she had received from the ACCESS staff.

Summary and Conclusions

Although traditional cognitive therapy approaches may not be well suited to reducing primary ADHD symptoms (i.e., inattention, hyperactivity–impulsivity), the manner in which ADHD presents itself clinically affords practitioners ample opportunities for incorporating cognitive therapy strategies in the clinical management of children and adolescents with ADHD. This chapter illustrated many of the ways in which such cognitive therapy opportunities might arise (see Table 9.3). There are likely many other ways in which cognitive therapy can be used, limited only by the clinical situations that present themselves. Our hope, therefore, is that readers are now more aware of, and more open to, incorporating cognitive therapy strategies in their provision of clinical services to children and adolescents with ADHD.

TABLE 9.3. Examples of Cognitive Distortions Related to ADHD

Unrealistic thoughts	Parent	Child/adolescent
About ADHD	"ADHD is just an excuse for bad behavior."	"I can't control myself because I have ADHD."
About oneself	"I must be a lousy parent because I cannot control my child."	"I never do anything right."
About others	"My child is just lazy; he never listens to me."	"My mom is always picking on me; no one likes me."
About future	"If this keeps up, my child will never get into college."	"I'll never get my homework done tonight so I won't even try."
About adherence to treatment	"We tried this before and nothing works; my spouse will never agree to this."	"I don't want to be different from the other kids."

References

Abikoff, H. (1985). Efficacy of cognitive training interventions: A critical review. *Clinical Psychology Review, 5,* 479–512.

Abikoff, H., Gallagher, R., Wells, K. C., Murray, D. K., Huang, L., Lu, F., et al. (2013). Remediating organizational functioning in children with ADHD: Immediate and long-term effects from a randomized controlled trial. *Journal of Consulting and Clinical Psychology, 81,* 113–128.

Achenbach, T. M. (2009). *The Achenbach System of Empirically Based Assessment (AESBA): Development, findings, theory, and applications.* Burlington: University of Vermont Research Center for Children, Youth, and Families.

American Psychiatric Association. (2013). *Diagnostic and statistical manual of mental disorders* (5th ed.). Arlington, VA: Author.

Anastopoulos, A. D., DuPaul, G. J., Weyandt, L. L., Morrissey-Kane, E., Sommer, J. L., Rhoads, L. H., et al. (2016). Rates and patterns of comorbidity among first-year college students with ADHD. *Journal of Clinical Child and Adolescent Psychology.* Available at *www.tandfonline.com/doi/abs/10.1080/15374 416.2015.1105137?journalCode=hcap20.*

Anastopoulos, A. D., & King, K. A. (2015). A cognitive-behavior therapy and mentoring program for college students with ADHD. *Cognitive Behavioral Practice, 22,* 141–151.

Anastopoulos, A. D., Rhoads, L. H., & Farley, S. E. (2006). Counseling and training parents. In R. A. Barkley, *Attention deficit hyperactivity disorder: A handbook for diagnosis and treatment* (3rd ed., pp. 453–479). New York: Guilford Press.

Anastopoulos, A. D., & Shelton, T. L. (2001). *Assessing attention-deficit/hyperactivity disorder.* New York: Kluwer Academic/Plenum.

Angold, A., Costello, E. J., & Erkanli, A. (1999). Comorbidity. *Journal of Child Psychology and Psychiatry, 40,* 57–87.

Angold, A., Prendergast, M., Cox, A., Harrington, R., Simonoff, E., & Rutter, M. (1995). The Child and Adolescent Psychiatric Assessment (CAPA). *Psychological Medicine, 25,* 739–753.

Bagwell, C. L., Molina, B., Pelham, W. E., & Hoza, B. (2001). Attention-deficit hyperactivity disorder and problems in peer relations: Predictions from childhood to adolescence. *Journal of the American Academy of Child and Adolescent Psychiatry, 40,* 1285–1292.

Barkley, R. A. (2013). *Defiant children: A clinician's manual for assessment and parent training* (3rd ed.). New York: Guilford Press.

Barkley, R. A. (Ed.). (2015). *Attention-deficit/hyperactivity disorder* (4th ed.). New York: Guilford Press.

Barkley, R. A., Anastopoulos, A. D., Guevremont, D. C., & Fletcher, K. E. (1992). Adolescents with attention deficit hyperactivity disorder: Mother–adolescent interactions, family beliefs and conflicts, and maternal psychopathology. *Journal of Abnormal Child Psychology, 20,* 263–288.

Barkley, R. A., Edwards, G., Laneri, M., Fletcher, K., & Metevia, L. (2001). The efficacy of problem-solving communication training alone, behavior management training alone, and their combination for parent–adolescent conflict in teenagers with ADHD and ODD. *Journal of Consulting and Clinical Psychology, 69,* 926–941.

Barkley, R. A., Guevremont, D. G., Anastopoulos, A. D., DuPaul, G. J., & Shelton, T. L. (1993). Driving-related risks and outcomes of attention deficit hyperactivity disorder in adolescents and young adults: A 3- to 5-year follow-up survey. *Pediatrics, 92,* 212–218.

Barkley, R. A., Guevremont, D. C., Anastopoulos, A. D., & Fletcher, K. E. (1992). A comparison of three family therapy programs for treating family conflicts in adolescents with attention-deficit hyperactivity disorder. *Journal of Consulting and Clinical Psychology, 60*(3), 450–462.

Barkley, R. A., Murphy, K. R., & Fischer, M. (2008). *ADHD in adults: What the science says.* New York: Guilford Press.

Barkley, R. A., & Robin, A. L. (2014). *Defiant teens: A clinician's manual for assessment and family intervention* (2nd ed.). New York: Guilford Press.

Chambless, D. L., & Hollon, S. D. (1998). Defining empirically supported therapies. *Journal of Consulting and Clinical Psychology, 66*(1), 7–18.

Conners, C. K. (2008a). *Conners 3rd edition.* North Tonawanda, NY: Multi-Health Systems.

Conners, C. K. (2008b). *Conners Comprehensive Behavior Rating Scales.* North Tonawanda, NY: Multi-Health Systems.

Conners, C. K. (2009). *Conners Early Childhood.* North Tonawanda, NY: Multi-Health Systems.

Cunningham, C. E., Bremner, R. B., & Secord-Gilbert, M. (1998). *COPE, the Community Parent Education Program: A school based family systems oriented workshop for parents of children with disruptive behavior disorders (Leader's manual).* Hamilton, Ontario, Canada: COPE Works.

DuPaul, G. J., Power, T. J., Anastopoulos, A. D., & Reid, R. (2016). *ADHD Rating Scale—5 for Children and Adolescents.* New York: Guilford Press.

DuPaul, G. J., & Stoner, G. (2015). *ADHD in the schools: Assessment and intervention strategies* (3rd ed.). New York: Guilford Press.

DuPaul, G. J., Weyandt, L. L., O'Dell, S. M., & Varejao, M. (2009). College students with ADHD: Current status and future directions. *Journal of Attention Disorders, 13*(3), 234–250.

Eddy, L. D., Canu, W. H., Broman-Fulks, J. J., & Michael, K. D. (2015). Brief cognitive behavioral therapy for college students with ADHD: A case series report. *Cognitive and Behavioral Practice, 22*(2), 127–140.

Elia, J., Ambrosini, P., & Berrettini, W. (2008). ADHD characteristics: I. Concurrent co-morbidity patterns in children and adolescents. *Child and Adolescent Psychiatry and Mental Health, 2*. Available at *https://capmh.biomedcentral.com/articles/10.1186/1753-2000-2-15*.

Evans, S. W., Owens, J. S., & Bunford, N. (2014). Evidence-based psychosocial treatments for children and adolescents with attention-deficit/hyperactivity disorder. *Journal of Clinical Child and Adolescent Psychology, 43*(4), 527–551.

Evans, S. W., Schultz, B. K., DeMars, C. E., & Davis, H. (2011). Effectiveness of the Challenging Horizons After-School Program for young adolescents with ADHD. *Behavior Therapy, 42*, 462–474.

Fleming, A. P., McMahon, R. J., Moran, L. R., Peterson, A. P., & Dreessen, A. (2015). Pilot randomized controlled trial of dialectical behavior therapy group skills training for ADHD among college students. *Journal of Attention Disorders, 19*(3), 260–271.

Flory, K., Molina, B. S. G., Pelham, W. E., Jr., Gnagy, E., & Smith, D. (2006). Childhood ADHD predicts risky sexual behavior in young adulthood. *Journal of Clinical Child and Adolescent Psychology, 35*, 571–577.

Gallagher, R., Abikoff, H., & Spira, E. G. (2014). *Organizational skills training for ADHD: An empirically supported treatment.* New York: Guilford Press.

He, J. A., & Antshel, K. M. (2016). Cognitive behavioral therapy for attention-deficit/hyperactivity disorder in college students: A review of the literature. *Cognitive and Behavioral Practice*. Available at *www.sciencedirect.com/science/article/pii/S1077722916300268*.

Johnston, C., & Mash, E. J. (2001). Families of children with attention-deficit/hyperactivity disorder: Review and recommendations for future research. *Clinical Child and Family Psychology Review, 4*, 183–207.

Kaufman, J., Birmaher, B., Brent, D., Rao, U., Flynn, C., Moreci, P., et al. (1997). Schedule for Affective Disorders and Schizophrenia in School-Age Children—Present and Lifetime Version (K-SADS-PL): Initial reliability and validity data. *Journal of the American Academy of Child and Adolescent Psychiatry, 36*, 980–988.

Kendall, P. C., & Braswell, L. (1982). Cognitive-behavioral self-control therapy for children: A components analysis. *Journal of Consulting and Clinical Psychology, 50*, 672–689.

Kern, R. M., Rasmussen, P. R., Byrd, S. L., & Wittschen, L. K. (1999). Lifestyle, personality, and attention deficit hyperactivity disorder in young adults. *Journal of Individual Psychology, 55*, 186–199.

Klimkeit, E., Graham, C., Lee, P., Morling, M., Russo, D., & Tonge, B. (2006). Children should be seen and heard. Self-report of feelings and behaviors in primary-school-age children with ADHD. *Journal of Attention Disorders, 10,* 181–191.

LaCount, P. A., Hartung, C. M., Shelton, C. R., Clapp, J. D., & Clapp, T. K. W. (2015). Preliminary evaluation of a combined group and individual treatment for college students with attention-deficit/hyperactivity disorder. *Cognitive and Behavioral Practice, 22*(2), 152–160.

LaCount, P. A., Hartung, C. M., Shelton, C. R., & Stevens, A. E. (2015). Efficacy of an organizational skills intervention for college students with ADHD symptomatology and academic difficulties. *Journal of Attention Disorders.* Available at *www.researchgate.net/profile/Patrick_Lacount2/publication/280867081_Efficacy_of_an_Organizational_Skills_Intervention_for_College_Students_With_ADHD_Symptomatology_and_Academic_Difficulties/links/55cb618e08aeb975674c71ae.pdf.*

Langberg, J. M., Epstein, J. N., Becker, S. P., Girio-Herrera, E., & Vaughn, A. J. (2012). Evaluation of the homework, organization, and planning skills (HOPS) intervention for middle school students with attention deficit hyperactivity disorder as implemented by school mental health providers. *School Psychology Review, 41,* 342–364.

Meichenbaum, D. H., & Goodman, J. (1971). Training impulsive children to talk to themselves: A means of developing self-control. *Journal of Abnormal Psychology, 77*(2), 115–126.

Molina, B. S., Flory, K., Bukstein, O. G., Greiner, A. R., Baker, J. L., Krug, V., et al. (2008). Feasibility and preliminary efficacy of an after-school program for middle schoolers with ADHD: A randomized trial in a large public middle school. *Journal of Attention Disorders, 12,* 207–217.

Molina, B. S., Marshal, M. P., Pelham, W. E., & Wirth, R. J. (2005). Coping skills and parent support mediate the association between childhood attention-deficit/hyperactivity disorder and adolescent cigarette use. *Journal of Pediatric Psychology, 30*(4), 345–357.

Norwalk, K., Norvilitis, J. M., & MacLean, M. G. (2009). ADHD symptomatology and its relationship to factors associated with college adjustment. *Journal of Attention Disorders, 13,* 251–258.

Pelham, W. J., & Fabiano, G. A. (2008). Evidence-based psychosocial treatments for attention-deficit/hyperactivity disorder. *Journal of Clinical Child and Adolescent Psychology, 37,* 184–214.

Pelham, W. J., Wheeler, T., & Chronis, A. (1998). Empirically supported psychosocial treatments for attention deficit hyperactivity disorder. *Journal of Clinical Child Psychology, 27*(2), 190–205.

Pliszka, S. R. (2015). Comorbid psychiatric disorders in children. In R. A. Barkley (Ed.), *Attention-deficit/hyperactivity disorder* (4th ed., pp. 140–168). New York: Guilford Press.

Prevatt, F., & Yelland, S. (2015). An empirical evaluation of ADHD coaching in college students. *Journal of Attention Disorders, 19,* 666–677.

Reich, W., Welner, Z., Herjanic, B., & MHS Staff. (1996). *Diagnostic Interview for Children and Adolescents—IV Computer Program (DICA-IV).* New York: MultiHealth Systems.

Reynolds, C. R. & Kamphaus, R. W. (2015). *Behavior Assessment System for Children, Third Edition.* Bloomington, MN: PsychCorp.

Robin, A. L., & Foster, S. (1989). *Negotiating parent–adolescent conflict.* New York: Guilford Press.

Scheithauer, M. C., & Kelley, M. L. (2014). Self-monitoring by college students with ADHD: The impact on academic performance. *Journal of Attention Disorders.* Available at *http://journals.sagepub.com/doi/abs/10.1177/1087054714553050.*

Shaffer, D., Fisher, P., Lucas, C., Dulcan, M., & Schwab-Stone, M. (2000). NIMH Diagnostic Interview Schedule for Children, Version IV (NIMH DISC-IV): Description, differences from previous versions, and reliability of some common diagnoses. *Journal of the American Academy of Child and Adolescent Psychiatry, 39,* 28–38.

Shaw-Zirt, B., Popali-Lehane, L., Chaplin, W., & Bergman, A. (2005). Adjustment, social skills, and self-esteem in college students with symptoms of ADHD. *Journal of Attention Disorders, 8,* 109–120.

Swanson, J. M. (1992). *School-based assessments and interventions for ADD students.* Irvine, CA: KC Publishing.

Wolraich, M. L., Feurer, I., Hannah, J. N., Pinnock, T. Y. & Baumgaertel, A. (1998). Obtaining systematic teacher reports of disruptive behavior disorders utilizing DSM-IV. *Journal of Abnormal Child Psychology, 26,* 141–152.

CHAPTER TEN

Treatment of Eating Disorders

Kristen M. Culbert
Kristen Anderson
Wayne A. Bowers
Daniel Le Grange

We review the clinical features and evidence-based treatments for eating disorders, with particular consideration to interventions that are developmentally appropriate for youth. Because there is relatively limited research on the treatment of eating disorders in youth, we briefly review empirical support for cognitive-behavioral therapy (CBT) for eating disorders in adults, followed by an overview of their application to youth. Empirical support for family-based treatment (FBT) for eating disorders is also reviewed, as FBT was specifically developed for children and adolescents.[1] Finally, we provide case examples within our presentation and discuss important future directions.

---

[1] FBT for eating disorders, as described herein, is not based on a family-systems approach. FBT focuses on behavioral recovery, which occurs as a result of the parents working together to eliminate the child's problematic eating disorder behaviors and, in the case of anorexia nervosa, to help their child achieve appropriate weight restoration. Although behavioral theory is not a formal component of FBT, the ways in which parents intervene may involve behavioral principles, and improvements in family functioning and cognitive changes often indirectly occur following the implementation of this treatment. Along these lines, FBT could be considered (albeit not in a strict sense) a behavioral-based therapy or variant of CBT that deemphasizes cognitive change.

Eating Disorder Diagnoses and Phenomenology

Eating disorders are broadly characterized by disturbances in eating behaviors and attitudes toward one's body shape and weight, which result in several psychosocial impairments and medical complications (American Psychiatric Association, 2013). Eating disorders typically onset during adolescence or early young adulthood and are more common in females than males (female-to-male prevalence ratio approximately 2:1–10:1; American Psychiatric Association, 2013). DSM-5 recognizes three primary eating disorder diagnoses—anorexia nervosa (AN), bulimia nervosa (BN), and binge-eating disorder (BED)—as well as residual diagnostic categories—other specified feeding or eating disorder (OSFED) and unspecified feeding or eating disorder (UFED)—that were previously referred to as eating disorder not otherwise specified (EDNOS) in DSM-IV-TR. The residual categories can encompass a wide variety of clinical presentations, such as subthreshold cases of AN, BN, or BED; individuals of normal weight status who engage in recurrent episodes of purging in the absence of binge eating; and individuals who endorse atypical eating behaviors (American Psychiatric Association, 2013).

AN is marked by disturbances in attitudes and perceptions toward body weight and shape and the maintenance of a low body weight (i.e., body weight less than minimally expected for one's age, gender, developmental trajectory, and physical health; American Psychiatric Association, 2013). Low body weight is often achieved via extreme caloric restriction and increased physical activity. Although disturbances in attitudes and perceptions toward weight and shape are also a key feature of BN, persons with BN have an average to elevated body weight (American Psychiatric Association, 2013). Core symptoms of BN include recurrent episodes of binge eating (i.e., consumption of an objectively large amount of food within a short amount of time and feeling loss of control during the episode) and the use of inappropriate compensatory behaviors (e.g., self-induced vomiting, excessive exercise, misuse of laxatives, diuretics, or enemas; American Psychiatric Association, 2013). The exclusionary criterion for BN (i.e., that diagnostic criteria for AN cannot be met) is important to ensure that individuals do not receive more than one current eating disorder diagnosis (American Psychiatric Association, 2013). Indeed, a substantial proportion of individuals with AN engage in binge eating and/or compensatory behaviors (e.g., AN binge–purge subtype; American Psychiatric Association, 2013; Eddy et al., 2002; Eddy, Dorer, et al., 2008), and thus low weight status can be a primary distinguishing difference between the diagnosis of AN versus BN. By definition, there are no specific diagnostic criteria for the residual eating disorder categories, but clinical features of persons diagnosed within these categories often resemble those of AN and BN and are of similar duration and severity (Allen, Byrne, Oddy, & Crosby, 2013; Le Grange et al., 2012). Notably, based on DSM-IV-TR criteria, approximately 40–70% of eating disorder cases received an EDNOS diagnosis. Modifications to criteria in DSM-5 (e.g., reducing the frequency requirement for recurrent binge eating and purging from twice a week to once a week; recognizing BED as a stand-alone disorder) have substantially reduced the number of cases falling within the residual diagnostic categories, but estimates are still quite high (i.e., 15–30%; Allen et al., 2013). An "unspecified/other" eating disorder diagnosis therefore is the most common but least studied eating disorder in adolescence (Allen et al., 2013; Eddy, Celio-Doyle, Rienecke Hoste, Herzog, & Le Grange, 2008) and adulthood (e.g., Keel, Brown, Holm-Denoma, & Bodell, 2011).

In addition to the diagnostic criteria, additional features may occur in persons with eating disorders. For example, distortion of body size and shape (Mohr et al., 2011), cognitive preoccupation with body weight and food (Brooks, Prince, Stahl, Campbell, & Treasure, 2011), frequent weighing of oneself or body-checking behavior (Kachani, Brasiliano, Cordás, & Hochgraf, 2013), and social withdrawal are commonly present (Wolff & Treasure, 2011). Medical consequences as a result of eating disorder symptoms (e.g., low heart rate and cardiovascular problems, dehydration, electrolyte and mineral disturbances, disruptions in bowel functioning, kidney dysfunction) are also frequently observed and may complicate treatment, particularly in outpatient treatment settings (Wolff & Treasure, 2011). Psychiatric comorbidities (e.g., Swanson et al., 2011; Wolff & Treasure, 2011), such as depression, anxiety, and obsessive–compulsive disorders, as well as personality vulnerabilities (e.g., impulsivity; Wonderlich, Connolly, & Stice, 2004), self-injurious behavior (e.g., cutting; Stein, Lilenfeld, Wildman, & Marcus, 2004), and suicidal ideation (Stein et al., 2004) are also common and often need to be addressed.

Persons with eating disorders often view their difficulties as ego-syntonic and thus may deny the seriousness of the illness and view their behavior as reasonable (Bowers, Evans, Le Grange, & Andersen, 2003). The ego-syntonic nature of eating disorders can complicate both assessment (e.g., denial or underreporting of symptoms) and treatment (e.g., interference with motivation and the development of a collaborative relationship). Moreover, the treatment of adolescents with eating disorders is often initiated by their parents, and thus the pursuit of therapy may be involuntary, and noncompliance or disengagement in the therapy can result (Bowers et al., 2003). It is perhaps not surprising that leading empirically supported treatments for adolescents with eating disorders stress the importance of parental involvement, either to aid in the facilitation of the goals of individual-based therapy (e.g., CBT; Cooper & Stewart, 2008; Wilson & Sysko, 2006) or as the primary mechanism for facilitating symptom change in FBT (Le Grange & Lock, 2010; Lock & Le Grange, 2013).

Diagnostic Assessment

The diagnostic assessment with an adolescent is largely similar to that with an adult, with the exception of parental involvement. The initial evaluation and diagnostic assessment aims to establish the presenting concerns, history of the problem, prior treatment and medical history, academic and social functioning, and, importantly, a detailed account of eating disorder symptoms and comorbid psychopathology. The assessment collects information about the presenting difficulties from the perspective of both the parents and the adolescent, as the adolescent may deny symptoms or be unable to accurately or fully describe her or his thoughts and behaviors (Gowers & Bryant-Waugh, 2004). Further, it is advisable that both parents be present for the initial assessment, because this can provide a more comprehensive account and description of the adolescent's difficulties. The presence of both parents also serves to indirectly communicate that there is collective concern about the child's well-being and desire to support her or him in treatment. Semistructured interviews, such as the Eating Disorder Examination (EDE) or Kiddie Schedule for Affective Disorders and Schizophrenia (K-SADS) and the modified version of the EDE for parents (PEDE), are useful for collecting detailed information regarding the youth's overall symptom presentation (Couturier, Lock, Forsberg, Vanderheyden, & Yen, 2007). Semistructured interviews ensure that the broad range of eating disorder symptoms (e.g., extent of dietary restriction, objective vs. subjective binge episodes, beliefs about body weight and shape, purging behavior) and comorbid diagnoses (e.g., anxiety, depression) are thoroughly assessed. Information obtained from clinical interviews can be integrated across informants to provide an overall picture of the youth's current and past difficulties and can serve to determine the most suitable treatment recommendations. Notably, parents may report more eating disorder symptoms or portray a more severe pattern of symptomatology than the child does (Couturier et al., 2007); however, it is also not uncommon for the teen to endorse symptoms (e.g., self-induced vomiting) that the parents were unaware of prior to the assessment. In addition to the psychological assessment, it is imperative for the adolescent to complete a medical evaluation and be deemed medically stable prior to the initiation of treatment (Cooper & Stewart, 2008; Le Grange & Lock, 2010).

Developmental Considerations

Several developmental issues are important in the treatment of youth with eating disorders. Normal developmental tasks, such as identity development, increases in autonomy, changes in interpersonal relationships (e.g., Meeus, Iedema, Helsen, & Vollebergh, 1999), and the physical, biological, and psychosocial changes associated with pubertal maturation (Klump, 2013), are often key issues relevant to the development, maintenance, and treatment of eating disorders. In addition, during an eating disorder, it is common for persons to show evidence of developmental regression. For example, teens may become more dependent on their parents and become socially withdrawn from their peers. Treatment will often need to address and facilitate the teen's return to normal adolescent development following symptom attenuation (Cooper & Stewart, 2008; Le Grange & Lock, 2010; Lock & Le Grange, 2013).

Given that social, emotional, and cognitive skills are less developed in children as compared with adults, a child's relative development on these skills is important in the selection and application of a treatment (Bowers et al., 2003). Indeed, formal thought and abstract reasoning skills develop during early to late adolescence. Adolescents may have difficulty articulating their internal experiences and difficulty linking their thoughts to their behavioral symptoms (Bravender et al., 2010; Gowers & Bryant-Waugh, 2004). Adolescents show substantial variation in their capacity for self-observation, self-reflection, and metacognitive abilities, as well as in their ability to integrate thoughts and emotions about themselves (Bowers et al., 2003; Rosso et al., 2004). Cognitive skills may be further hindered by cognitive deficits that arise secondary to the illness (e.g., being underweight), such as increased rigidity of beliefs or decreased capacity for self-reflection (Fairburn, 2008). Clinical practice with adolescents, therefore, requires careful consideration of individual differences in social, emotional, and cognitive ability levels.

The inclusion of parents and others (e.g., siblings, other caregivers) is often emphasized in the treatment of youth with eating disorders. Parents and family members can play a helpful role in recovery (Le Grange & Lock, 2010), and, if family-related issues become an obstacle to change, these issues can be addressed in treatment (Bowers et al., 2003). Moreover, it may be beneficial to acknowledge the ways in which a person's social system (e.g., parents, siblings, peers) may negatively (e.g., comments regarding dieting and body weight) or positively (e.g., eating meals as a family and providing support) influence recovery. It may also be helpful to discuss the ways in which a youth's eating disorder symptoms affect her or his social system, including disruptions in academic performance or family and social relationships. For example, prospective data have shown that parent–child conflict (e.g., hostility or discontent) can arise as a consequence of eating pathology (Spanos, Klump, Burt, McGue, & Iacono, 2010). Parents often describe dramatic changes in their child's thoughts, feelings, and behaviors, such as engaging in "devious" behavior to avoid weight gain (e.g., hiding food, lying about what was eaten; Cottee-Lane, Pistrang, & Bryant-Waugh, 2004). Managing these mood and behavioral challenges can result in caregivers' feeling increased sadness, distress, and frustration, as well as a diminished quality of life (e.g., putting family and personal activities on hold; Kyriacou, Treasure, & Schmidt, 2008). Thus efforts to reduce caregiver strain can be an important treatment consideration.

Identifying ways that the youth can use her or his social system to promote adaptive change and symptom reduction can be important in treatment (Cooper & Stewart, 2008; Le Grange & Lock, 2010). For example, the school may be identified as a resource for the facilitation of treatment goals, such as approving and monitoring the consumption of daily snacks and allowing parents to monitor and support their child during lunch. During treatment, the adolescent's siblings and friends can play a supportive role (e.g., providing comfort or distraction during or before and after meals). For example, in FBT, the therapist engages the family in conversations about how each member of the family is coping with the eating disorder and what can be done to provide support for their family member. In families in which there are no siblings or all siblings are living outside of the home, friends can play a similar role to siblings, if desired by the adolescent and her or his family. Similar conversations could also occur in CBT, and, if deemed suitable (by all involved parties), friends or siblings could be invited to attend a session if their involvement fits with an identified goal (e.g., to increase understanding and facilitate ways they may be able to provide support; Waller et al., 2007). Overall, the specific ways in which developmental considerations are taken into account may depend upon the therapeutic modality, but leading treatments (e.g., CBT, FBT) agree that parents can play a critical role in their child's recovery.

Empirically Supported Treatments

Emphasis is often placed on diagnostic distinctions between the eating disorders (e.g., AN vs. BN); however, crossover between eating disorder diagnoses is common (e.g., Eddy, Dorer, et al., 2008), and some researchers have begun to highlight similarities in symptoms shared across the diagnostic categories rather than focusing on the differences (see Table 10.1). Moreover, regardless of diagnosis, individuals with eating disorders often share a "core cognitive psychopathology" in that their self-worth is unduly tied to their body weight and shape and the perceived ability (or inability) to control them (Fairburn, 2008; Waller et al., 2007). Other eating disorder symptoms (e.g., dietary restriction, excessive exercising, binge eating, purging behaviors) typically develop secondary to this core cognitive psychopathology (Fairburn, 2008; Waller et al., 2007; see Table 10.1).

Conceptualizing eating disorders as a spectrum of presenting features that share a common core psychopathology has implications for etiology, maintenance, and treatment; this conceptualization also fits within the research domain criteria (RDoC) system in that etiological and maintenance

TABLE 10.1. Cognitive, Behavioral, and Physical Features of Eating Disorders

Eating disorder symptoms	AN	BN	BED	Unspecified/other diagnosis
Cognitive features				
Body dissatisfaction Dissatisfaction with the size and/or shape of one's body and/or specific body parts (e.g., stomach, thighs)	Yes (T)	Yes (T)	Yes (S)	Yes (S)
Weight concerns A preoccupation with one's body weight, a desire to lose weight, and the pursuit of thinness	Yes (T)	Yes (T)	Yes (S)	Yes (S)
Fear of weight gain Intense fear of weight gain or becoming fat	Yes (C)	Yes (T)	Yes (S)	Yes (S)
Overevaluation of body shape and weight Body shape and weight unduly influence one's scheme for self-evaluation	Yes (C)	Yes (C)	Yes (S)	Yes (S)
Behavioral features				
Binge eating The act of eating a large amount of food within in short period of time (e.g., 2 hours) and experiencing a lack of control over eating during the binge episode	Yes (S)	Yes (C)	Yes (C)	Yes (S)
Compensatory weight-control behaviors The use of inappropriate behaviors to compensate for food consumed, typically in an attempt to prevent weight gain (e.g., self-induced vomiting, laxative or diuretic misuse, fasting, excessive exercise)	Yes (S)	Yes (C)	No	Yes (S)

Symptom present? is the column group header spanning AN, BN, BED, and Unspecified/other diagnosis.

(continued)

TABLE 10.1. (continued)

Eating disorder symptoms	Symptom present?			
	AN	BN	BED	Unspecified/other diagnosis
Low weight status Body weight less than minimally expected given one's age, sex, developmental trajectory, and health status	Yes (C)	No	No	Yes (S)
Overweight status Body weight higher than expected given one's age, sex, and health status	No	Yes (S)	Yes (S)	Yes (S)

Note. Yes, the corresponding symptom is present in the eating disorder; No, the corresponding symptom is not present in the eating disorder; C, the corresponding symptom is a core feature of the eating disorder and thus is part of the diagnostic criteria; T, the corresponding symptom is typically present in patients who present with the eating disorder but is not part of the diagnostic criteria; S, the corresponding symptom is sometimes present in patients who present with the eating disorder but is not part of the diagnostic criteria. Notably, DSM-5 criteria for AN include "or" statements, such that a patient must have the intense fear of weight gain *or* persistent behavior that interferes with weight gain *and* overevaluation of body shape or weight, disturbances in how her or his body weight or shape is experienced, or lack of recognition of the seriousness of her or his low weight status.

processes (e.g., biological, affective, and cognitive mechanisms) may be more closely linked to component symptoms of eating disorder psychopathology than to diagnostic categories (Insel et al., 2010). Consequently, the same treatment modality that is effective for one eating disorder (e.g., AN or BN) may be applicable across the eating disorder spectrum, with treatment strategies adapted as needed depending on current symptom presentation (e.g., focus on weight gain in persons with low-weight status; Fairburn, 2008). Along these lines, treatment approaches effective for full-syndrome cases (AN or BN) will likely be effective for individuals who exhibit similar symptoms, but perhaps at a lower frequency or duration (e.g., those diagnosed with OSFED).

Two of the empirically supported treatment modalities for eating disorders, CBT and FBT, have been adapted for a range of eating disorder diagnoses. A transdiagnostic perspective led to the modification of CBT for BN (CBT-BN), the previous leading treatment for adults with BN, and resulted in the development of alternative forms of CBT (e.g., CBT "Enhanced" [CBT-E]; Fairburn, 2008)[2] that can be used with the broad spectrum of eating disorders. CBT-E was developed as a treatment for *eating disorder psychopathology* as opposed to being limited to a specific eating disorder diagnosis (Fairburn, Cooper, & Shafran, 2008). It is considered to be "enhanced" given its transdiagnostic approach and the incorporation of new treatment strategies (Fairburn, 2008). For example, CBT-E includes modules that can be used to target additional factors (e.g., low self-esteem, clinical perfectionism, interpersonal difficulties) in treatment that, if not addressed, might hinder recovery (Fairburn, 2008). Although a transdiagnostic perspective is not a tenet of FBT, careful consideration of both the shared and distinct clinical features between AN and BN has led to the extension and adaptation of FBT for AN to adolescents with BN (Le Grange & Lock, 2010; Lock & Le Grange, 2013).

Cognitive-Behavioral Therapy

Empirical Support in Adults

CBT-BN was established as the treatment of choice for adults with BN (Fairburn, 2008; Wilson & Pike, 2001), whereas the efficacy of CBT in the treatment of AN has remained limited (for review, see Bulik, Brownley, Shapiro, & Berkman, 2012). Specifically, CBT-BN was found to be significantly more effective in the alleviation of BN symptoms than interpersonal therapy (IPT; Agras, Walsh, Fairburn, Wilson, & Kraemer, 2000; Fairburn

---

[2]Other transdiagnostic CBT approaches for eating disorders have also been developed (e.g., see Waller et al., 2007), but, to our knowledge, treatment-outcome research for these alternative approaches have not been published. Thus our general focus on CBT-E is based on the fact that empirical data are available for this approach.

et al., 1991; Fairburn, Jones, Peveler, Hope, & O'Connor, 1993; Fairburn, Peveler, Jones, Hope, & Doll, 1993; Wilson et al., 2002), behavioral therapy (BT; Fairburn et al., 1991; Fairburn, Jones, et al., 1993), and psychodynamic or supportive psychotherapies (Garner et al., 1993; Walsh, Wilson, Loeb, Devlin, & Pike, 1997; Wilson et al., 1999). IPT has been accepted as an appropriate evidence-based alternative to CBT for persons with BN, as symptom reductions were achieved more rapidly with CBT-BN, but both approaches (CBT-BN and IPT) showed similar therapeutic efficacy at 1 year and 6 years posttreatment (Agras et al., 2000; Fairburn, Peveler, et al., 1993; Fairburn et al., 1995). For AN, data suggest that CBT may reduce relapse risk for adults who first undergo weight restoration (Pike, Walsh, Vitousek, Wilson, & Bauer, 2003), but the extent to which CBT is more helpful than alternative treatment approaches (e.g., BT, IPT; Channon, De Silva, Hemsley, & Perkins, 1989; McIntosh et al., 2005; McIntosh et al., 2006) in the underweight state of AN has been less clear (Bulik et al., 2012).

Importantly, less than ideal treatment outcome rates (e.g., < 50%) *and* recognition of high diagnostic crossover and shared symptomatology across eating disorders drove efforts to modify and enhance the therapeutic effectiveness of CBT so that it could be applied to the broad spectrum of eating disorders (Fairburn, 2008; Waller et al., 2007). As noted earlier, such efforts resulted in the development of transdiagnostic treatments, including the "enhanced" version of CBT (CBT-E) for eating disorders (Fairburn, 2008). Data suggest that CBT-E is a more effective treatment than CBT-BN (e.g., Fairburn et al., 2009) and that CBT-E is effective in the treatment of persons with a range of eating disorder diagnoses, including AN (Byrne, Fursland, Allen, & Watson, 2011; Fairburn et al., 2013), BN (Fairburn et al., 2009), and "unspecified/other" eating disorders (i.e., individuals who were diagnosed with DSM-IV EDNOS; Fairburn et al., 2009). For example, at the end of treatment, as well as at a 60-week follow-up, individuals treated with CBT-E showed a substantial reduction in eating disorder symptoms (e.g., scoring less than 1 standard deviation of community norms on validated measures of eating pathology; Byrne et al., 2011; Fairburn et al., 2009; Fairburn et al., 2013), and in persons with low weight, substantial increases in body weight were obtained (e.g., achievement of body mass index [BMI] $\geq$ 18.5; mean weight gain approximately 7.5 kg [16.5 pounds]; Byrne et al., 2011; Fairburn et al., 2013). Notably, persons with substantial co-occurring problems (e.g., mood intolerance, perfectionism, low self-esteem) have been shown to respond better to the broad version of CBT-E (i.e., CBT-Eb; a version that targets eating disorder symptoms and addresses co-occurring problems), whereas those without substantial co-occurring problems respond well to the focused version of CBT-E (i.e., CBT-Ef; a version that exclusively targets eating disorder symptomatology; Fairburn et al., 2008; Fairburn et al., 2009).

To our knowledge, only one randomized controlled trial compared CBT-E with an alternative treatment—integrative cognitive-affective therapy (ICAT; Wonderlich et al., 2014). ICAT is a therapy that incorporates motivational interviewing and targets self-oriented cognition (i.e., self-discrepancies: actual self vs. ideal self), emotion, and maladaptive coping within the context of nutritional rehabilitation (Wonderlich et al., 2014). Results indicated that ICAT is a suitable alternative to CBT-E for persons with BN. Both treatments resulted in significant reductions in bulimic symptoms and other outcomes (e.g., self-oriented cognitions, mood symptoms); no significant differences were observed between the treatments at the end of treatment or at 4-month follow-up (Wonderlich et al., 2014). Taken together, although strong conclusions about CBT-E await longer-term outcome data (e.g., approximately 5–6 years posttreatment) and direct comparison of CBT-E to other alternative treatment modalities (e.g., IPT), the initial data for CBT-E in the treatment of adults with eating disorders are promising. Additional exploration of ICAT, in particular its effectiveness with other eating disorder diagnoses and longer-term outcomes, remains an important future direction.

Empirical Support in Adolescents

Controlled trials of CBT in the treatment of adolescents with eating disorders are scarce. However, the use of CBT for adolescents with other disorders (e.g., depression, anxiety) indirectly suggests that this therapeutic approach may be feasible and effective for adolescents with eating disorders (Gowers, 2006). To date, four published studies have examined the use of various CBT approaches in adolescents with eating disorders, one of which used CBT-E.

Gowers et al. (2007) found no substantial between-treatment differences (inpatient vs. individual CBT with parental feedback vs. general child and adolescent mental health services) in outcomes of adolescents with AN (mean age approximately 15 years) at 1 or 2 years follow-up. Across the treatments, teens made progress at 1 year and additional improvements at 2 years (e.g., mean improvements in weight, global measures of psychopathology), but full recovery rates were rather poor across adolescents in all treatments (i.e., 33% fully recovered and 27% continued to meet criteria for AN at 2-year follow-up; Gowers et al., 2007).

In a somewhat older adolescent sample (mean age approximately 17.5 years), Schmidt et al. (2007) compared an adapted version of FBT with CBT-guided self-care in adolescents with BN symptomatology. Adolescents in the CBT-guided self-care group showed significantly greater reductions in binge eating at 6 months but no differences in binge-eating frequency were observed between the two treatments at 12 months (Schmidt et al., 2007). There were no significant differences between FBT or CBT-guided self-care for reductions in vomiting or other behavioral or attitudinal symptoms of eating disorders at 6 and 12 months (Schmidt et al., 2007). Both treatments, therefore, resulted in good outcomes (e.g., approximately 50% reported abstinence of objective binge eating and purging and reductions in food-related fears and dietary restriction at 12 months), but CBT-guided self-care showed a slight advantage in the faster reduction of binge eating, as well as lower overall treatment cost (Schmidt et al., 2007). Conversely, in a slightly younger sample of adolescents with BN (mean age = 15.8 years, SD = 1.5), a recent randomized controlled trial found that FBT was superior to an adapted version of CBT (i.e., modified for adolescents) in promoting abstinence from binge eating and purging at the end of treatment and at the 6-month follow-up; however, abstinence rates did not significantly differ at the 12-month follow-up (Le Grange, Lock, Agras, Bryson, & Booil, 2015). These data suggest that both FBT and CBT are viable treatment options for adolescents with BN, but abstinence may occur more quickly via FBT.

The effectiveness of CBT-E in adolescents with eating disorders was examined in adolescents with AN (mean age = 15.5 years, SD = 1.3; Dalle Grave, Calugi, Doll, & Fairburn, 2013). Adolescents showed substantial weight gain (i.e., mean increase approximately 8.6 kg [18.9 pounds]; 32.1% reached 95% of expected body weight) and significant reductions in eating disorder psychopathology (i.e., 96.6% scored below 1 SD of the community mean on a validated measure of eating pathology) at the end of the 40-session treatment (Dalle Grave et al., 2013). At the 60-week follow-up, weight gain was maintained or continued (i.e., 44.8% reached 95% of expected body weight) and 89.7% of teens continued to show minimal residual eating disorder symptoms (Dalle Grave et al., 2012). These results provide initial support for the utility and effectiveness of CBT-E in adolescents with AN (Dalle Grave et al., 2012) and indirectly suggest that CBT-E may be more effective than alternative CBT approaches (e.g., Gowers et al., 2007). The extent to which CBT-E is effective for other eating disorders (e.g., BN) and whether it is more effective than alternative treatments (e.g., FBT) remains to be evaluated.

Cognitive-Behavioral Theory of Eating Disorders

A transdiagnostic cognitive-behavioral conceptualization of eating disorders and their component symptoms (see Figure 10.1) was adapted from the models presented in Fairburn (2008) and Waller et al. (2007). Broadly, transdiagnostic models focus on the current state of the disorder and the cognitions, moods, and behaviors that contribute to the maintenance of the eating disorder symptomatology. The processes denoted inside the circle highlight how component symptoms of eating disorder psychopathology could work together to maintain the expression of the disorder. The core cognitive feature (i.e., overvalued beliefs of body shape and weight), is contained at the top of the model given that it is a central symptom for the maintenance of eating disorders; the arrow leading to dieting symptomatology is the strongest (i.e., largest in size) to represent that the overvalued beliefs–dieting relationship is present in most eating disorder cases. The symptoms contained within dashed boxes or connected with dashed arrows are those that are more individualized and thus may *or* may not be present in a particular person; it is the different combination of these symptoms or interconnected processes that give rise to a particular eating disorder phenotype (e.g., AN restricting type vs. AN binge–purge type vs. BN). We have included an outer circle to reiterate that eating disorder symptoms occur within a larger contextual framework: A wide range of individual differences (e.g., biological systems, learned beliefs or expectancies, personality) transact to further contribute to the "person-specific" expression of eating pathology. Notably, these individual-difference variables contained around the outside of the circle could also be subsequently affected by eating disorder symptoms (hence, bidirectional arrows in Figure 10.1) and thus may be important factors to consider within treatment.

As suggested above, the transdiagnostic cognitive-behavioral theory presented by Fairburn (2008) posits that overvalued beliefs of body shape and weight and one's control over them is central to the development and maintenance of eating psychopathology; other co-occurring eating disorder symptoms stem from this core cognitive feature (see Figure 10.1). Dietary restriction and associated cognitive (e.g., preoccupation with thoughts about body weight and eating) and behavioral (e.g., body and weight checking behaviors; noncompensatory methods of weight control) weight-control features subsequently lead to the development and maintenance of other eating disorder symptoms, in particular low weight status and/or the development of binge eating (Fairburn, 2008; Murphy et al., 2010). Thus binge eating is presumed to occur, not as a direct expression of the core cognitive psychopathology, but, rather, as a result of intermediary factors such as attempts at dietary restriction (Fairburn, 2008; Murphy et al., 2010). For example, the breaking of dietary rules or the experience of hunger due to dietary restriction may result in negative self-evaluations (e.g., perceived evidence of failure or poor self-control) or physiological vulnerability, which could serve to trigger objective (e.g., consumption of a large amount of food and experience of loss of control) or subjective (e.g., self-perceived as a large amount of food, but actually small or moderate, and loss of control) binge-eating episodes (see Figure 10.1). Binge eating may also occur in response to other internal (e.g., negative mood) or external triggers (e.g., daily stressors; Fairburn, 2008; see Figure 10.1). Although binge eating may temporarily reduce negative mood states (Haedt-Matt & Keel, 2011), a person with an eating disorder often experiences subsequent increases in concerns about body weight and shape, eating, and her or his ability to control these factors (Fairburn, 2008). In addition, binge

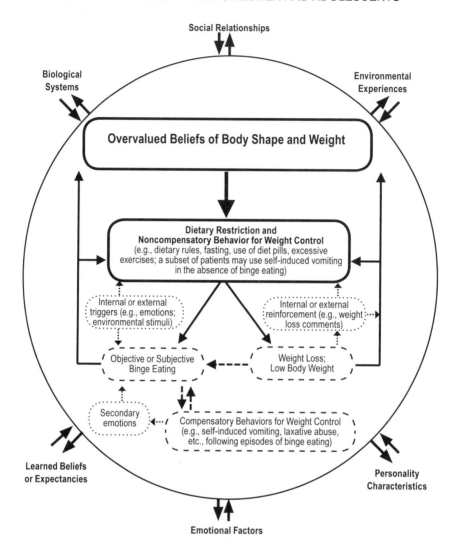

FIGURE 10.1. A transdiagnostic cognitive-behavioral theory of eating disorder psychopathology. This figure integrates transactional processes and transdiagnostic theories of eating pathology from Fairburn (2008) and Waller et al. (2007).

eating may be followed by behavioral attempts at weight control, such as increased dietary restriction and compensatory behaviors (e.g., self-induced vomiting). This cycle of restriction, binge eating, and purging may further disrupt the physiological regulation of food intake and further increase risk for binge eating. Inaccurate beliefs about the effectiveness of compensatory behaviors, such as self-induced vomiting and laxative abuse, may also serve to maintain binge eating, particularly for individuals who are unaware that vomiting retrieves only a fraction of the food consumed and laxatives have little to no effect (Fairburn, 2008; Kaye, Weltzin, Hsu, McConaha, & Bolton, 1993; Roerig, Steffen, Mitchell, & Zunker, 2010). When dietary restriction predominates or occurs in the absence of binge eating, extreme weight loss and a low body weight can result, such as in persons with AN (Fairburn, 2008; see Figure 10.1). Several eating disorder features, both cognitive and behavioral in nature, are considered to be maintained as a result of the physical and psychosocial consequences of a low body weight. For example, underweight individuals may become increasingly preoccupied with food, eating, and body weight and shape; they may also experience feelings of fullness or discomfort when eating and may show more cognitive inflexibility and social withdrawal (Fairburn, 2008). Such symptoms will serve to maintain and perpetuate the disorder, such as increasing efforts toward dietary restriction (e.g., internal reinforcement mechanisms; see Figure 10.1).

An alternative transdiagnostic model presented by Waller et al. (2007) uses the Fairburn model as a starting point prior to considering more complex paradigms. Specifically, Waller et al. (2007) place a primary importance on the relationship between emotional states and the use of eating disorder behaviors, arguing that emotional regulation is one of the key functions of the eating disorder. Restrictive and bulimic behavior may therefore result from primary and secondary emotion or avoidance of such emotion (e.g., affective internal triggers; see Figure 10.1; Waller et al., 2007). Primary avoidance of emotion involves the avoidance of affect arising in the first place and secondary avoidance of emotion involves the reduction of affect once affect has been triggered (see Figure 10.1). Notably, positive regard from others may also be received following one's dieting behaviors and weight loss, which could serve to reinforce dieting behaviors and further enhance overvalued beliefs regarding body weight and shape (e.g., external reinforcement mechanisms; see Figure 10.1; Waller et al., 2007).

Similar to Fairburn (2008) and Waller et al. (2007), Gowers and Green (2009) identify a transdiagnostic model that points to an overvaluation of weight and shape and the need for control in an adolescent's world as maintaining factors for eating disorder symptoms. For those individuals who develop BN or binge eating, severe dietary restraint is used to enhance the idea of being in control, while extreme concerns about shape and weight foster and influence continued dietary restriction (Gowers & Green, 2009). Dietary restraint and compensatory mechanisms (e.g., purging) are conceptualized as methods used to cope with moderate interpersonal conflict, intense stress, and negative moods (Gowers & Green, 2009). These methods of coping are played out within the influence of relevant early experiences (Gowers & Green, 2009).

The aforementioned transdiagnostic cognitive-behavioral conceptualizations provide a description of the many processes that might be present and serve to maintain the eating disorder symptoms; however, individual differences in the presence and operation of these mechanisms are to be expected. Identifying which factors and how these factors are interlinked for a specific person is a key component of all transdiagnostic models and versions of CBT for eating disorders. Indeed, the interventions developed by Fairburn (2008), Waller et al. (2007), and Gowers and Green (2009) are all designed to create a treatment that fits the individual's specific psychopathology while maintaining a flexible case formulation. Each of these therapeutic CBT approaches stresses a collaborative working relationship based on the individual's needs that is active and transparent and that imbues the individual with the responsibility for change; however, each of these models suggests somewhat different pathways to change.

Treatment and Intervention

CBT consists of many "moving parts" (Wilson & Zandberg, 2012): It uses both cognitive and behavioral techniques, integrated with psychoeducation, to help persons with eating disorders to reestablish patterns of eating and to decrease concerns with body weight and shape (Wilson & Pike, 2001; Fairburn, 2008). The use of CBT for adolescents with eating disorders is largely similar to that in adults, with a few exceptions (Cooper & Stewart, 2008). Modifications primarily aim to address the developmental issues discussed earlier, such as involvement of parents and adjusting treatment to suit the teen's emotional and cognitive level (Cooper & Stewart, 2008). It has been suggested that CBT may not be appropriate for persons under the age of 13 or 14 (Cooper & Stewart, 2008; Dalle Grave et al., 2013) and that younger persons may instead benefit from FBT. However, no study has empirically explored whether age influences the effectiveness of CBT for eating disorders. When age has been evaluated in the treatment of children and adolescents with anxiety disorder, the findings indicate no differences in outcomes (Kendall & Peterman, 2015).

Consistent with the principles of CBT (e.g., Beck, 2011), establishment of a collaborative therapeutic relationship is critical to assisting the adolescent in overcoming the eating disorder. This collaborative individual-based approach to treatment means that the relative role of parents in treatment is largely guided by the adolescent and his or her needs. Parental involvement is openly discussed and collaboratively determined by the therapist and teen throughout treatment (Cooper & Stewart, 2008). The individual, collaborative, structured, and goal-oriented approach of CBT fits well with the increased desire for autonomy and independence that coincides with adolescent development (Bowers et al., 2003; Cooper & Stewart, 2008). The egalitarian and empirical approach of CBT can also help to engage the adolescent in treatment and aid in the formation of an effective collaboration (Bowers et al., 2003). At the start of treatment, it can therefore be useful for therapists to heavily emphasize that treatment involves working together as a collaborative "team," to convey a genuine interest in getting to know the teen and his or her struggles, and to acknowledge the teen's potential experience of treatment (e.g., some components of treatment may be difficult or unpleasant but will be beneficial in the long term) using an honest and empathic approach (Waller et al., 2007.) For example, a therapist might say:

> "The work we do together may be challenging at times. You may experience some components of treatment to be difficult or even unpleasant—I want you to know that such an experience is normal; you would not be the first person to feel that way. I merely ask that you let me know when you find activities to be difficult or unpleasant because then we can talk more about that, and, if necessary, figure out how to make the activity most relevant or effective for you. At times, you may also become frustrated with me or what I am asking you to do; it is OK for you to feel that way, too. I want us to be a team and to work effectively together to best understand your struggles, but I don't expect you to always "like" me or the things that I ask you to do. If you do have these types of reactions, I only hope that you will share them with me—again, so we can talk more about it and to ensure that these reactions do not interfere with treatment progress. . . . Ultimately, I recognize that treatment can be hard, uncomfortable, and time-consuming; I would not push you to engage in this treatment if I did not truly think it could be helpful to you. Research studies have demonstrated the effectiveness of this treatment, and other adolescents I have worked with have found treatment to be quite valuable."

We next provide an overview of CBT-E, which, as noted previously, targets eating disorder psychopathology and is not limited to a particular eating disorder diagnosis (Fairburn, 2008). We focus on the application of CBT-E for the treatment of adolescents with eating disorders because, to our knowledge, this is currently the CBT approach that has the strongest empirical support with adolescents and has published corresponding treatment resources.[3] We provide a general overview of CBT-E as outlined by Fairburn (2008), with a particular focus on suggested modifications for youth by Cooper and Stewart (2008). We interject clinical descriptions and examples of the use of many of these CBT techniques from our clinical

---

[3] Again, we acknowledge that alternative transdiagnostic CBT interventions for children and adolescents with eating disorders have also been developed (see comprehensive treatment guides: Gowers & Green, 2009; Waller et al., 2007).

experience with adolescents. Although we have not received formal training in CBT-E, the CBT approach we have implemented with youth follows a relatively similar treatment structure and includes many of the same procedures.

CBT-E generally follows four phases over 20 sessions; however, a longer treatment duration (e.g., 40 sessions; Cooper & Stewart, 2008; Dalle Grave et al., 2013; Fairburn, 2008) is recommended for underweight persons (e.g., AN). We discuss the 20-session CBT-E approach, followed by a brief overview of recommended modifications for the underweight adolescent. Readers are encouraged to access treatment resources (see Fairburn, 2008, for more details).

Stage 1: Sessions 0–7

Setting Up Treatment

Contact with the family should be initiated quickly. A substantial delay in treatment could have adverse effects (e.g., interference with the youth's engagement; change in the presenting symptoms) and may interfere with establishing symptom change as quickly as possible (Fairburn, 2008). Contraindications to immediate initiation of treatment include compromised physical health, severe clinical depression or suicide risk, persistent substance misuse, or life events that may interfere with treatment.

Establishing the Role of Parents

Parental involvement begins at the start of treatment (Cooper & Stewart, 2008), and, given that parents will often be transporting the teen to treatment, it is important that parents understand treatment expectations and the therapeutic approach. Because a main goal of Stage 1 is to promote early change, appointments are scheduled twice a week during the first 4 weeks (Fairburn, 2008). We schedule a collateral session with parents at least once during the initial stage of treatment (but these can occur as often as needed) to provide parents with education about the treatment, eating disorders, and their anticipated role in their child's treatment. Parental involvement typically occurs more regularly early in treatment as a means of facilitating and assisting the youth in making necessary changes. It is expected that parental involvement will decrease as the youth's symptoms are attenuated and the youth is capable of taking a more independent role (Cooper & Stewart, 2008).

Moreover, parents are informed that they will be asked to support the individual in ways that are agreed upon by the therapist and youth, and thus they will be involved in the facilitation of treatment on an as-needed basis. It should be made clear to parents that their child will be asked to complete "homework" assignments throughout treatment, such as self-monitoring forms, but that these records are considered private (Cooper & Stewart, 2008). We have found that it can be helpful for adolescents to share the constructed formulation (see "Creating the Symptom Formulation" below; Figures 10.2 and 10.3) with their parents (if they are willing), as this can serve to initiate parent–child discussions about the eating difficulties and may provide the parents with a better understanding of their child's current struggles with eating and body concerns. A therapist may say to parents:

"Your support of your adolescent's efforts may be very useful. Thus, throughout the course of treatment, I will be working with [*youth's name*] to determine how you might be able to best support [*youth's name*]."

The First Face-to-Face Meeting

In the first session, the therapist should aim to demonstrate an understanding of the adolescent's presenting problems, to identify any ambivalence that she or he may have about treatment, to engage the youth in treatment, and to work to increase or facilitate her or his motivation for change (Cooper & Stewart, 2008; Fairburn, 2008). The CBT model is introduced and the structure and goals of treatment are reviewed, including the regular use of homework assignments.

Creating the Symptom Formulation. The therapist and adolescent jointly create a personalized formulation (e.g., a hypothesized maintenance model) of the eating disorder symptoms (Cooper & Stewart, 2008; Fairburn, 2008). This formulation is used to identify the person's key symptoms and the bidirectional associations between these symptoms (Fairburn, 2008). This process begins to model the collaborative nature of the therapeutic relationship and creates a foundation for understanding the youth's eating disorder symptomatology. In our experience, it can be helpful to show an example formulation (e.g., a simplified version linking body shape and weight concerns → dieting → binge eating) before engaging in this activity, as this provides the teen with a conceptual framework for the task which otherwise may seem abstract.

To initiate this task, the therapist might say something like:

"In order to better understand your current eating and weight-related attitudes and behaviors, I would like us to spend some time creating a diagram today. As we work to create this diagram, we will try to think through how your thoughts and behaviors may be working together to maintain your current eating difficulties . . . here is an example of a diagram linking up various eating disorder symptoms [show an example similar to Figure 10.1]. I am showing you this merely as a general visual template of what we want to try to create; since every person is different, our goal is to understand your attitudes and behaviors and the specific ways they may be interconnected to lead to your day-to-day experiences."

Upon completion, the therapist explains that treatment will target and "break" the interacting mechanisms that are maintaining the cycle of eating disorder symptoms and that this formation will be adapted, as needed, throughout treatment (e.g., when more is learned or as changes in symptoms occur; Cooper & Stewart, 2008; Fairburn, 2008). The formulation serves as an initial conceptualization of the youth's difficulties and can create a sense of hope for change. Consequently, it is important that the formulation accurately represents the eating problem using the youth's own words and that sufficient time is devoted to this activity (Fairburn, 2008). Case examples are presented in Figures 10.2 and 10.3a (later in the chapter).

Introducing Self-Monitoring. Self-monitoring of eating behaviors (e.g., recording food and drinks consumed; time and location of consumption) in between treatment sessions is a key component of treatment that is introduced in the first session (Cooper & Stewart, 2008; Fairburn, 2008). Explaining the rationale is important for enhancing the adolescent's "buy-in" and adherence. Self-monitoring provides a detailed picture of the youth's daily eating patterns and associated difficulties, will increase her or his self-awareness, and, ultimately, will serve to promote change. Formal instructions and self-monitoring templates are available in the treatment manual (see Fairburn, 2008). The clinician could introduce self-monitoring as follows:

> "Self-monitoring is a central component of treatment. It will be an important tool that will allow you to gain a better understanding of your eating difficulties. Enhancing your understanding of your in-the-moment behaviors, as well as your corresponding thoughts and feelings, will allow you to become an expert on your eating difficulties, and, ultimately, to overcome them!"

Consistent with any CBT intervention, it is imperative that the therapist discusses any anticipated problems the adolescent may foresee in the completion of self-monitoring logs prior to embarking on this assignment. The therapist and adolescent would collaboratively problem-solve around any anticipated challenges. For example, the teen may anticipate feeling embarrassed to pull out paper versions of the self-monitoring logs at school, in which case the therapist and adolescent could brainstorm alternative options, such as the use of other recording devices (e.g., mobile phone) or finding a more private setting (e.g., classroom, counselor's office).

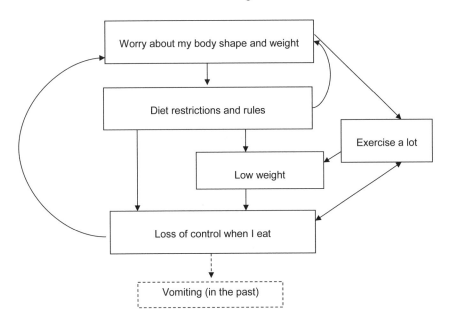

FIGURE 10.2. An example symptom formulation of an AN case using the patient's own words.

Additional Components of Treatment

Psychoeducation regarding nutrition, normal weight regulation, and the medical and psychological consequences of eating disorders are provided to the adolescent and caregivers early in treatment (Cooper & Stewart, 2008; Fairburn, 2008). We have found that psychoeducation often has a powerful effect on symptom reduction, particularly if the individual experiences increased concern about the medical side effects of the illness or a new understanding of the ineffectiveness and dangers of weight-control behaviors (e.g., self-induced vomiting, laxative abuse).

Remaining Stage 1 interventions are largely behavioral in nature, although cognitive shifts may indirectly result from these behavioral interventions. Self-monitoring logs are reviewed in each session, and the therapist and adolescent work together to address any difficulties or problematic patterns of eating behavior (Fairburn, 2008). For example, if the self-monitoring forms reveal that the adolescent has a pattern of consuming relatively few calories from morning to early afternoon and a history of binge episodes in the evening, then the therapist and adolescent would work together to determine possible ways to intervene to break this pattern (e.g., eating more frequently throughout the day, eating larger meals and snacks). The therapist can also use such information as a means of reiterating the purpose and utility of other key components of treatment, such as the establishment of regular eating (see the following subsection). Careful review of self-monitoring forms can also be helpful to identify the extent to which the person is: (1) consuming a variety of foods and (2) engaging in other eating disorder behaviors (e.g., consuming only a half of an apple or sandwich) that, without detailed recording or probing by the therapist, may not become apparent in treatment. Self-monitoring will also serve to heighten the youth's "in-the-moment" awareness to facilitate her or his initiation of different behavioral choices (Fairburn, 2008). In addition to the ongoing completion and review of self-monitoring logs, two key CBT-E procedures are also introduced: the establishment of regular eating and in-session weekly weighing (Cooper & Stewart, 2008; Fairburn, 2008).

Regular Eating. The individual is introduced to regular eating in Session 2 or 3 (Fairburn, 2008). Regular eating requires the adolescent to alter her or his eating patterns, such that she or he eats three planned meals and two to three planned snacks each day. A clinician could explain regular eating by saying something like:

"Up until this point I have not asked you to make any changes regarding your eating, and I think reviewing your self-monitoring forms prior to asking you to make any changes has been quite helpful. Would you agree? . . . For example, we were able to learn that you try to avoid eating anything until 2 P.M., but that frequently means that [*insert information that was learned—examples follow*] (1) you spend a lot of that time thinking about food, and (2) you feel so hungry that you eat more than you intended or planned. It is now time to start making changes with your eating, but I want to clarify that at this point, the focus is on changing when you eat, not what you eat. The goal is for you to begin eating at regular intervals in the day, as this has been found to be a very helpful intervention for people with eating difficulties. What are your initial thoughts and feelings about giving this new approach a try? . . . Now let's take a look at your weekly schedule and identify the times of the day you would eat your meals and snacks."

Once the concept and rationale of regular eating (e.g., three meals and two to three snacks) is introduced, it is useful to discuss how regular eating can be integrated into the youth's daily routine. Given that an adolescent's school schedule may vary from day to day, the plan for meals and snacks may need to be slightly adjusted for each day. In addition, the therapist may begin to model the use of problem-solving skills to aid in the facilitation of behavioral changes, including the implementation of regular eating. For example, if the adolescent reports that she or he is not consuming snacks because she or he forgets to do so, then the therapist and adolescent can spend time generating a list of possible ways to help her or him remember and determine which method(s) the adolescent will try—for example, setting an alarm on a mobile phone or watch, getting formal permission from teachers and school to consume a snack or determining a location (e.g., school nurse's or counselor's office) to eat the snack, and establishing how parents may be able to help, such as ensuring that the adolescent has a lunch and snacks packed for school. An adolescent may also report that meals or snacks are not being regularly consumed because she or he is uncertain about what to eat or has difficulty making that decision "in the moment." If so, we have found that it can be useful to spend time in session collaboratively creating a list of possible meals or snacks. Creating a list can decrease the amount of "thinking" necessary in the moment and can serve to reiterate the regular eating goal of planning ahead for meals and snacks (e.g., knowing when to eat and generally what will be consumed).

Weekly In-Session Weighing. Weekly in-session weighing, and the elimination of weight-checking behavior in between sessions, are primary components of treatment. In-session weighing provides concrete data about what is happening (or not happening) to a youth's body weight and provides an opportunity for psychoeducation about normal fluctuations in body weight (e.g., normal changes due to degree of hydration, bloating, constipation; Fairburn, 2008). In-session weighing also helps the therapist determine the extent to which an adolescent may negatively interpret inconsequential fluctuations in weight and make inaccurate assumptions (e.g., "My weight is up 0.3 pounds! I knew my weight was going to be up this week because I had ice cream twice last weekend"), and thus it can serve to facilitate an open dialogue regarding the adolescent's reaction to her or his body weight. Over time, weekly in-session weighing serves to promote cognitive changes in the ways in which individuals think about their weight and the effects of eating on their body weight (Fairburn, 2008). For example, individuals with an eating disorder often assume that eating a feared food (e.g., a cookie) and eating regularly will make them gain substantial amounts of weight; some will assume that weight gain will never stop. The use of concrete data (e.g., weekly weight logs) and ongoing communication about what is happening to their weight serves to diminish and alter these inaccurate assumptions (Fairburn, 2008). Further, if the adolescent is not fully grown, in-session weighing can also be used to initiate conversations about normal growth and the expectation that her or his weight will increase during the natural developmental process (e.g., the therapist can explain that body weight should continue to increase until the adolescent is fully grown, following her or his weight and height trajectory). In-session weighing could be introduced as follows, although for underweight persons the discussion would address their expected and necessary weight gain:

"Most people with an eating disorder worry that their weight will substantially increase if they begin to change their eating patterns. It is often feared that weight gain will occur and never stop. We are going to monitor your weight across treatment—your weight will be taken and recorded at the beginning of every session, and I am going to ask you to refrain from weighing yourself in between our sessions. Monitoring your weight on a weekly basis will provide us with data that can allow us to find out whether or not your weight drastically changes when you start changing your eating behaviors. In-session weighing will also allow us to discuss and work through any reactions you have to your weight in the moment."

In response to an adolescent's reactions to inconsequential fluctuations in weight, a clinician might say:

"You commented that you knew your weight was going to be up this week because you had ice cream last weekend. Let's talk more about that. . . . Do you remember when I explained that one's body weight will naturally fluctuate, and thus many 'changes' in weight are trivial? We had discussed that there is a natural fluctuation range of about 6 pounds around one's body weight. Taking this information into account, as well as looking at your patterns of weight over the past month, is there another way to think about your weight being 'up 0.3 pounds' from last week? . . . [additional prompts, if needed] Looking at these data, has your weight substantially changed in the past month? . . . or would you say that it has stayed pretty much the same?"

Additional Strategies. Additional strategies to alter problematic eating behaviors (e.g., binge eating, purging, or excessive exercising) include the use of incompatible behaviors to resist the urge to binge or purge or to make these behaviors less likely to occur. The adolescent could be encouraged to think about the ways in which her or his parents may be able to provide support in the extinguishing of eating disorder behaviors. For example, if agreed upon by the adolescent, parents could be asked to temporarily avoid purchasing foods that have been identified as triggering for binge eating or to provide guidance and support in the establishment of regular eating. If purging is prominent, the parent could be asked to play a supportive role by engaging in an activity with the adolescent for a period of time following meals or snacks.

Several goals are expected to be achieved by the end of the first stage, including the adolescent's being actively engaged in treatment (e.g., completing self-monitoring forms), exposed to in-session weighing, informed about normal weight fluctuation, aware of the consequences of weight avoidance and frequent weight checking, and learning to eat regularly (Cooper & Stewart, 2008; Fairburn, 2008). If there are problems with compliance or engagement, it is recommended that these issues be directly addressed with the adolescent (Fairburn, 2008). For example, the therapist can help the adolescent evaluate negative thoughts (e.g., "This treatment is not helping"; "These interventions are going to make me gain weight"; "I feel worse than I did a month ago") that may be interfering with treatment. Our experience is that the facilitation of such discussions typically sheds light on the problem(s) and continues to communicate that the therapist has a genuine concern for and interest in the adolescent and her or his circumstances. Open conversations about treatment challenges can also encourage youth to actively reflect upon and problem-solve ways to address such issues. Ongoing concerns regarding treatment progress can also be discussed during Stage 2.

Stage 2: Sessions 8 and 9

In Stage 2, the therapist and adolescent review treatment progress, discuss any barriers to change, review and modify the formulation as needed, and plan for Stage 3 (Fairburn, 2008). Individuals who are actively engaged, committed to treatment, and making good progress should be positively reinforced via explicit praise and acknowledgement of the important changes they have made. If an individual has not made good progress, then this stage of treatment will aim to collaboratively identify, understand, and address potential barriers (Fairburn, 2008). Moreover, this second stage encourages therapists to consider any changes to the youth's eating disorder and to adjust the treatment as necessary (Fairburn, 2008). Reflection and consideration of the person's treatment progress is important, because subsequent treatment sessions are highly individualized based on their presenting difficulties. For example, if issues of perfectionism appear to be interfering with treatment progress, then the broad version of CBT-E may be deemed necessary at this point (for details, see Fairburn, 2008). Appointments occur on a weekly basis for the remainder of treatment, unless the individual is underweight (Fairburn, 2008).

Stage 3: Sessions 10–17

Although behavioral interventions are largely the focus of treatment in the first two stages, Stage 3 addresses the other factors (as identified in the youth's formulation) that are maintaining the eating disorder (Fairburn, 2008). There is considerable flexibility in terms of the topics explored and strategies implemented (Fairburn, 2008; Murphy et al., 2010). The youth's overevaluation of body shape and weight should be addressed in this stage, which may include:

- Exploring the consequences of overvalued beliefs about body shape and weight on the adolescent's self-worth and self-esteem.
- Exploring the role of these beliefs in the perpetuation of eating disorder behaviors (e.g., dieting, binge eating, purging).
- Helping the adolescent to increase the number or significance of other areas in her or his life that can promote positive self-evaluation, such as reengaging in activities or hobbies she or he previously enjoyed.
- Addressing body checking or avoidance behaviors (e.g., if the adolescent is trying on last summer's clothing and negative emotions are triggered when clothes do not fit, create a plan for removing these clothes from her or his closet).
- Exploring the origins of the adolescent's overevaluation of body weight and shape and working toward a reappraisal.

To begin identifying overvalued beliefs about body weight and shape (and the consequences of such), a "self-evaluation" pie chart can be developed in session (Fairburn, 2008). This activity could be introduced as follows:

"Today we will spend some time thinking about how you evaluate yourself as a person—for example, people often judge themselves based on many aspects of their lives (relationships with friends, school achievements, hobbies, etc.). In our work together, we have learned [*therapist can refer to the person's formulation diagram*] that concerns about your body shape and weight play a really important role in how you evaluate yourself, so we'll definitely want to consider that within this activity; however, I want you to think of other aspects that may be relevant, too. . . . Let's start by developing a list of all the aspects of your life that factor into how you judge yourself as a person. What are the things that make you feel good about yourself when they are going well or bad about yourself when they are not going well? . . . You've done a great job identifying these factors. Now we are going to try to fill in this circle, like a pie, such that each slice represents the relative proportion or influence of each factor on your overall self-evaluation—that means that together, the components have to total 100%. Out of all the factors you've identified, which one do you think we should start with? . . . And how big should we make this slice of the pie? . . . Now looking at the completed pie, what does it suggest to you about how you judge yourself? . . . In what ways is it helpful to think like this? . . . In what ways may it be unhelpful to think like this? . . . Since we've now identified that it is quite risky to have so much of your self-evaluation based on how you feel about your body weight and shape, let's brainstorm some ways you might be able to modify this. How might you 'shrink' the slice of pie that is focused on your body weight and shape? . . . [*additional prompts, if needed*] Is there any way to enhance these other areas you've identified?"

Treatment will likely need to address dietary rules and food avoidance (e.g., feared foods) and the effects of these rules and beliefs on the adolescent's eating behavior (Fairburn, 2008; Murphy et al., 2010). To begin to tackle the problem of food avoidance, the therapist and adolescent may collaboratively establish a list of the avoided foods and systematically reintroduce such foods back into her or his diet (Fairburn, 2008; Murphy et al., 2010). We have found that parents can be helpful in providing support for such changes, such as helping the adolescent to think about activities she or he might join or providing support and guidance in the consumption of feared foods (e.g., establishing a plan about when and what will be reintroduced, ensuring the food is available, and providing the adolescent with emotional support and aiding in the prevention of a binge episode).

Problem-solving and coping skills may also be formally discussed and enhanced during this stage as a means of helping the adolescent to more effectively deal with a range of events or situations that may affect her or his eating behavior (Cooper & Stewart, 2008). Notably, while this stage aims to address more cognitive-based symptoms of the eating disorder, the treatment interventions do not formally teach cognitive restructuring skills (Fairburn, 2008). Fairburn (2008) and others (e.g., Waller et al., 2007) suggest that fostering behavioral change and discussing the outcomes of those changes is one of the most powerful ways to create cognitive change. This approach, along with the active use of problem-solving skills, is also likely more suitable for the adolescent's developmental capabilities (Cooper & Stewart, 2008).

Stage 4: Sessions 15–20

Stage 4 focuses on reviewing treatment progress and the maintenance of change. Individuals may begin to do weekly weighing at home, rather than in session (Fairburn, 2008). To minimize relapse, the therapist and adolescent review the strategies in treatment that were helpful, establish realistic expectations for the future, prepare for setbacks, and discuss the difference between a "lapse" and a "relapse" (Fairburn, 2008; Murphy et al., 2010). Therapy appointments are spaced out, occurring biweekly or monthly.

Treatment Considerations and Adaptations for Underweight Individuals

If an adolescent is underweight, it is first imperative to determine whether starting with CBT-E is clinically appropriate (Cooper & Stewart, 2008; Fairburn, 2008). Specifically, in addition to the contraindicators of treatment previously listed (e.g., severe depression or suicidality, events that would interfere with regular treatment attendance), if an adolescent's weight loss is too great (e.g., $\geq$ 20% of body weight), then a preliminary intervention may be required before the initiation of outpatient CBT-E (Cooper & Stewart, 2008). Preliminary interventions would aim to facilitate weight restoration and thus could include FBT (i.e., an alternative evidence-based outpatient treatment; see later in the chapter) or an inpatient or intensive day program (Cooper & Stewart, 2008). CBT-E could then begin after the completion of these interventions.

Several key components of the 20-session version of CBT-E for non-underweight individuals are also implemented in this 40-session version, including collaboratively creating a formulation of the youth's eating disorder symptoms, in-session weekly weighing, real-time self-monitoring, and establishment of regular eating that will aim to reduce dieting or long delays between meals and snacks (Fairburn, 2008). Modifications to the treatment primarily include: increases in the time that may be needed to enhance motivation and engage the person in treatment, psychoeducation about the side effects and consequences of being underweight, and a focus on weight regain and the ways in which this can be achieved (e.g., addition of snacks and types of food eaten; Fairburn, 2008). A primary goal is to have the individual decide that regaining weight will be helpful, and thus a considerable amount of time in treatment may be devoted to helping the youth consider the pros and cons of change, evaluating her or his list of reasons for change, and establishing how she or he might go about regaining weight (Fairburn, 2008). For example, the therapist could work with the adolescent to develop a list of the types of foods she or he may eat, how she or he will go about eating more on a daily basis, and the ways in which physical activity could be reduced. The ways in which parents may be able to help the adolescent achieve these goals can also be explored, such as no longer prepping alternative meals that are driven by the child's requests or sitting with the youth during meals and snacks.

It is recommended that the person's progress in treatment be frequently reviewed, including any changes in her or his weight status and level of motivation and commitment to change (Fairburn, 2008). When the individual achieves a healthy weight range, then efforts are made to help the adolescent accept and maintain this weight (Fairburn, 2008). However, as noted above, it is important to review the necessity of continual weight gain in youth who will continue to grow, as the "healthy weight range" will be a moving target until their growth is complete.

Case Example

The following case represents a typical clinical presentation and our general CBT treatment approach for an adolescent with BN. To preserve confidentiality and anonymity, case material has been disguised, and much of the included information is fictional.

Presenting Concerns and Initial Assessment

Sarah was a 15-year-old female who presented to our eating disorders program to address several symptoms consistent with a diagnosis of BN. Sarah's parents were concerned about her changes in eating patterns, preoccupation with body weight, and corresponding weight loss (approximately 5 pounds). Sarah was evaluated by our multidisciplinary treatment team, including medical and psychiatric examinations. At the time of her evaluation, Sarah endorsed an undue influence of body weight and shape on her self-evaluation, restrictive eating behaviors (e.g., skipping meals, eliminating "junk food" from her diet) and strict dietary rules (e.g., skipping meals, calorie limits, time schedule), fear of weight gain, objective binge-eating episodes (10 episodes in the previous 28 days; about two to three times a week for the past 3 months), subjective binge-eating episodes (10 episodes in the previous 28 days; about two to three times a week for the past 3 months), self-induced vomiting (20 episodes in the previous 28 days; about four to six times a week for the past 3 months), and laxative misuse (four episodes in the previous 28 days, no prior use). In addition, Sarah engaged in body checking, as her mother reported that she had frequently observed Sarah looking in the mirror and pinching the skin on her face, arms, and thighs. Sarah disclosed that she was weighing herself two to three times per day and that thoughts about eating and weight gain preoccupied her mind. She also reported feeling guilty when she ate, particularly after violating dietary rules. These symptoms had been occurring for approximately 6 months, which coincided with the start of her swim season. Sarah indicated that she "felt fat" in her bathing suit and believed that losing a few pounds would make her look more attractive and allow her to become a better swimmer. Sarah presented to the clinic at 100.49% of her expected body weight (height in inches: 68.4, weight in pounds: 133), and her scores on the EDE interview were elevated and consistent with individuals diagnosed with an eating disorder (see Figure 10.3). Sarah did not meet DSM-IV-TR criteria for any other Axis I or Axis II disorder and had no previous eating disorder or other psychological treatment.

She lived with her parents and had one older sibling. She was a straight-A student and a top competitor on the school swim team. Sarah's parents stated that she had always been a "high achiever." Sarah reported that self-discipline and meeting her eating and weight goals instilled feelings of success; however, daily mishaps (e.g., breaking dietary rules, weight gain) tended to trigger negative automatic thoughts, such as "I am a failure" and "I can't do anything right."

Formulation

Sarah met diagnostic criteria for BN. The initial onset of dieting coincided with the start of the swim season, when Sarah began to feel uncomfortable with her body weight and desired to lose weight. Given information obtained from the initial assessment and Sarah's symptom formulation (see Figure 10.3), her difficulties could be conceptualized as follows:

Sarah may have started to diet as a way to cope with the core belief "I am not good enough"; this belief was likely activated via her engagement in social comparison with her peers in the domains of body weight/shape and athletic ability. As she began to restrict her eating behavior, Sarah experienced heightened preoccupation with food and her body weight. Initially, Sarah may have recognized that restrictive eating provided her with a sense of accomplishment and thus provided her with some relief from negative thoughts and feelings. However, concurrently, her restrictive eating behaviors likely resulted in physiological disruptions and intense feelings of hunger, which made it more difficult to follow dietary rules and made her more vulnerable to experiencing a loss of control when eating. Sarah put substantial pressure on herself to meet unrealistic and high expectations. Thus, as the development of binge eating ensued, Sarah had several negative thoughts (e.g., "I completely failed"; "My mistakes will make me gain weight") that resulted in negative emotions (e.g., anxiety, worry, sadness, frustration). Sarah likely developed several inappropriate compensatory behaviors (e.g., self-induced vomiting, laxative misuse, excessive exercise) and "checking behaviors" (e.g., frequently weighing herself, evaluating herself in the mirror, pinching her skin) to maladaptively cope and reduce her distress; however, engaging in these behaviors often exacerbated, as opposed to reduced, her levels of distress. The combination of these psychological and physiological factors were expected to underlie and maintain Sarah's eating disorder symptoms.

Treatment Summary

CBT for eating disorder symptoms was implemented. Sarah attended a total of 18 outpatient individual psychotherapy sessions. The clinician also met separately with Sarah's mother and father once at the beginning of treatment. During Phase I of treatment, Sarah and her parents were provided with psychoeducation regarding the CBT model, therapy structure, and likely treatment outcome. Medical problems associated with eating disorder symptoms were also reviewed. Treatment initially focused on identifying Sarah's problematic eating disorder behaviors and collaboratively creating a CBT maintenance model of her symptoms (see Figure 10.3).

At the start of treatment, Sarah reported eating only two meals and one snack on most days. She frequently skipped lunch at school, reportedly due to a desire to lose weight, feeling uncomfortable eating in front of others,

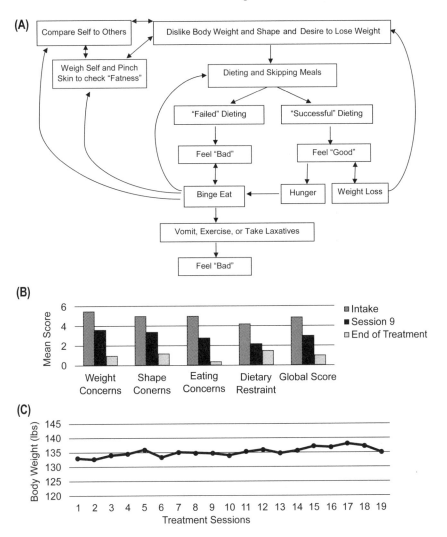

FIGURE 10.3. Assessment and treatment data for case example (Sarah), including (A) symptom formulation of BN symptoms, (B) Eating Disorder Examination (EDE) interview scores, and (C) body weight tracking.

and fears of being negatively judged or evaluated by her peers. The importance and benefits of self-monitoring and regular eating (e.g., three meals and three to four snacks a day) were explained. Sarah was encouraged to engage in regular eating and to complete food logs throughout the course of treatment. Food logs were reviewed in session to identify eating patterns and to make connections between Sarah's reported feelings of hunger, food choices, and overall consumption. Sarah was somewhat inconsistent with her completion of food logs at the start of treatment. Through discussion, it was discovered that Sarah's reluctance to engage in regular eating and to complete food logs largely stemmed from fears of weight gain. Additional psychoeducation was provided, and, following discussion, Sarah agreed to give regular eating and self-monitoring "a try" for 1 week. Over the course of treatment, she became more open to discussing her eating patterns and independently acknowledged the benefits of engaging in regular eating and the completion of self-monitoring. Sarah began to complete her food logs regularly and thoroughly. She started to come prepared to identify and discuss possible "problem" behaviors (e.g., dietary rules, feared foods, anxiety related to eating, feelings of hunger, grazing/picking at food), and she was eager to brainstorm possible ways she might intervene to help herself overcome such difficulties.

Sarah challenged herself to start eating in front of others, including her peers at school (for lunch) and family (for dinner). The adverse effects of dieting and food restrictions were continuously discussed, particularly in regard to serving as "triggers" for binge eating or urges to binge eat. Through self-monitoring and weekly discussions, it was discovered that Sarah was more prone to binge eat when she skipped meals, had limited structure, felt anxious, grazed/picked at food in between meals or snacks, and/or felt "bored" in an environment with "junk food" freely available. Sarah also determined that utilizing her mother for support was helpful. For example, Sarah discussed the challenges she faced with eating and her thoughts and feelings about weight/shape with her mother, and together they would aim to work through possible solutions or alternative ways of thinking. She also began planning ahead and engaged in incompatible behaviors (e.g., reading a book, calling a friend, going for a walk with her mother) when she felt the urge to graze or binge eat.

Sarah also admitted to engaging in body checking (e.g., staring at herself in the bathroom mirror to check her chin, pinching the skin on her arms when sitting in class), which she noted often increased her negative self-evaluation and negative mood symptoms. Notably, Sarah was also observed engaging in body checking during sessions, such as being preoccupied with examining her thighs; this behavior allowed for in-the-moment identification of automatic thoughts, feelings, and thought restructuring. Sarah also brainstormed ways she could help herself to overcome body checking, which included removing mirrors in her bedroom, aiming to sit with her hands clasped, and asking for support persons (e.g., her mother, a close friend) to either verbally speak up or nonverbally acknowledge (e.g., tap her shoulder) when they observed the behavior.

Phases II and III of treatment introduced cognitive interventions, including problem-solving techniques, distorted/maladaptive thinking, and thought restructuring. Sarah was also encouraged to eat a range of foods, including feared foods (e.g., ice cream, cake, pasta, coffee creamer). Sarah made active attempts to engage in feared food behavioral experiments, particularly with the support of her mother. She noted that her cognitive thoughts/fears about "bad" foods decreased when she observed minimal changes in her weight and engaged in thought restructuring (e.g., "This one piece of cake cannot realistically make me gain 5 pounds"). Sarah completed several automatic thought logs, which were reviewed in session. Thought logs were often completed based on difficult eating situations (e.g., going out to eat with her family) or body image (e.g., putting on her swimsuit in the locker room, getting dressed to go out with her friends). Sarah was able to effectively challenge and restructure many of her distorted negative thoughts, often resulting in decreased negative affect and a more positive outlook. Sarah discussed several conclusions she came to throughout the course of treatment, including:

> "It is not hard to get back into my eating routine after 'bad' days."
> "Rules about eating do not help me. Setting absolute rules tends to set me up for challenges, and ultimately failure."
> "Physical appearance is just one aspect of me; it doesn't define or determine my friendships or success in life."

Weekly weighing occurred in each session. Sarah was informed of her weight in order to have accurate knowledge of what was happening to her weight throughout treatment. The importance of understanding weight as a range, rather than a set number, was frequently discussed. Emphasis was also placed on not focusing on inconsequential day-to-day fluctuations in weight, and Sarah was encouraged to refrain from weighing herself in between therapy sessions. Having a scale easily accessible in the home presented challenges for Sarah, and thus she asked her mother to support her in efforts to reduce "weight-checking" behaviors by getting rid of the scale. Notably, Sarah's weight showed minimal and appropriate fluctuation throughout treatment, ranging from 132 to 138 pounds (see Figure 10.3). Sarah's preoccupation with the number on the scale waxed and waned; however, after about 2 months of treatment, Sarah began to exhibit substantial changes in her thoughts regarding body weight that further aided in her eating disorder symptom remittance. For example, she concluded:

> "My weight is a function of a general lifestyle and is not meaningfully influenced by a single food decision."
> "Changes in my body weight and shape will not get me as much in life [in terms of positive outcome expectations] as I sometimes imagine."
> "Any upward or downward change in my weight does not mean my weight is on a new trajectory (i.e., it is not indicative of weight gain); it is merely normal weight fluctuation."

In addition to cognitive interventions, Phase III of treatment continued to focus on altering maladaptive behaviors. Of particular note was Sarah's tendency to engage in exercise more than once per day, skipping meals, and/or avoiding eating in front of others. She was encouraged to engage in behavioral experiments (e.g., limiting exercise to once per day, no exercising on weekends, eating in front of others and observing outcomes). The pros and cons of these behavioral changes were discussed, and Sarah frequently concluded that taking days off or limiting exercise (e.g., refraining from additional exercise outside of swim practice) often resulted in her feeling physically better, despite somewhat increased levels of anxiety in the short term. She also acknowledged that eating in front of others had some benefits, as she was less likely to experience a loss of control over her eating and could pace her eating with those around her. She also recognized that others were often self-focused during meals and thus were likely not being evaluative or judgmental of Sarah.

Phase IV of treatment consisted of reviewing Sarah's progress and relapse prevention. Sarah reported that she benefited from treatment, as treatment helped her to (1) identify and challenge distorted assumptions and thoughts; (2) think differently about her body weight/shape, eating, and exercise; (3) recognize and accept the concept of normal weight fluctuation; (4) problem-solve, particularly on "bad" days or when urges to binge eat increased; (5) accept that her weight was a process and function of a lifestyle, not one behavioral choice (e.g., eating a cookie, skipping a workout); and (6) learn to "wait out" urges to binge eat or purge because they will go away. She also stated that treatment helped her to recognize that eating regularly would not cause her to gain weight and that structure in her day and eating patterns is helpful in reducing binge eating. She acknowledged that she gained more "flexibility in her thinking" and gained more trust in "listening to [her] body" (when hungry or tired). She intended to continue to use several of the skills she learned in treatment, including focusing on planning ahead for the day, engaging in regular eating, focusing on eating more slowly (e.g., stopping to drink water throughout the meal, pacing her eating based on the speed of others, taking a break if "urges" to binge eat occurred), aiming for a structured daily schedule, using her mother for support, and completing thought and/or problem-solving logs as needed, with a particular emphasis on the prompt "What would you tell a friend?" Sarah reported feeling positive about ending treatment and expressed feeling hopeful about her ability to continue to effectively manage eating disorder symptoms.

Taken together, Sarah appeared to greatly benefit from CBT for the reduction of eating disorder symptoms (see Figure 10.3). She maintained a healthy weight, integrated feared foods back into her diet, began to eat regularly on a consistent basis, and reduced body- and weight-checking behaviors. Sarah also showed a large and sustained reduction in the frequency of objective binge eating, subjective binge eating, and inappropriate compensatory behaviors (e.g., self-induced vomiting, excessive/driven exercise, laxative misuse). The majority of binge-eating and/or compensatory behaviors over the last 2 months of treatment were isolated instances and occurred during particularly stressful weeks. Further, during periods in which her eating disorder symptoms were exacerbated, Sarah had insight into the triggers of her eating disorder behaviors (e.g., stress, irregular eating schedule, lack of adequate sleep). As a result of her success in treatment, Sarah was not referred for additional treatment; however, she agreed that she would seek additional treatment if her disordered eating symptoms returned and were deemed unmanageable on her own.

Family-Based Treatment

Empirical Support

FBT has received strong empirical support for the treatment of adolescents with AN and, more recently, for adolescents with BN (Le Grange, Crosby, Rathouz, & Leventhal, 2007; Le Grange et al., 2015), particularly when symptom duration is relatively short (<1–3 years; Le Grange & Lock, 2010; Lock & Le Grange, 2013). In adolescents with AN, specifically those with an age of onset at 18 years or younger (mean age = 16.6 years, SD = 1.7) and duration of illness less than 3 years, FBT has emerged as superior to individual supportive psychotherapy (SPT; Russell, Szmukler, Dare, & Eisler, 1987), and its effectiveness was maintained at a 5-year follow-up (Eisler et al., 1997). Similarly, adolescents with AN (ages 12–19; mean age approximately 14.3 years, SD approximately 2.4) who received behavioral family systems therapy (BFST), which was modeled after the FBT approach, showed better BMI outcomes at posttreatment and at 1-year follow-up than those who received an ego-oriented treatment (Robin, Siegel, Koepke, Moye, & Tice, 1994). Such effects were subsequently replicated in an independent sample spanning a slightly wider age range (ages 11–20; mean age approximately 15 years; Robin, Siegel, & Moye, 1995; Robin et al., 1999). One of the largest randomized trials of FBT for AN replicated and extended these results (Lock et al., 2010; N = 121; ages 12–18, mean age = 14.6 years, SD = 1.6), as adolescents who received FBT versus adolescent-focused therapy (AFT, based on the ego-oriented treatment) showed similar full remission (>95% expected body weight and within 1 SD of the community mean on a validated measure of eating pathology) rates at the end of treatment, but FBT was superior to AFT in terms of the number of youth who achieved partial remission (>85% expected body weight), total BMI percentile changes, and improvements in eating disorder psychopathology. Further, a greater number of youth who received FBT were fully remitted at 6-month and 12-month follow-ups, as compared with those who received AFT (Lock et al., 2010). Adolescents with AN who had more severe cognitive eating disorder symptoms at baseline showed greater remission rates when treated with FBT than AFT (Le Grange et al., 2012). Additionally, adolescents with AN who show early weight gain (approximately 5–7 pounds) by Session 4 are more likely to be in remission at the end of treatment, irrespective of whether they received FBT or AFT, although FBT was superior to AFT in terms of greater weight gain outcomes at follow-up (Le Grange, Accurso, Lock, Agras, & Bryson, 2014). Finally, in a large (N = 164; ages 12–18; mean age = 15.3 years, SD = 1.8) study that compared FBT to systemic family therapy (SyFT; a treatment that addresses general family processes), FBT emerged as the preferred treatment for adolescents with AN given that it resulted in significantly faster weight gain, significantly fewer days in the hospital, and lower overall treatment costs per patient (Agras et al., 2014). However, adolescents with more severe obsessive–compulsive symptoms achieved greater weight gain with SyFT (Agras et al., 2014).

Modifications to the standard implementation of FBT have shown promising results. In an examination of the dose of FBT (i.e., 10 vs. 20 sessions) for AN, Lock, Agras, Bryson, and Kraemer (2005) found no significant differences in BMI outcomes at the end of treatment, but youth who received 20 sessions of FBT showed significantly greater reductions on eating pathology and internalizing symptom scales than those who received only 10 sessions (mean age = 15.2 years, SD approximately 1.6). However, there were no differences on outcome measures of BMI or measures of eating disorder symptom changes between the short- and long-term versions of FBT at long-term follow-up (average approximately 4 years posttreatment; Lock, Couturier, & Agras, 2006). Both a conjoint (i.e., adolescent and her or his family together) and separated (i.e., parents and adolescent receive separate sessions) form of FBT have also been shown to be effective for adolescents with AN (mean age approximately 15 years) in terms of reductions in eating pathology and increases in self-esteem and body weight (Eisler et al., 2000; Le Grange, Eisler, Dare, & Russell, 1992), and no long-term differences in treatment outcomes were observed at a 5-year follow-up, with the exception that families high on maternal criticism at pretreatment showed better outcomes with the separated format (Eisler, Simic, Russell, & Dare, 2007).

Fewer studies have investigated the utility and effectiveness of FBT for adolescents with BN, but existing data support its use. In a small sample (N = 23) composed of adolescents and young adults (mean age = 24 years, SD = 8.4), individuals with BN were found to do equally well in FBT as in individual SPT at the end of treatment and at a 5-year follow-up (Russell et al., 1987; Eisler et al., 1997). However, in a larger randomized controlled trial of adolescents with BN (N = 41; ages 12–19, mean age = 16.1 years, SD = 1.6), a greater percentage of youth who received FBT reported abstinence from bulimic behaviors at the end of treatment and at the 6-month follow-up than did those who received individual SPT (Le Grange et al., 2007). Faster reductions in overall eating pathology were also observed in adolescents with BN who received FBT as compared to SPT (Le Grange et al., 2007). Interestingly, symptom reduction at Session 6 predicted remission at posttreatment and 6-month follow-up, regardless of treatment type (Le Grange, Doyle, Crosby, & Chen, 2008). Additional analyses point to some treatment moderations. Specifically, youth who reported lower eating disorder cognitions and depressive symptoms at baseline showed better remission-related outcomes, particularly when treated with FBT as compared with SPT (Le Grange, Crosby, & Lock, 2008). Adolescents with BN who showed greater baseline purging also showed a faster change in eating concerns when treated with FBT than with SPT; adolescents who showed lower rates of purging at baseline did equally well in FBT and SPT (Ciao, Accurso, Fitzsimmons-Craft, & Le Grange, 2015). In addition, younger individuals who received FBT (rather than SPT) showed a greater reduction in eating concerns, whereas similar changes in eating concerns were observed in older adolescents regardless of treatment type (Ciao et al., 2015). These data suggest that, in general, FBT may be more efficacious than SPT for adolescents with BN who are younger, exhibit more frequent purging, and report lower eating disorder cognitions and depressive symptoms.

As described previously (see the section "Empirical Support in Adolescents," pp. 231–232), FBT has also shown relatively similar outcomes to CBT in the treatment of adolescents with BN; however, only two studies have been conducted. In the first study, no significant differences were observed between treatments for reductions in eating disorder symptomatology at 6 or 12 months, although CBT resulted in faster reductions in binge eating and lower direct treatment costs at the end of treatment (Schmidt et al., 2007). In the most recent study, there were no treatment outcome differences between FBT and CBT at 12-month follow-up, but FBT resulted in fewer hospitalizations and greater abstinence from binge eating and purging at end of treatment and 6-month follow-up (Le Grange et al., 2015). FBT also resulted in greater reductions in depressive symptoms at the end of treatment (Le Grange et al., 2015). Nonetheless, family pathology was a significant moderator of treatment, with data suggesting that FBT may be the treatment of choice for low-conflict families, whereas FBT and CBT may be equally suitable for high-conflict families (Le Grange et al., 2015).

Family-Based Theory

FBT is theoretically agnostic regarding the cause of the eating disorder (Le Grange, 1999; Le Grange & Lock, 2010; Lock & Le Grange, 2013), and, similar to CBT, FBT is an approach that focuses on the current presenting symptoms rather than exploration of the etiology. It differs from more traditional family therapy models, which often aim to counteract the effects of external causative factors (e.g., familial dynamics) in the development of a problem and, instead, focuses on abolishing the individual's eating disorder symptoms by empowering parents to help their child overcome the eating disorder (Ciao, Anderson, & Le Grange, 2015). Further, rather than emphasizing an adolescent's desires for autonomy and control, FBT emphasizes that adolescents with eating disorders are imbedded in their families, are often regressed, and are very much out of control (i.e., the eating disorder is considered to be in control of the adolescent; Le Grange & Lock, 2010; Lock & Le Grange, 2013). Normal adolescent development and the youth's ability to independently comply with the demands of treatment (e.g., weight gain, reductions in purging, consumption of feared foods) are conceptualized as being arrested due to the complex nature of the eating disorder (Le Grange & Lock, 2010; Lock & Le Grange, 2013). Thus the involvement of parents is considered necessary to help the youth recover and resume normal adolescent development as quickly as possible (Le Grange & Lock, 2010; Lock & Le Grange, 2013).

Treatment Approach and Intervention

The basic premise of FBT is that parents should be considered the most useful resource in the treatment of adolescents with eating disorders. It is believed that most families can help their children and have the necessary skills for doing so. The therapist, therefore, serves as an expert consultant who can provide the parents with support, suggestions, ideas, information, and feedback, yet the parents are encouraged to independently determine the strategies they will employ (Le Grange & Lock, 2010; Lock & Le Grange, 2013). Parents may therefore navigate their way through treatment in a trial-and-error fashion, with strategies altered or adapted as needed, as this process facilitates their learning, problem solving, and empowerment in their child's treatment and recovery. Two additional fundamental tenets underlie the FBT approach, specifically: (1) neither the child nor the parents should be blamed for the cause of the illness, and (2) the illness should be externalized and separated from the child (Le Grange & Lock, 2010; Lock & Le Grange, 2013). It is important to clarify with all members of the family that many of the youth's current behaviors, reactions, emotions, and so forth are a direct consequence of the eating disorder and not reflective of who she or he is as a person (Le Grange & Lock, 2010; Lock & Le Grange, 2013). In addition, although the family is seen as a critical resource to helping the adolescent to achieve recovery and to facilitate behavioral changes, once the influence of the eating disorder on the adolescent's life is substantially reduced, the youth resumes gradual autonomy and is actively encouraged to return to normal adolescent developmental tasks (Le Grange & Lock, 2010; Lock & Le Grange, 2013).

Herein, we describe FBT, which is a highly focused and staged treatment that targets eating disorder psychopathology and emphasizes the role of the family in the recovery of children and adolescents with AN and BN. We briefly review FBT, as it is described by Lock and Le Grange (2013) for AN and by Le Grange and Lock (2010) for BN. Readers are referred to these manuals for more details; formal training is also commercially available.

FBT for AN and BN follows three phases that occur over the duration of 20 sessions. In contrast to CBT, the treatment duration of FBT is similar for persons with AN and BN (and therefore tends to be shorter than the recommended length, i.e., 40 sessions, of CBT-E for underweight persons). FBT is conducted within a treatment-team approach (ongoing medical monitoring by a physician and medication management by a psychiatrist, as needed), with the therapist serving as the team leader (Le Grange & Lock, 2010; Lock & Le Grange, 2013). FBT emphasizes behavioral recovery rather than youth insight or cognitive changes.

Furthermore, although behavioral theory is not a formal component of FBT, parental interventions may align with behavioral principles, and improvements in family functioning and cognitive changes often indirectly occur following the implementation of this treatment (Le Grange & Lock, 2010; Lock & Le Grange, 2013). Along these lines, FBT could be considered (albeit not in a strict sense) a behavioral-based therapy or a variant of CBT that deemphasizes cognitive change.

Phase I: Sessions 1–10

Setting Up Treatment

FBT is a time-limited treatment, and its success is said to be affected by early symptom change (Le Grange et al., 2008). Thus the therapist's connection with the family and early communication of treatment expectations and goals is critical. The first contact with the family to set up the initial treatment appointment should establish the role of the parents in their child's treatment. It is also important to effectively communicate the importance of the entire family's involvement in treatment (Le Grange & Lock, 2010; Lock & Le Grange, 2013). Contact with the family is made quickly following the referral, as this responsiveness underscores the message that there is a crisis in the family that is in need of immediate attention (Le Grange & Lock, 2010; Lock & Le Grange, 2013). It may, however, also be helpful for the therapist to acknowledge that the parents might feel overwhelmed, demoralized, and skeptical about their ability to play a key role in their child's recovery. If such feelings are endorsed, the therapist should aim to normalize these reactions and to convey a sense of confidence in the parents' ability to help their child. The therapist aims to use a warm but grave and concerned tone in all communication with the family (Le Grange & Lock, 2010; Lock & Le Grange, 2013).

In the initial contact, the therapist has three primary goals: (1) to stress the seriousness of the eating disorder and thus establish that there is a crisis within the family, (2) to set the foundation for parental involvement and management of the crisis, and (3) to provide information about the multidisciplinary treatment approach and establish the role of the team, such as ongoing medical monitoring by the pediatrician and psychiatric consultation for medication management, if needed (Le Grange & Lock, 2010; Lock & Le Grange, 2013). The therapist stresses that all family members living in the household, or even those not living in the household but with whom the adolescent spends a significant amount of time (e.g., grandparent), should be involved in treatment and attend the first session (Le Grange & Lock, 2010; Lock & Le Grange, 2013). The therapist may need to insist that consultation with the entire family is the only way to effectively address the crisis.

The First Face-to-Face Meeting

The first face-to-face meeting with the family aims to reiterate the seriousness of the youth's eating problem, as well as to begin to engage the entire family in treatment. Specific goals include:

1. Obtaining a history of the problem and how it has affected the family.
2. Assessing family functioning (e.g., coalitions or conflicts), primarily those that would interfere with the ability to work together in the achievement of treatment goals (e.g., lack of parental alignment or a disengaged parent).
3. Conveying the seriousness of the illness and attaining an optimal level of anxiety—for example, if parental anxiety is too high, the therapist should aim to reduce it; if parental anxiety is low, then the therapist should aim to increase the anxiety. This is achieved via reviewing medical consequences and mortality rates of eating disorders and discussing the long-term outcomes of early intervention and the effectiveness and utility of parental involvement.
4. Acknowledging potential feelings of self-blame within the parents and adolescent and aiming to reduce such blame (e.g., agnostic stance).
5. Helping to instill confidence in the parents and their ability to help their child (e.g., "You have a long history of being able to effectively feed your other children").
6. Externalizing or separating the illness from the adolescent (e.g.,

aiming to seek acknowledgment that there was a time when things were different).

7. Establishing weekly weighing, which will occur at the beginning of every appointment and serve to set the tone of the session, particularly if the adolescent is underweight (Le Grange & Lock, 2010; Lock & Le Grange, 2013).

In the treatment of BN, a binge-eating and purging log will also be established and completed at the beginning of every appointment (Le Grange & Lock, 2010).

For the adolescent with AN, the first session will conclude with the therapist charging the parents with the task of helping their child through recovery from the eating disorder, beginning with weight restoration (Lock & Le Grange, 2013). Siblings are also provided with a clear definition of their role in treatment—for example, to find ways to support their sibling, not to serve as an additional parent. Instructions for the family meal are also reviewed. Specifically, parents are asked to bring a meal that they collaboratively decide will help their child gain weight (Lock & Le Grange, 2013). Importantly, decisions about the meal should not occur in consultation with the adolescent or be limited to what the adolescent has been willing to eat. At the end of this session a therapist might say something like:

"It is clear from all of the information you provided as a family that [youth's name] is very ill and is suffering from anorexia nervosa. We know this illness will continue to worsen if something isn't done about this urgently. As parents you have already begun the process of helping [youth's name], and your support and decision making concerning food and exercise is essential at this time. What I would like you to do in anticipation of our next session is to discuss, as parents, a meal that will renourish your starving child. Please bring that meal to our next visit."

For the adolescent with BN, treatment is slightly modified such that parents are encouraged to collaborate with their son or daughter in terms of how to best confront the eating disorder symptoms (Le Grange & Lock, 2010). This more collaborative approach for BN cases, as compared with AN cases, is largely due to the fact that many adolescents with BN experience the binge-eating and purging symptoms as undesirable (Le Grange & Lock, 2010). The parental involvement in the treatment of adolescents with BN is largely focused on helping the child to overcome her or his problematic eating behaviors and to reinforce healthy eating patterns. The first session will conclude with the therapist charging the parents and the adolescent with the task of establishing regular eating, without episodes of binge eating and purging (Le Grange & Lock, 2010). Similar to FBT for AN, the supportive role that siblings will play within treatment is explained, and instructions for the family meal are reviewed. However, rather than focusing on foods that would help an individual regain weight (as in the case of persons with AN), parents are asked to bring a typical family meal with the inclusion of a food that is difficult for the adolescent to eat (Le Grange & Lock, 2010). For example, the family could bring an item from the adolescent's forbidden or feared food list or a food item that the youth may find triggering for binge eating.

The Family Meal

The second session begins with weighing the adolescent (and collecting information on binge and purge episodes in persons with BN) and then proceeding to the family meal. The purpose of the family meal is to provide an opportunity for the therapist to observe and assess the family structure, patterns around eating (food preparation, serving, etc.), and discussions about food choices and mealtimes (Le Grange & Lock, 2010; Lock & Le Grange, 2013). For individuals with AN, the family meal provides the parents with an opportunity to practice using a united parental front and to gain confidence in their abilities to successfully help their child eat more than the youth intended, in particular, supporting and convincing their child to eat "one more bite" (Lock & Le Grange, 2013). For individuals with BN, the family meal provides parents with the opportunity to experience success in their ability to help their child eat feared or forbidden food and, thus, to begin to reestablish a healthy pattern of eating and to attenuate binge-eating and purging behaviors (Le Grange & Lock, 2010). This in-the-moment experience of consuming a difficult food item also provides the adolescent with the unique opportunity to convey his or her thoughts that make it difficult to eat a forbidden or feared food. The therapist helps to facilitate a strong parental alliance, as well as to concurrently align the adolescent with his or her siblings (Le Grange & Lock, 2010; Lock & Le Grange, 2013). Both parents and siblings are complimented by the therapist on their positive efforts to support the adolescent during this meal. During a family meal, the therapist might say something like:

> "Based on the meal you have brought in today, it appears that the eating disorder may be influencing some of your decisions about what [youth's name] eats. For example, I noticed you brought sandwiches that had condiments and cheese for everyone else in the family, but the sandwich for [youth's name] only consisted of turkey and bread. Let's talk a bit about how those decisions were made. . . . I also want to acknowledge that you were very successful at getting [youth's name] to eat more of the potatoes, and you did this by working together as parents and staying persistent. This persistence coupled with an increased

focus on the caloric needs of [*youth's name*] will go very far in eradicating this illness."

The Remainder of Phase I

The remainder of Phase I focuses exclusively on the attenuation of eating disorder symptoms and, in the case of AN, on weight restoration. Parents are therefore continuously encouraged to figure out the best way to refeed their underweight child and to evaluate their efforts in treatment (Lock & Le Grange, 2013). For individuals with BN, parents are continuously encouraged to take charge of reestablishing healthy eating habits and to employ strategies that will limit or prevent binge-eating and purging episodes (Le Grange & Lock, 2010). The therapist continues to provide support to the family, aims to modify any apparent criticism toward the adolescent, reiterates the importance of externalizing the illness, and helps the family to evaluate the ways in which siblings are serving to support the adolescent (Le Grange & Lock, 2010; Lock & Le Grange, 2013). It is imperative that the focus of treatment remains on food and eating and, therefore, the therapist may need to direct or redirect the family back to these issues (Le Grange & Lock, 2010; Lock & Le Grange, 2013). Throughout Phase I, the adolescent is weighed at the beginning of each session, her or his weight is plotted on a graph, and this information is shared with the family in treatment to ensure transparency about the relative weekly progress. Binge-and-purge tracking logs are also reviewed at the beginning of every session for persons with BN. In regard to initiating discussions about the youth's weight and eating, a therapist might say:

> "[*Youth's name*] has gained 6 pounds in the last three sessions, due to your extensive efforts at nourishment, including supervising all of her meals and ensuring she is eating a rich variety of foods; however, it appears that this past week, the eating disorder has gotten a bit stronger. As parents, how would you like to approach this next week to ensure that we continue moving forward at eradicating the eating disorder?"

Phase II: Sessions 11–16

The shift from Phase I to Phase II typically occurs around Session 11; however, prior to making this transition, it is expected that youth with AN will have demonstrated substantial weight gain (approximately 90% of expected body weight for age and height) and be able to eat without substantial struggles and that youth with BN should have demonstrated an absence of binge eating and purging and regular eating without the need of excessive parental involvement (Le Grange & Lock, 2010; Lock & Le

Grange, 2013). The parents should also be feeling relieved, empowered, and confident in their abilities to manage the illness. If these guidelines are met, then control of food and eating will be slowly transferred back to the adolescent in a gradual manner (Le Grange & Lock, 2010; Lock & Le Grange, 2013). The therapist assists the family in navigating this transition. For example, initial steps may include the adolescent's dishing out her or his own food under parental supervision (in the case of AN). The therapist will continue to weigh the adolescent at every session, and weight gain or weight maintenance is discussed (Le Grange & Lock, 2010; Lock & Le Grange, 2013). Binge-eating and purge logs also continue to be reviewed weekly for individuals with BN (Le Grange & Lock, 2010). Treatment sessions often transition from weekly to every second to third week during this treatment phase, and toward the end of Phase II, time within treatment sessions can begin to be devoted to other, more general issues of adolescence (e.g., peer relations), presuming they are directly related to the eating disorder symptoms (Le Grange & Lock, 2010; Lock & Le Grange, 2013). The spacing of sessions should reflect clinical progress and match the level of support the family needs. At this point in treatment, a therapist might say something along the lines of:

> "[*Youth's name*] is doing an excellent job choosing her snacks, and it sounds like you have continued to feel that she is making good progress. What would you consider to be the next step for [*youth's name*] in furthering her independence related to eating?"

Phase III: Sessions 17–20

Transition to Phase III of treatment occurs when the youth's eating disorder symptoms have largely dissipated and weight restoration has been achieved (minimum expected body weight approximately 95%; Le Grange & Lock, 2010; Lock & Le Grange, 2013). Within Phase III, treatment aims to modify the parent–child relationship, as the eating disorder should no longer be the basis of the parent–child relationship (Le Grange & Lock, 2010; Lock & Le Grange, 2013). A primary goal is to get the individual back on a normal adolescent trajectory of development. This will typically require conversations about normal adolescent development (e.g., puberty, social identity and roles, leaving home for college) and the ways in which the illness temporarily disrupted the youth's life and development (Le Grange & Lock, 2010; Lock & Le Grange, 2013). The parents and adolescent are encouraged to discuss adolescent issues (e.g., friends, rules, dating) relevant to the teen's developmental stage. The therapist can facilitate parent–child discussions, such as how the parents might help the teen face and solve adolescent-related issues. During these discussions, it may be helpful to ask the parents to reflect upon what they recall about the struggles of being an adolescent, as doing so may allow the parents to more easily relate to the dilemmas faced by their child (fitting in with peers, identity, etc.). Finally, treatment progress is reviewed and relapse prevention is discussed. If the adolescent is in need of additional treatment (e.g., to address comorbidities, such as anxiety), relevant referrals are made at this time. Notably, sessions are typically spaced out toward the end of treatment (approximately monthly), as this may further aid to instill confidence in the family regarding the adolescent's recovery and her or his ability to manage the illness, as well as ease the transition associated with the final termination (Le Grange & Lock, 2010; Lock & Le Grange, 2013).

Summary and Future Directions

Although eating disorders often develop during adolescence, research on the treatment of children and adolescents with eating disorders has largely lagged behind that of adults. There are publications that establish guidelines for treatment, but these too are primarily focused on treatment of adults. Moreover, until recently there have been few published manuals that a clinician could rely upon to treat youth with an eating disorder. When looking at the treatment of adolescents and children with eating disorders to date, the most promising and extensive treatment data have involved the family.

Results from treatment outcome studies of CBT and FBT for adolescents with eating disorders are indeed promising. FBT is currently considered the first-line outpatient treatment for adolescents with AN. FBT results in fast symptom reductions, which are important given the substantial number of medical complications that correspond to AN. Nonetheless, it is important to acknowledge that some of the differences favoring FBT for AN diminish at longer-term follow-up, and other treatments may be suitable alternatives. Along these lines, emerging data suggest that CBT-E may be an efficacious alternative treatment for AN (at least for adolescents ≥ 13 years old). In the case of BN, both CBT and FBT have produced favorable outcomes in the reduction of eating disorder symptomatology, although findings have been mixed as to which treatment produces faster reductions in binge eating and purging (see Le Grange et al., 2015, vs. Schmidt et al., 2007). These initial results do not indicate one specific treatment for BN over another but provide a foundation in support of both CBT and FBT in the treatment of BN.

When considering the complexity of factors that can maintain eating disorder symptoms for adolescents (e.g., developmental phase; ego-syntonic nature of AN; binge–purge cycles), it is important that parents support their children in treatment. Although the role of parents may differ in CBT versus FBT, it is clear that the inclusion of parents in treatment can be helpful to the recovery of adolescents with eating disorders. The beneficial role of parents is notable, as the inclusion of parents in child/adolescent treatment for anxiety is less clear-cut (Kendall, Hudson, Gosch, Flannery-Schroeder, & Suveg, 2008).

Direct comparisons between CBT-E (or other forms of CBT, as well as alternative treatments such as IPT) and FBT in the treatment of adolescents with eating disorders are scarce, but necessary. Findings from additional studies can build upon current evidence and better elucidate which treatment to use and for whom. Treatment expectations (e.g., hope, perceptions of efficacy) have yet to be investigated as a factor for adolescents with eating disorders, but they may be beneficial to explore in future research. Indeed, positive recovery expectations have been shown to enhance parent and child engagement in treatment and treatment outcomes for other health conditions (Mondloch, Cole, & Frank, 2001). In addition, nonresponders to treatment are evident in both CBT and FBT studies, and additional work is needed to modify and enhance treatment for these persons. As treatments continue to be refined, studies regarding dissemination of treatment are needed. Indeed, it is our impression that once outside a research site the consistency or rigor of treatment protocols drops meaningfully. Alternative formats for treatment, such as group-based treatments, either with individual or family-based programs, may merit exploration.

References

Agras, W., Rossiter, E., Arnow, B., Telch, C., Raeburn, S., Bruce, B., et al. (1994). One-year follow-up of psychosocial and pharmacologic treatment for bulimia nervosa. *Journal of Clinical Psychiatry, 55,* 179–183.

Agras, W. S., Walsh, B. T., Fairburn, C. G., Wilson, G. T., & Kraemer, H. C. (2000). A multicenter comparison of cognitive-behavioral therapy and interpersonal psychotherapy for bulimia nervosa. *Archives of General Psychiatry, 57,* 459–466.

Allen, K. L., Byrne, S. M., Oddy, W. H., & Crosby, R. D. (2013). DSM-IV-TR and DSM-5 eating disorders in adolescents: Prevalence, stability, and psychosocial correlates in a population-based sample of male and female adolescents. *Journal of Abnormal Psychology, 122,* 720–732.

American Psychiatric Association. (2013). *Diagnostic and statistical manual of mental disorders* (5th ed.). Arlington, VA: Author.

Beck, J. S. (2011). *Cognitive behavior therapy: Basics and beyond* (2nd ed.). New York: Guilford Press.

Bowers, W. A., Evans, K., Le Grange, D., & Andersen, A. E. (2003). Treatment of adolescent eating disorders. In M. A. Reinecke, F. M. Dattilio, & A. Freeman (Eds.), *Cognitive therapy with children and adolescents: A casebook for clinical practice* (pp. 247–280). New York: Guilford Press.

Bravender, T., Bryant-Waugh, R., Herzog, D., Katzman, D., Kriepe, R. D., Lask,

B., et al. (2010). Classification of eating disturbance in children and adolescents: Proposed changes for the DSM-V. *European Eating Disorders Review, 18*, 79–89.

Brooks, S., Prince, A., Stahl, D., Campbell, I. C., & Treasure, J. (2011). A systematic review and meta-analysis of cognitive bias to food stimuli in people with disordered eating behaviour. *Clinical Psychology Review, 31*, 37–51.

Bulik, C. M., Brownley, K. A., Shapiro, J. R., & Berkman, N. D. (2012). Anorexia nervosa. In P. Sturmey & M. Hersen (Eds.), *Handbook of evidence-based practice in clinical psychology: Vol. 1. Child and adolescent disorders* (pp. 575–597). Hoboken, NJ: Wiley.

Byrne, S. M., Fursland, A., Allen, K. L., & Watson, H. (2011). The effectiveness of enhanced cognitive behavioural therapy for eating disorders: An open trial. *Behaviour Research and Therapy, 49*(4), 219–226.

Channon, S., De Silva, P., Hemsley, D., & Perkins, R. (1989). A controlled trial of cognitive-behavioural and behavioural treatment of anorexia nervosa. *Behaviour Research and Therapy, 27*(5), 529–535.

Ciao, A. C., Accurso, E. C., Fitzsimmons-Craft, E. E., & Le Grange, D. (2015). Predictors and moderators of psychological changes during the treatment of adolescent bulimia nervosa. *Behaviour Research and Therapy, 69*, 48–53.

Ciao, A. C., Anderson, K., & Le Grange, D. (2015). Family approaches to treatment. In L. Smolak & M. P. Levine (Eds.), *Wiley handbook of eating disorders* (pp. 828–842). Hoboken, NJ: Wiley.

Cooper, Z., & Stewart, A. (2008). CBT-E and the younger patient. In C. G. Fairburn, *Cognitive behavior therapy and eating disorders* (pp. 221–230). New York: Guilford Press.

Cottee-Lane, D., Pistrang, N., & Bryant-Waugh, R. (2004). Childhood onset anorexia nervosa: The experience of parents. *European Eating Disorders Review, 12*, 169–177.

Couturier, J., Lock, J., Forsberg, S., Vanderheyden, D., & Yen, H. L. (2007). The addition of a parent and clinician component to the Eating Disorder Examination for children and adolescents. *International Journal of Eating Disorders, 40*, 472–475.

Dalle Grave, R., Calugi, S., Doll, H. A., & Fairburn, C. G. (2013). Enhanced cognitive behaviour therapy for adolescents with anorexia nervosa: An alternative to family therapy? *Behaviour Research and Therapy, 51*, R9–R12.

Eddy, K. T., Celio Doyle, A., Rienecke Hoste, R., Herzog, D. B., & Le Grange, D. (2008). Eating disorder not otherwise specified in adolescents. *Journal of the American Academy of Child and Adolescent Psychiatry, 47*, 156–164.

Eddy, K. T., Dorer, D. J., Franko, D. L., Tahilani, K., Thompson-Brenner, H., & Herzog, D. B. (2008). Diagnostic crossover in anorexia nervosa and bulimia nervosa: Implications for DSM-V. *American Journal of Psychiatry, 165*, 245–250.

Eddy, K. T., Keel, P. K., Dorer, D. J., Delinsky, S. S., Franko, D. L., & Herzog, D. B. (2002). Longitudinal comparison of anorexia nervosa subtypes. *International Journal of Eating Disorders, 31*, 191–201.

Eisler, I., Dare, C., Russell, G. F., Szmukler, G., Le Grange, D., & Dodge, E. (1997). Family and individual therapy in anorexia nervosa: A 5-year follow-up. *Archives of General Psychiatry, 54*, 1025–1030.

Eisler, I., Dare, C., Hodes, M., Russell, G., Dodge, E., & Le Grange, D. (2000).

Family therapy for adolescent anorexia nervosa: The results of a controlled comparison of two family interventions. *Journal of Child Psychology and Psychiatry, 41,* 727–736.

Eisler, I., Simic, M., Russell, G. F., & Dare, C. (2007). A randomised controlled treatment trial of two forms of family therapy in adolescent anorexia nervosa: A five-year follow-up. *Journal of Child Psychology and Psychiatry, 48,* 552–560.

Fairburn, C. G. (2008). *Cognitive behavior therapy and eating disorders.* New York: Guilford Press.

Fairburn, C. G., Cooper, Z., Doll, H. A., O'Connor, M. E., Bohn, K., Hawker, D. M., et al. (2009). Transdiagnostic cognitive-behavioral therapy for patients with eating disorders: A two-site trial with 60-week follow-up. *American Journal of Psychiatry, 166,* 311–319.

Fairburn, C. G., Cooper, Z., Doll, H. A., O'Connor, M. E., Palmer, R. L., & Dalle Grave, R. (2013). Enhanced cognitive behaviour therapy for adults with anorexia nervosa: A UK–Italy study. *Behaviour Research and Therapy, 51,* R2–R8.

Fairburn, C. G., Cooper, Z., & Shafran, R. (2008). Enhanced cognitive behavior therapy for eating disorders ("CBT-E"): An overview. In C. G. Fairburn, *Cognitive behavior therapy and eating disorders* (pp. 23–34). New York: Guilford Press.

Fairburn, C. G., Jones, R., Peveler, R. C., Carr, S. J., Solomon, R. A., O'Connor, M. E., et al. (1991). Three psychological treatments for bulimia nervosa: A comparative trial. *Archives of General Psychiatry, 48,* 463–469.

Fairburn, C. G., Jones, R., Peveler, R. C., Hope, R. A., O'Connor, M. E., et al. (1993). Psychotherapy and bulimia nervosa: Longer-term effects of interpersonal psychotherapy, behavior therapy, and cognitive behavior therapy. *Archives of General Psychiatry, 50,* 419–428.

Fairburn, C. G., Norman, P. A., Welch, S. L., O'Connor, M. E., Doll, H. A., & Peveler, R. C. (1995). A prospective study of outcome in bulimia nervosa and the long-term effects of three psychological treatments. *Archives of General Psychiatry, 52,* 304–312.

Fairburn, C. G., Peveler, R. C., Jones, R., Hope, R. A., & Doll, H. A. (1993). Predictors of 12-month outcome in bulimia nervosa and the influence of attitudes to shape and weight. *Journal of Consulting and Clinical Psychology, 61,* 696–698.

Garner, D. M., Rockert, W., Davis, R., Garner, M. V., Olmsted, M. P., & Eagle, M. (1993). Comparison of cognitive-behavioral and supportive–expressive therapy for bulimia nervosa. *American Journal of Psychiatry, 150,* 37–46.

Gowers, S. G. (2006). Evidence based research in CBT with adolescent eating disorders. *Child and Adolescent Mental Health, 11,* 9–12.

Gowers, S., & Bryant-Waugh, R. (2004). Management of child and adolescent eating disorders: The current evidence base and future directions. *Journal of Child Psychology and Psychiatry, 45*(1), 63–83.

Gowers, S. G., Clark, A., Roberts, C., Griffiths, A., Edwards, V., Bryan, C., et al. (2007). Clinical effectiveness of treatments for anorexia nervosa in adolescents: Randomized controlled trial. *British Journal of Psychiatry, 191,* 427–435.

Gowers, S. G., & Green, L. (2009). *Eating disorders: Cognitive behavioral therapy with children and young people*. London: Routledge.

Haedt-Matt, A. A., & Keel, P. K. (2011). Revisiting the affect regulation model of binge eating: A meta-analysis of studies using ecological momentary assessment. *Psychological Bulletin, 137*, 660–681.

Insel, T., Cuthbert, B., Garvey, M., Heinssen, R., Pine, D. S., Quinn, K., et al. (2010). Research domain criteria (RDoC): Toward a new classification framework for research on mental disorders. *American Journal of Psychiatry, 167*, 748–751.

Kachani, A. T., Brasiliano, S., Cordás, T. A., & Hochgraf, P. B. (2013). Body checking and associated cognitions among Brazilian outpatients with eating disorders and nonpsychiatric controls. *Body Image, 10*, 127–130.

Kaye, W. H., Weltzin, T. E., Hsu, L. K. G., McConaha, C. W., & Bolton, B. (1993). Amount of calories retained after binge eating and vomiting. *American Journal of Psychiatry, 150*, 969–969.

Keel, P. K., Brown, T. A., Holm-Denoma, J., & Bodell, L. P. (2011). Comparison of DSM-IV versus proposed DSM-5 diagnostic criteria for eating disorders: Reduction of eating disorder not otherwise specified and validity. *International Journal of Eating Disorders, 44*, 553–560.

Kendall, P. C., Hudson, J., Gosch, E., Flannery-Schroeder, E., & Suveg, C. (2008). Cognitive-behavioral therapy for anxiety disordered youth: A randomized clinical trial evaluating child and family modalities. *Journal of Consulting and Clinical Psychology, 76*, 282–297.

Kendall, P. C., & Peterman, J. (2015). CBT for anxious adolescents: Mature yet still developing. *American Journal of Psychiatry, 172*, 519–530.

Klump, K. L. (2013). Puberty as a critical risk period for eating disorders: A review of human and animal studies. *Hormones and Behavior, 64*, 399–410.

Kyriacou, O., Treasure, J., & Schmidt, U. (2008). Understanding how parents cope with living with someone with anorexia nervosa: Modelling the factors that are associated with carer distress. *International Journal of Eating Disorders, 41*, 233–242.

Le Grange, D. (1999). Family therapy for adolescent anorexia nervosa. *Journal of Clinical Psychology, 55*, 727–740.

Le Grange, D., Accurso, E. C., Lock, J., Agras, S., & Bryson, S. W. (2014). Early weight gain predicts outcome in two treatments for adolescent anorexia nervosa. *International Journal of Eating Disorders, 47*(2), 124–129.

Le Grange, D., Crosby, R. D., & Lock, J. (2008). Predictors and moderators of outcome in family-based treatment for adolescent bulimia nervosa. *Journal of the American Academy of Child and Adolescent Psychiatry, 47*(4), 464–470.

Le Grange, D., Crosby, R. D., Rathouz, P. J., & Leventhal, B. L. (2007). A randomized controlled comparison of family-based treatment and supportive psychotherapy for adolescent bulimia nervosa. *Archives of General Psychiatry, 64*, 1049–1056.

Le Grange, D., Doyle, P., Crosby, R. D., & Chen, E. (2008). Early response to treatment in adolescent bulimia nervosa. *International Journal of Eating Disorders, 41*, 755–757.

Le Grange, D., Eisler, I., Dare, C., & Russell, G. (1992). Evaluation of family treatments in adolescent anorexia nervosa: A pilot study. *International Journal of Eating Disorders, 12,* 347–357.

Le Grange, D., & Lock, J. (2010). Family-based treatment for adolescents with bulimia nervosa. In C. M. Grilo & J. E. Mitchell (Eds.), *The treatment of eating disorders: A clinical handbook* (pp. 372–387). New York: Guilford Press.

Le Grange, D., Lock, J., Agras, W. S., Bryson, S. W., & Booil, J. (2015). Randomized clinical trial of family-based treatment and cognitive-behavioral therapy for adolescent bulimia nervosa. *Journal of the American Academy of Child and Adolescent Psychiatry, 54,* 886–894.

Le Grange, D., Lock, J., Agras, W. S., Moye, A., Bryson, S. W., Jo, B., et al. (2012). Moderators and mediators of remission in family-based treatment and adolescent-focused therapy for anorexia nervosa. *Behaviour Research and Therapy, 50,* 85–92.

Lock, J., Agras, W. S., Bryson, S., & Kraemer, H. C. (2005). A comparison of short- and long-term family therapy for adolescent anorexia nervosa. *Journal of the American Academy of Child and Adolescent Psychiatry, 44,* 632–639.

Lock, J., Couturier, J., & Agras, W. S. (2006). Comparison of long-term outcomes in adolescents with anorexia nervosa treated with family therapy. *Journal of the American Academy of Child and Adolescent Psychiatry, 45,* 666–672.

Lock, J., & Le Grange, D. (2013). *Treatment manual for anorexia nervosa: A family-based approach.* New York: Guilford Press.

Lock, J., Le Grange, D., Agras, W. S., Moye, A., Bryson, S. W., & Jo, B. (2010). Randomized clinical trial comparing family-based treatment with adolescent-focused individual therapy for adolescents with anorexia nervosa. *Archives of General Psychiatry, 67,* 1025–1032.

McIntosh, V., Jordan, J., Carter, F., Luty, S., McKenzie, J., Bulik, C., et al. (2005). Three psychotherapies for anorexia nervosa: A randomized controlled trial. *American Journal of Psychiatry, 162,* 741–747.

McIntosh, V. V., Jordan, J., Luty, S. E., Carter, F. A., McKenzie, J. M., Bulik, C. M., et al. (2006). Specialist supportive clinical management for anorexia nervosa. *International Journal of Eating Disorders, 39,* 625–632.

Meeus, W., Iedema, J., Helsen, M., & Vollebergh, W. (1999). Patterns of adolescent identity development: Review of literature and longitudinal analysis. *Developmental Review, 19,* 419–461.

Mohr, H. M., Röder, C., Zimmermann, J., Hummel, D., Negele, A., & Grabhorn, R. (2011). Body image distortions in bulimia nervosa: Investigating body size overestimation and body size satisfaction by fMRI. *NeuroImage, 56,* 1822–1831.

Mondloch, M. V., Cole, D. C., & Frank, J. W. (2001). Does how you do depend on how you think you'll do?: A systematic review of the evidence for a relation between patients' recovery expectations and health outcomes. *Canadian Medical Association Journal, 165*(2), 174–179.

Murphy, R., Staebler, S., Cooper, Z., & Fairburn, C. G. (2010). Cognitive behavioral therapy for eating disorders. *Psychiatric Clinics of North America, 33,* 611–627.

Pike, K. M., Walsh, B. T., Vitousek, K., Wilson, G. T., & Bauer, J. (2003). Cognitive behavior therapy in the posthospitalization treatment of anorexia nervosa. *American Journal of Psychiatry, 160,* 2046–2049.

Robin, A. L., Siegel, P. T., Koepke, T., Moye, A. W., & Tice, S. (1994). Family therapy versus individual therapy for adolescent females with anorexia nervosa. *Journal of Developmental and Behavioral Pediatrics, 15,* 111–116.

Robin, A. L., Siegel, P. T., & Moye, A. (1995). Family versus individual therapy for anorexia impact on family conflict. *International Journal of Eating Disorders, 17,* 313–322.

Robin, A. L., Siegel, P. T., Moye, A. W., Gilroy, M., Dennis, A. B., & Sikand, A. (1999). A controlled comparison of family versus individual therapy for adolescents with anorexia nervosa. *Journal of the American Academy of Child and Adolescent Psychiatry, 38,* 1482–1489.

Roerig, J. L., Steffen, K. J., Mitchell, J. E., & Zunker, C. (2010). Laxative abuse: Epidemiology, diagnosis, and management. *Drugs, 70,* 1487–1503.

Rosso, I. M., Young, A. D., Femia, L. A., & Yurgelun-Todd, D. A. (2004). Cognitive and emotional components of frontal lobe functioning in childhood and adolescence. *Annals of the New York Academy of Sciences, 1021*(1), 355–362.

Russell, G. F., Szmukler, G. I., Dare, C., & Eisler, I. (1987). An evaluation of family therapy in anorexia nervosa and bulimia nervosa. *Archives of General Psychiatry, 44,* 1047–1056.

Schmidt, U., Lee, S., Beecham, J., Perkins, S., Treasure, J., Yi, I., et al. (2007). A randomized controlled trial of family therapy and cognitive behavior therapy guided self-care for adolescents with bulimia nervosa and related disorders. *American Journal of Psychiatry, 164,* 591–598.

Spanos, A., Klump, K. L., Burt, S. A., McGue, M., & Iacono, W. G. (2010). A longitudinal investigation of the relationship between disordered eating attitudes and behaviors and parent–child conflict: A monozygotic twin differences design. *Journal of Abnormal Psychology, 119,* 293–299.

Stein, D., Lilenfeld, L. R., Wildman, P. C., & Marcus, M. D. (2004). Attempted suicide and self-injury in patients diagnosed with eating disorders. *Comprehensive Psychiatry, 45,* 447–451.

Swanson, S. A., Crow, S. J., Le Grange, D., Swendsen, J., & Merikangas, K. R. (2011). Prevalence and correlates of eating disorders in adolescents: Results from the national comorbidity survey replication adolescent supplement. *Archives of General Psychiatry, 68*(7), 714–723.

Waller, G., Cordery, H., Corstorphine, E., Hinrichsen, H., Lawson, R., Mountford, V., et al. (2007). *Cognitive behavioral therapy for eating disorders: A comprehensive treatment guide.* Cambridge, UK: Cambridge University Press.

Walsh, B. T., Wilson, G. T., Loeb, K. L., Devlin, M. J., & Pike, K. M. (1997). Medication and psychotherapy in the treatment of bulimia nervosa. *American Journal of Psychiatry, 154,* 523–531.

Wilson, G. T., Fairburn, C. C., Agras, W. S., Walsh, B. T., & Kraemer, H. (2002). Cognitive-behavioral therapy for bulimia nervosa: Time course and mechanisms of change. *Journal of Consulting and Clinical Psychology, 70*(2), 267.

Wilson, G. T., Loeb, K. L., Walsh, B. T., Labouvie, E., Petkova, E., Liu, X., et al. (1999). Psychological versus pharmacological treatments of bulimia nervosa: Predictors and processes of change. *Journal of Consulting and Clinical Psychology, 67,* 451–459.

Wilson, G. T., & Pike, K. M. (2001). Eating disorders. In D. Barlow (Ed.), *Clinical *handbook of psychological disorders* (3rd ed., pp. 332–375). New York: Guilford Press.

Wilson, G. T., & Sysko, R. (2006). Cognitive-behavioural therapy for adolescents with bulimia nervosa. *European Eating Disorders Review, 14,* 8–16.

Wilson, G. T., & Zandberg, L. J. (2012). Cognitive–behavioral guided self-help for eating disorders: Effectiveness and scalability. *Clinical Psychology Review, 32*(4), 343–357.

Wolff, G., & Treasure, J. (2011). Medical and psychological consequences of eating disorders. In J. Morris (Ed.), *ABC of eating disorders* (pp. 20–25). Hoboken, NJ: Wiley.

Wonderlich, S. A., Connolly, K. M., & Stice, E. (2004). Impulsivity as a risk factor for eating disorder behavior: Assessment implications with adolescents. *International Journal of Eating Disorders, 36,* 172–182.

Wonderlich, S. A., Peterson, C. B., Crosby, R. D., Smith, T. L., Klein, M. H., Mitchell, J. E., et al. (2014). A randomized controlled comparison of integrative cognitive-affective therapy (ICAT) and enhanced cognitive-behavioral therapy (CBT-E) for bulimia nervosa. *Psychological Medicine, 44,* 543–553.

CHAPTER ELEVEN

Addressing Academic Skills Problems

Matthew K. Burns
Melissa Coolong-Chaffin
Rebecca Kanive

There is a pandemic in U.S. schools. Gutkin (2012) pointed out that our rate of failure for children in this country is alarming and called it a "pandemic." Approximately one-third of the nation's fourth and eighth graders' scores demonstrated proficiency in reading, and approximately 35–40% were proficient in math (U.S. Department of Education, 2015). Although those numbers are alarming, one could wonder about their relevance in a book about cognitive therapy. Our reply is twofold.

First, there is a clear link between academic skills deficits and behavior difficulties, so much so that it seems that "sometimes the best mental health intervention is to teach a student how to read" (A. Canter, personal communication, September 2006). Academic difficulties can lead to frustration, escape-maintained behavior, and other behavior difficulties (Hagan-Burke, Gilmour, Gerow, & Crowder, 2015). The relationship between academic and behavior difficulties is relatively stable throughout development (Bub, McCartney, & Willett, 2007; Morgan, Farkas, Tufis, & Sperling, 2008; Reinke, Lewis-Palmer, & Merrell, 2008), and co-occurring academic and behavior problems early in development led to greater risk of being diagnosed with a disability and dropping out of school later in life (Darney, Reinke, Herman, Stormont, & Ialongo, 2013).

Second, the current approach in schools is not working. In addition to the alarmingly low percentage of students proficient in reading and math, approximately 50% of adolescents in U.S. schools are diagnosed with a mental disorder, with one-third of the adolescent population being diagnosed with anxiety disorders (Merikangas et al., 2010). Gutkin (2012) attributed much of the poor outcome for students to mental health service providers' acceptance of the medical model explanation for student difficulties that attributes the difficulties to internal states of disease and pathology. Gutkin (2009, 2012; Sheridan & Gutkin, 2000) argued for an ecological approach that modifies the environment in which students function because " 'curing' internal pathologies and then returning children to unchanged environments that either created or supported the creation of these pathologies in the first place would seem to be an act of futility that invites recidivism and poor generalization" (Gutkin, 2009, p. 482).

Cognitive therapy provides an alternative to less successful approaches for two reasons. First, cognitive therapy focuses on one's set of beliefs, attitudes, and expectations and teaches how to use them in adaptive way (Reinecke, Dattilio, & Freeman, 2003). In other words, cognitive therapy focuses on internal states but also recognizes that the internal states are malleable. Second, cognitive therapy teaches strategies to solve problems, communicate, and interact with others while framing efforts within a developmental perspective (see Kendall, Chapter 1, this volume), which are core tenets of ecological systems theory. Most readers are likely familiar with Bronfenbrenner's (1979) framework for understanding development, but more contemporary views of ecological systems theory stress the "person–context interrelatedness" (Tudge, Mokrova, Hatfield, & Karnik, 2009, p. 199) of the systems. An ecological approach to intervention considers the developmental phase of the person and the processes of interaction within the multiple contexts, which is also a goal of cognitive therapy.

Cognitive Therapy and Academic Skills Problems

Because cognitive therapy focuses on problem-solving and coping strategies through assessment, teaching, and self-monitoring (Reinecke et al., 2003), it provides a unique method to reshape inefficient or ineffective student approaches to learning. Next, we discuss strategies used in reading and math, methods to assess and teach them, and self-monitoring.

Reading Strategies

Reading is a complex process that entails numerous skills and strategies. Afflerbach, Pearson, and Paris (2008) defined reading strategies as goal-directed attempts to control how a reader decodes text, reads words, and understands text, but skills are much more automatic and result in decoding and comprehending text with speed and efficiency. Students with severe reading problems do not read strategically and do not self-monitor their understanding (Gersten, Fuchs, Williams, & Baker, 2001). Moreover, research has consistently demonstrated the positive effects of strategy instruction for students with reading difficulties (Berkeley, Mastropieri, & Scruggs, 2011).

Many strategic approaches to reading have been shown to be effective. For example, reciprocal teaching teaches students to apply cognitive strategies while reading to improve comprehension (Brown & Palincsar, 1989). The student is taught to generate questions, summarize, clarify word meanings or confusing text, and predict what might appear in the following text. This method has consistently led to improvements in reading comprehension with students who decode adequately but do not read with high comprehension (Spörer, Brunstein, & Kieschke, 2009; Lysynchuk, Pressley, & Vye, 1990). However, students must also be aware of the strategies they are using and how well they use them, regardless of the strategy being implemented. Instruction in reading comprehension is most effective if it develops readers' understanding of their own cognitive processes involved in reading (National Reading Panel, 2000)

Mathematics Strategies

Strategic competence in math is "the ability to formulate mathematical problems, represent them, and solve them" (Kilpatrick et al., 2001, p. 124), and, much like reading, it is dependent on skills such as conceptual understanding and procedural fluency (Lemaire & Siegler, 1995). Development of strategic competence follows a process in which basic computational calculations are solved using procedural strategies (e.g., counting on fingers) with a gradual shift toward being solved by retrieval, which is a more efficient strategy (Price, Mazzocco, & Ansari, 2013). Students with mathematics difficulties have persistent difficulties in computing problems due to immature strategies (Geary, 2004; Jordan, Hanich, & Kaplan, 2003). Teaching effective strategies (e.g., mature and efficient) to struggling students to improve mastery and fluency is an important contributor to a student's ability to solve problems (Baker, Gersten, & Lee, 2002; Gersten, Jordan, & Flojo, 2005). Moreover, strategy choice on addition problems significantly correlated ($r = .71$, $p < .01$) with performance on mathematical achievement measures (Geary & Burlingham-Dubree, 1989). The most prevalent strategy types included and studied within research are discussed next.

Counting

Counting strategies are considered the slowest and least accurate of strategies that children use to solve arithmetic problems. Barrouillet, Mignon, and Thevenot (2008) examined strategies in subtraction problem solving in children and suggested that using the algorithmic strategy of counting may prevent reinforcement of facts. Students directly model the problem, sometimes by representing the multiplicand by sets of tally marks and then counting each individual tally mark or with pictures representing sets and objects in each set. Although basic, modeling of a problem demonstrates conceptual understanding.

Repeated Addition

Repeated addition involves representing the multiplicand (first number) the number of times indicated by the multiplier (second number) and then adding these numbers. For example, to solve 3×7, a student would set up the problem as $3 + 3 + 3 + 3 + 3 + 3 + 3 =$ and then add the digits to find the sum of 21. Finding the product may rely on a student's competency with counting by digits such as 2's or 5's. Multiplication is commonly thought of as repeated addition, bit multiplication requires higher-order multiplicative thinking, which develops out of but is not equal to knowledge of addition (Clark & Kamii, 1996).

Decomposition

More mature strategies such as decomposition involve use of rules and/or derived facts to solve problems. Decomposition relies on a student's retrieval of specific, easily retrieved multiplication (e.g., doubles or facts with factors of 2 or 5) and adding or subtracting. For example, if attempting to solve a problem such as 4×5, a student may know the doubles fact that $4 \times 4 = 16$ and then add an additional 4 to that product to find the answer of 20.

Direct Retrieval

Learned associations of pairs of factors with their product, in which response is rapid and no visible computation is identified, is considered to be direct retrieval and is often a product of development due to the strength of association between the problem and the answer increasing with practice (Lemaire & Siegler, 1995). Direct retrieval is considered a mature approach to completing computation, and fluent retrieval of facts significantly predicted more advanced mathematical skills (VanDerHeyden & Burns, 2009).

Word Problems

The strategies described above are useful for computation, especially multiplication and division, but a different strategy is used for word problems and other applications. Montague (1992) combined cognitive and metacognitive elements into the Say–Ask–Check prompt that was tied to the seven cognitive strategy steps including (1) reading the problem (the student reads and studies the problem before proceeding), (2) paraphrasing the problem (the student restates the problem in order to demonstrate understanding), (3) drawing the problem (the student creates a drawing of the problem to consolidate understanding), (4) creating a plan to solve the problem (the student generates a plan to solve the problem), (5) predicting/estimating the answer (the student uses estimation or other strategies to predict or estimate the answer), (6) computing the answer (the student follows the plan to solve the problem), and (7) checking the answer (the student reviews the computation steps to verify the answer).

Homework

The word "homework" has a specific application to cognitive therapists, but it has a different application for academic problems. Homework is independent practice of recently taught objectives in a setting that is different from the one in which they were initially learned, which has been shown to be an effective component of cognitive therapy (Kazantzis, Whittington, & Dattillio, 2010) and of learning new academic skills (Dettmers, Trautwein, Lüdtke, Kunter, & Baumert, 2010; Gustafsson, 2013). However, the effects of homework in an academic task may also have implications for cognitive therapy, because homework completion has been linked to increased self-regulation, such as setting goals, self-efficacy, self-reflection, time management, and delayed gratification (Ramdass & Zimmerman, 2011).

Langberg, Epstein, Becker, Girio-Herra, and Vaughn (2012) implemented the homework, organization, and planning skills (HOPS) intervention with 47 middle school students with attention problems and found that it led to more organized action, better managed materials, more effective planning, and improved homework completion behavior. HOPS teaches school materials organization, homework recording and management, and planning/time management in daily 20-minute sessions that involve (1) book bag, school binder, and locker organization, (2) an organization system for transferring homework materials to and from school, (3) accurate and consistent recording of homework assignments, (4) breaking projects and studying for tests down into smaller, more manageable pieces, (5) self-monitoring, and (6) a point system for implementing the system (Langberg, 2011).

Researchers have effectively used other approaches to improve completion of school homework, including parental consultation with collaborative goal setting and teaching management strategies (Raggi, Chronis-Tuscano, Fishbein, & Groomes, 2009), group contingencies (Lynch, Theodore, Bray, & Kehle, 2009), and self-monitoring and self-management of behavior

(Axelrod, Zhe, Haugen, & Klein, 2009). Therefore, it seems that cognitive therapists may support therapeutic goals related to self-regulation if they work with students to better complete homework through some combination of goal setting, self-monitoring, contingencies for completing homework, and instruction in organizational strategies.

Assessment

Assessment is a critical aspect of any intervention model and is crucial to effective cognitive therapy because therapists use the assessment data to better understand the problem (Reinecke et al., 2003). Researchers have spent decades attempting to identify sources of data to better understand reading and math problems. Cronbach dedicated much of his career to finding an aptitude-by-treatment interaction (ATI) in which data from assessments of underlying cognitive processes (e.g., working memory, short-term memory, and spatial reasoning) could be used to identify interventions with differential effects (Cronbach, 1957). However, research found no special benefit of those data for understanding reading and math problems (Cronbach & Snow, 1977).

Recent attempts to identify interventions based on data from cognitive assessments have not fared much better, as meta-analyses of more than 200 studies since 2009 have found small effects ($d = 0.27$; Burns, 2016). The meta-analysis by Burns et al. (2016) also reported small effects for interventions derived from cognitive processing data ($g = 0.17$), but measures that directly assessed the skill (decoding skill or reading fluency) led to much larger effects ($g = 0.43$ and 0.50, respectively), which was presented as evidence for a skill-by-treatment interaction (STI). An STI is defined as systematically identifying and manipulating environmental conditions that are directly related to the problem in order to isolate skill deficits and suggest appropriate interventions matched to student skill needs (Burns, Codding, Boice, & Lukito, 2010). In addition, a previous meta-analysis found a low correlation between student reading growth and IQ ($r = .11$) but a significantly stronger correlation between reading growth and baseline measures of reading fluency ($r = .37$) and word attack ($r = .36$; Scholin & Burns, 2012). Moreover, word reading correlated with IQ at $r = .35$ and with memory at $r = .31$ but with word attack at $r = .61$, spelling at $r = .70$, and reading comprehension at $r = .64$ (Swanson, Trainin, Necoechea, & Hammill, 2003).

Given that direct measures of the skill lead to more effective interventions, cognitive therapists can benefit from an assessment of the skill involved in the problem. Of course, the therapist will need to assess not only the strategy that students are using but also underlying skills to be certain that the deficit is not more fundamental. Table 11.1 lists measures for various skill deficits to assess underlying skills. The numbered items in the table are designed to show a sequence. For example, start by assessing overall reading, then examine comprehension skill, and then fluency/decoding skills. The measures included in Table 11.1 are commonly used by schools, and there is a strong chance that the required data already exist. The table also includes sample criteria with which the data can be compared. Next, we discuss an assessment framework to determine an instructional level (an appropriate level of change) for students as a way to begin assessments and methods to assess reading and mathematics strategies used by the student.

Instructional Level

Teachers and other school personnel often talk about the importance of teaching students at their instructional level, or the appropriate balance between task expectations and student performance that results in the best learning (Burns & Parker, 2014). In fact, the term "instructional level" is probably one of the most used, and most important, in all of education. Curriculum-based assessment for instructional design (CBA-ID) is a quick and easy way to determine whether a student's assigned task represents an instructional level. Assessors implement CBA-ID for reading by having the student read for 1 minute from classroom reading material (e.g., basal reader, chapter book, content area book) while recording the number of words read correctly. The total number of words read correctly is then divided by the total number of words in the sample to create a percentage of words read correctly, which is then compared with an instructional level criterion of 93–97%.

Specific assessment procedures for reading involve placing the reading material in front of the student and instructing him or her to (1) start at the top of the page and read out loud, (2) do his or her very best reading, and (3) keep reading until he or she is told to stop. The student is told to try his or her best but that, if he or she comes to a word that is not known, then the word will be provided for him or her (Burns & Parker, 2014). The student is timed for 1 minute as he or she reads out loud, and errors are recorded. Any word that is not read correctly within 2 seconds is counted as an error. At the end of 1 minute, the number of words read correctly is counted, divided by the total number of words (words correctly read plus number of errors), and multiplied by 100. If the percentage falls within 93–97%, then the passage represents an instructional level. More challenging material (less than 93% correct) represents a frustration level, and more than 97% correct represents an independent level. We recommend repeating this process two additional times and selecting the median.

CBA-ID for math begins by selecting the objective to assess. In practice, it is often the objective (topic) being covered in class at that point. Once the objective is identified, then the interventionist can use a measure of that objective or can create her or his own with one of a number of free Web-based systems (e.g., *www.mathfactscafe.com*; *www.*

TABLE 11.1. Examples of Assessments of Skills to Identify Student Deficits

Skill	Measures	Data	Sample criteria
Reading			
Overall reading	Star Reading (2006b)	Standard score and percentile rank	40th percentile
	Measures of Academic Progress—Reading (Northwest Evaluation Association, 2004b)	Standard score and percentile rank	40th percentile
Reading comprehension	Group Reading Assessment and Diagnostic Evaluation (Williams, 2001)	Standard score and percentile rank	40th percentile
	Gray Oral Reading Test (Bryant, Wiederholt, & Bryant, 2004)	Standard score and percentile rank	40th percentile
Reading code	Curriculum-based measure (CBM) of oral reading fluency	Number and percentage of words read correctly	*https://dibels. uoregon.edu*: 93% correct
	CBM of letter–sound fluency or nonsense-word fluency	Number and percentage of sounds read correctly	*https://dibels. uoregon.edu*: 90% correct
Math			
Overall math	Star Math (2006a)	Standard score and percentile rank	40th percentile
	Measures of Academic Progress—Math (Northwest Evaluation Association, 2004a)	Standard score and percentile rank	40th percentile
Math procedures	CBM of math fluency	Number of problems correct per minute	*https://dibels. uoregon. edu/research/ techreports/#math*

TABLE 11.1. (*continued*)

	Curriculum-based assessment (CBA) of a single skill (e.g., single-digit multiplication)	Number and % of digits correct per minute (dcpm)	14 dcpm (second and third grade), 24 dcpm (fourth grade and above; Burns, VanderHeyden, & Jiban, 2006); 90% correct
Math concepts	CBM concepts and applications	Number or problems correct per minute	*www.easycbm.com*
	CBA of conceptual understanding (see Burns & Parker, 2014)	% of problems correct	90% correct

worksheetworks.com/math.html; *www.interventioncentral.org/teacher-resources/math-work-sheet-generator*). The probe should contain at least 25 problems, depending on the curriculum difficulty, and the order of the problems should be randomly determined.

After the probes are constructed, the student is given 2–4 minutes to complete as many items as he or she can, after which the probe is scored by computing digits correct per minute (DCPM). Most teachers would see 4 × 6 = 24 and 5 ×8 = 40 as two correct out of two (100%), but with DCPM, the student would receive credit for two digits for each answer (2 and 4, and 4 and 0), which would be four out of four. The following set of answers—2 × 5 = 12, 3 × 6 = 15, and 5 × 5 = 25—would be four out of six digits correct instead of one out of three. The student would receive credit for the "1" in "12" because that digit is correct and in the correct place, and the "1" in the second problem would also receive credit, but the "2" and "5," respectively, would be scored as incorrect. The student would also receive two out of two for the answer "25" because both digits are correct and in the correct place. In order to determine DCPM, the total number of digits correct in the probe is divided by the length of the administration (e.g., 40 digits correct in a 4-minute administration would result in 10 DCPM). The data are then compared to fluency criteria for an instructional level of 14–31 DCPM for second and third graders and 24–49 DCPM for older students (Burns, VanDerHeyden, & Jiban, 2006). Scores below the lowest end of the instructional level range fall within the frustration level and suggest that the skill is too difficult for the child, and those that exceed the highest score of the instructional level range fall within the independent range.

Using CBA-ID data to determine a student's instructional level has consistently led to increased reading fluency (Burns, 2007; Roberts & Shapiro,

1996), math skills (Burns, 2002), and student time on task (Gickling & Armstrong, 1978; Treptow, Burns, & McComas, 2007). Data from CBA-ID have also demonstrated sufficient reliability (Burns, Tucker, Frame, Foley, & Hauser, 2000; Burns et al., 2006; Parker, McMaster, & Burns, 2011) and resulted in valid decisions (Burns, 2007; Burns & Mosack, 2005).

Reading Strategies

Reading is not an observable process. Therefore, interventionists often interview students to discover their approaches to reading. We suggest asking students the 14 questions included in Table 11.2 to determine whether they predict (two questions), summarize (six questions), question (three

TABLE 11.2. Questions to Assess Use of Reading Strategies

Predicting

1. Do you ever find yourself making predictions as you read? If so, when?
2. Before you started reading, did you guess what the passage was going to be about? Why did you make that guess?

Summarizing

1. Throughout the reading, did you find yourself stopping and asking in the middle whether or not you understood what you just read?
2. Did you stop yourself at any point during the reading and sum up what you had read so far? If so, when?
3. Did you ask yourself what the passage was mostly about after reading?
4. Did you ask yourself what the important parts of the passage were before answering the questions?
5. Are you able to describe the most important ideas of what you just read to another person? If so, what are they?
6. Are you able to describe what the passage was about in one to two sentences? If so, will you describe it to me?

Generating questions

1. Did you wonder about the reasons why something happened at any point while reading? If so, when?
2. Do you want to know more about anything you read? If so, what?
3. Did you find yourself asking "why?" about anything in the story? If so, what?

Clarifying

1. Is there a part of this passage that you realized seemed fuzzy, so you went back and read it again? If so, what part?
2. Did you go back and reread any parts of what you read to better understand? If so, what parts?
3. At any time during reading, did you read a sentence that you didn't understand? If so, did you then read before and after that sentence to help you understand the meaning?

questions), and clarify (three questions) while reading. The data do not result in correct or incorrect responses but instead provide information about how the student is going about reading tasks. The questions are worded as "yes/no" to facilitate clarity in interpretation. If the student provides a response that suggests the affirmative for at least two-thirds of the items, then it is reasonable to assume that the student engages in that strategy at least a portion of the time. If the student provides mostly negative replies, then the student does not engage in that strategy, and the resulting intervention could focus on that goal.

Math Strategies

Math is also a cognitive function that is not easily observable, but, unlike reading, it can result in a visual product. Strategy use can also be assessed for math, once a basic skill deficit is ruled out, by (1) giving the student a problem that represents the specific type of problem with which the student struggles, (2) asking the student to show his or her work as he or she completes the problem, and (3) asking the student how what he or she wrote represents the problem. As shown in Table 11.3, student responses can suggest the type of strategy being used. Direct retrieval is usually the goal and could be set up as a strategy if the student used a less strategic approach.

Self-Monitoring

Once the interventionist has assessed the strategies, determined an intervention, and set a goal for performance, student progress should be monitored

TABLE 11.3. Common Strategies Used with Computation

Strategy Type	Definition	Example
Counting	Representations and pictures drawn to model the problem and count how many in total	Model the problem with representation (tallies, pictures, graphs) and count representation
Repeated addition	Repeatedly adding one factor for as many times as the other factor	$3 \times 4 = 4 + 4 + 4$ or $3 + 3 + 3 + 3$
Decomposition	Breaking down one or both factors and referring to known problems to create simpler problems to solve	$7 \times 8 = 7 \times 7 + 7$ or $6 \times 7 = 3 \times 7 \times 2$ or $8 \times 7 = 2 \times 7 \times 2 \times 2$ (e.g., doubles, doubles plus one)
Retrieval	Accurate numerical responses with or without an accurate number sentence	Problem: $3 \times 8 =$ Student response: 24

toward the goal, and self-monitoring should be used to continuously assess strategy use. Self-monitoring is most helpful for strategies that involve cognitive processes that cannot be directly observed, such as reading and math (Perry, Albeg, & Tung, 2012). Previous research found that self-monitoring not only increased behavioral variables such as increasing time on task (Wood, Murdock, Cronin, Dawson, & Kirby, 1998) and decreasing problem behavior (Rock, 2005) but also helped students appreciate the importance of the strategies that they are implementing (Pressley, Borkowski, & O'Sullivan, 1985). A meta-analysis of 13 studies found that self-monitoring was effective, but it was more effective when it was coupled with instruction in the strategies being monitored (Perry et al., 2012).

Self-monitoring is usually accomplished in reading and math by giving the students a response sheet that they fill out after they complete the target task. For example, Crabtree, Alber-Morgan, and Konrad (2010) asked students to complete a response sheet about answers to reading comprehension questions based on narrative story elements as they read, and they found an immediate increase in story recall. Falkenberg and Barbetta (2013) asked students to self-monitor their implementation of 10 basic guidelines to better complete homework and again saw an immediate effect. Interventionists can also just ask students to keep a record of the number of times they worked on a task, the amount of time spent on a task, or the strategies they used (Zumbrunn, Tadlock, & Roberts, 2011).

Treatment Strategies

Several different strategies exist (as described earlier), but all are generally taught with a similar process. First, remember that strategies are a student's deliberate attempts to control and modify efforts, and skills are automatic actions that result in successful completion of tasks that underlie reading and math (Afflerbach et al., 2008). Therefore, the interventionist determines whether the student needs additional support in learning the skill before learning a strategy. For example, can the student decode text or complete basic computation? Both of these are skills that should first be directly taught with explicit modeling, immediate corrective feedback, and sufficient opportunities to practice (Burns, VanDerHeyden, & Boice, 2008) to the point of automaticity.

Strategy instruction also has common attributes. Interventionists first model the strategy with explicit metacognition (Afflerbach et al., 2008). In other words, the interventionist implements every step of the strategy while orally describing what he or she is thinking so that the learning process and strategy implementation become visible. Second, the student is allowed to implement the strategy with careful scaffolding provided by the interventionist. During the scaffolding, the student would also orally report his or her metacognition, and the interventionist would provide immediate corrective feedback as needed. After completing the strategy with scaffolding, the student would then be allowed to implement the strategy on his or her own in a brief sample, for which the interventionist gives immediate feedback. Finally, the student uses the strategy independently in order to practice the strategy with a visual cue or reminder of the steps.

After the strategy has been taught, it is important for the student to self-monitor his or her use of it. Some of the examples provided here may be helpful, or the interventionist can create a self-monitoring tool by converting the steps in the strategy into dichotomous ("yes/no") choices that the student can complete after finishing a relevant academic task. It may also be beneficial to set goals and to have the student keep track of progress toward those goals.

The Role of Parents

As mentioned previously, cognitive therapy is consistent with an ecological approach to intervention that contextualizes problems, and thus solutions, as nested within a set of interrelated systems that interact and evolve across time. Inherent in this approach is a need to consider the critical contexts in which a child is learning and developing, including the family and broader cultural contexts.

Family Context

The positive impact of family involvement in children's education has long been recognized (Christenson, 2003). To maximize the effectiveness of interventions, it makes sense to capitalize on students' opportunities to learn in the multiple environments in which they function. In addition to the school contexts, the context of the home, as well as the relationship between school and home, are critical for student development (Christenson, 2003). Many terms are used to describe the contributions of the family to students' learning, including "parent involvement," "home–school collaboration," and "family–school partnerships," but the goal is always "promoting strong bonds between families and educators to enhance learning for all students" (Esler, Godber, & Christenson, 2008, p. 917).

Parent Involvement

Parent involvement in education has been defined as parents' dedication of resources to engage in activities at home and school, to provide a stimulating home environment, and to understand the child's progress in learning (Grolnik, Benjet, Kurowski, & Apostleria, 1997). There are six types of parent involvement in education that have helped shape research in the field—namely, parenting, communicating with the school, volunteering, learning at home, participating in decision making at the school, and collaborating with community (Epstein, 1995). All of these factors, with the exception of the last, collaborating with the community, were empirically validated as distinct factors within a multidimensional conceptualization of parent involvement (Fantuzzo, Tighe, & Childs, 2000). Examining the relationship between these factors and student outcomes has shown that home-based family involvement is related to student behaviors (e.g., motivation to learn, attention and persistence to tasks, receptive vocabulary, and lower levels of classroom behavior problems; Fantuzzo, McWayne, Perry, & Childs, 2004), to parent reports of student behavior (e.g., self-control, responsibility, and cooperative behavior in the home setting; McWayne, Hampton, Fantuzzo, Cohen, & Sekino, 2004), and to teacher-reported reading and math achievement, intellectual functioning, and overall classroom behavior (McWayne et al., 2004). In general, there is strong empirical evidence to support actively involving parents in the education process (Christenson & Carlson, 2005; Christenson, Rounds, & Gorney, 1992). Family factors that correlated with positive academic outcomes for students were high expectations for performance, attributing performance to effort as opposed to ability, home structure and support for learning, positive emotional interactions between parents and children, authoritarian parenting style, and parent involvement in education at home and school (Christenson et al., 1992).

Meta-analyses of family involvement interventions have shown small to large effects on reading (Fan & Chen, 2001; Senechal, 2006) and math achievement (Fan & Chen, 2001; Graue, Weinstein, & Walberg, 1983) in the elementary grades. The most promising findings have been found in studies that involved parent home tutoring of specific academic skills. For example, studies involving at-home tutoring by parents have shown increased academic gains for students in areas including math computation (Heller & Fantuzzo, 1993), word recognition (Vinoguard-Bausell, Bausell, Proctor, & Chandler, 1986), oral reading fluency (Gortmaker, Daly, McCurdy, Persampieri, & Hergenrader, 2007; Hook & DuPaul, 1999; Murad & Topping, 2000), and reading comprehension (Murad & Topping, 2000). Special populations have included students with attention-deficit/hyperactivity disorder (Hook & DuPaul, 1999) and students receiving special education services for cognitive and learning disabilities (Vinoguard-Bausell et al., 1986), as well as students displaying low achievement (Heller & Fantuzzo, 1993; Powell-Smith, Shinn, Stoner, & Good, 2000; Murad & Topping, 2000).

Home–School Collaboration

Home–school collaboration is closely related to, but distinct from, the concept of parent involvement. The difference lies in the conceptualization of the relationship. Parent involvement often implies a one-way flow of information between schools and parents, whereas home–school collaboration emphasizes a bidirectional exchange, with shared involvement, goals, and power (Christenson, 1995). Thus home–school collaboration can be conceptualized as parents and schools working together as equals to achieve academic and social outcomes for children (Cox, 2005). It is another category of intervention with proven effectiveness. Specifically, interventions involving a two-way exchange of information across home and school and those involving regular communication about student progress were effective in increasing academic performance and social behavior at school (Cox, 2005).

Family–School Partnerships

The concept of family–school partnerships encompasses the types of activities described previously, termed "parent involvement" and "home–school collaboration," but moves beyond these ideas, recognizing the partnership as more than something to strive for but as an absolutely essential component of education (Christenson, 2003, 2010). According to ecological system theory, the child functions within the discrete *microsystems* of home and school but is also affected by the *mesosystemic* influences of the transactional relationship between the home and school environments. The mesosystem has often been forgotten by those trying simply to "involve" parents. Christenson and Sheridan (2001) describe several key features of family–school partnerships including (1) a *student-focused philosophy* by which educators and parents work together to enhance development academically, socially, emotionally, and behaviorally; (2) *shared responsibility,* in which all parties are seen as essential, not simply desired, and a range of options exists for participation; (3) a *constructive relationship* whereby parties work together in meaningful ways toward shared goals; and finally (4) a *preventative, solution-oriented* focus, in which conditions are created to promote student success.

Multicultural Issues

The achievement gap between white and minority children has been a persistent and well-documented problem in the United States. It is tempting to conclude that the different outcomes experienced by members of different groups indicates that different learning needs are present and thus different teaching strategies are needed. However, in the same way that attempting to develop interventions based on ATI has failed to result in better outcomes (Burns et al., 2016), research has not shown that matching interventions to students based on their cultural backgrounds is effective (see Kane & Boan, 2005, for a review). In addition, the research literature is replete with methodological problems, including failing to clearly define fundamental constructs such as learning styles and culture, using measures with poor or unsubstantiated technical properties, and the fact that confounds such as age and cognitive ability are not controlled (Kane & Boan, 2005). Such issues make interpreting results tenuous at best and impossible in the worst-case scenario.

Fortunately, the intervention strategies described herein are generally effective for learners across backgrounds. Students for whom English is not their first language have a special set of unique needs that should be considered. Research has shown that many of the measures that are used to assess early literacy skills, including those described in this chapter, result in valid decisions about students who are English learners, and typical reading interventions are effective for this population as long as they also include a focus on academic language and vocabulary (Socie & Vanderwood, 2016). Other techniques, in addition to the interventions mentioned here, are especially appropriate for students who are English learners, including previewing and reviewing books used in school in the students' first language, engaging in therapeutic and instructional conversations that permit some use of the home language, and using bilingual glossaries for targeted vocabulary (August, McCardle, & Shanahan, 2014). Finally, frequent and specific feedback about performance and close monitoring of student progress seems especially important for students for whom English is not their first language (Socie & Vanderwood, 2016).

Case Examples

Reading: Fatima

Fatima was an African American female student in seventh grade who was referred because she was failing all of her classes and teachers reported that she had significant difficulties answering comprehension questions about text that she had just read.

Assessment

Fatima scored at the 20th percentile on the Measures of Academic Progress for reading (Northwest Evaluation Association, 2004b), which was the district-administered nationally normed test of reading comprehension. Her reading skills were then assessed with grade-level curriculum-based measures of reading (CBM-R) from the Aimsweb system, which resulted in a score of 132 words read correctly per minute, which was well below the 25th percentile on national norms, but read with 99.25% accuracy. Therefore, the seventh-grade reading material appeared to be an instructional level or even a mastery level for Fatima (Burns & Parker, 2014). Both of these measures were completed by Fatima's school.

Fatima was then assessed by asking her to read three short stories from her English 7 course and to answer the 14 questions outlined in Table 11.2. She responded positively to five questions for the first passage and four each for the second and third passages. She also correctly answered 20–30% of the comprehension questions that were provided by the textbook for each short story. She did not appear to be engaging in any strategy with consistency.

Intervention

Fatima participated daily in an English 7 course. She was taught the four reading comprehension strategies (predicting, summarizing, questioning, and clarifying). One comprehension strategy was taught each day for 4 days through modeling, guided practice, and independent practice. Each lesson used the following format: (1) The strategy was introduced to the participant; (2) the interventionist explained how the strategy would help her with reading comprehension; (3) the interventionist modeled how to use the strategy by reading two paragraphs of a passage aloud and thinking aloud as they implemented the strategy; (4) Fatima then practiced using the strategy aloud with guidance while reading paragraphs as the interventionist followed along and provided feedback; (5) Fatima independently practiced using the strategy; and (6) the interventionist discussed how Fatima used the strategy during independent practice to better understand what she read. The interventionist and Fatima also set a goal that she would independently read for at least 15 minutes each day and that she would record the number of minutes read in a journal.

Self-Monitoring

In addition to recording the number of daily minutes spent reading, Fatima answered the questions in Table 11.1 in a self-response sheet. She completed the sheet once each day in response to reading that was assigned for class, or for her independent reading if no reading was assigned for class. The self-monitoring began after all of the strategies were taught to her. She self-reported that she completed an average of 78% of the items on the response sheet. On her first rating, she indicated that she completed 50% of the items, but that number increased to 65, 79, 86, 86, and 93% on subsequent days.

Monitoring Progress

Fatima completed a comprehension assessment every day for 4 weeks. She read a page-long narrative story that was created for her using *www.readworks.org*. The reading passages were at her instructional level and included 10 comprehension problems. She completed the comprehension questions, which were scored by her classroom teacher, and she graphed the results, which are displayed in Figure 11.1. As can be seen in the figure, she scored low on the comprehension questions (average = 29%) throughout the instruction in the strategies, but her scores immediately increased (average = 87%) once she added in the self-monitoring of strategy use.

Mathematics: Jim

Jim was a white male fourth grader who attended a suburban elementary school in the upper Midwest. He was recently exited from speech and language special education services for articulation difficulties but did have a Section 504 Intervention Plan in place to accommodate attention difficulties. He was referred for support because of the reported attention problems, for which he was not taking any medications, and because of reported difficulties with mathematics. His elementary school served 510 students in kindergarten through fifth grade, 55% of whom were white and 45% of whom were eligible for the federal free or reduced-price lunch program. The district used enVisionMATH (2011) as their fourth-grade mathematics curriculum.

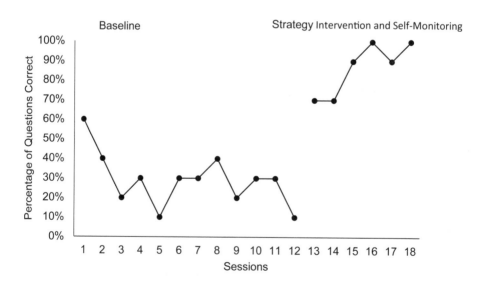

FIGURE 11.1. Percentage of comprehension questions answered correctly by Fatima before and after intervention.

Assessment

Jim scored at the 12th percentile on a district-administered group measure of mathematics skills. His computation skills were assessed with the Mathematics-Computation (M-Comp) curriculum-based measure published by Aimsweb (Mathematics Computation Administration and Scoring Guide, 2012), which is an 8-minute assessment of fluency with mathematics operations. Each item is awarded a number of points that range from 1 to 3. Jim earned 58 points, which scored at the 52nd percentile for his grade on a national norm and suggested adequate computational fluency. Moreover, he completed the probe with 25 DCPM, which was within the instructional level for a fourth-grade student.

Next, Jim was given three story problems that all involved single-digit multiplication, and he was asked to draw a picture that goes with the problem, to use the picture to solve the problem, and then to explain how the two go together. One of his drawings is displayed in Figure 11.2. He completed the answer by writing down 35 without apparently counting and correctly explained that the numbers represented five sets of seven items. He appeared to demonstrate an understanding of the problem and solved the problem with retrieval. Therefore, the interventionist decided to focus on a strategy for solving word problems and for attention.

Intervention

Jim participated in instruction regarding a strategy for solving word problems three times per week for approximately 3 weeks. Each intervention session required approximately 15 minutes to complete. During each session, Jim was taught the strategies for completing a word problem. He was given the student response sheet shown in Figure 11.3 as a visual prompt,

Tom's dresser has 5 drawers, and there are 7 shirts in each drawer. How many shirts does Tom have?

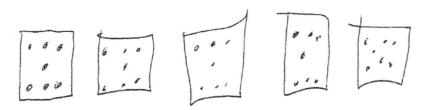

FIGURE 11.2. Jim's drawing of the corresponding story problem.

and then the interventionist modeled each step while completing a word problem that contained single-digit multiplication. The interventionist modeled the steps by "thinking out loud"; she orally stated what she was thinking for each step while completing it. Next, Jim and the interventionist completed a second word problem while working on the steps together. The interventionist would ask Jim to orally state what he thought at each step and then give feedback. If he did not complete the problem correctly, then he returned to Step 1, and the process was modeled again. If he did complete the problem correctly with help, then he completed a third story problem while thinking out loud and receiving feedback from the interventionist. At the completion of these three steps, Jim was given five more story problems to complete and was asked to fill in the response sheet in Figure 11.3 for each one.

Self-Monitoring

Self-monitoring for Jim consisted of two activities. First, any time he was asked to complete a word problem in class, he was instructed to use the response sheet in Figure 11.3 as a visual prompt but also to complete one sheet when he finished all of the problems that were assigned. Second, Jim was given a self-report of on-task behavior. Every 10 minutes that he worked independently on mathematics, he was instructed to stop and determine whether he was doing what he was supposed to be doing and paying attention. If so, he marked a *yes*, and if not, then he marked a *no*. He was allowed to take a break and engage in a choice of activity for 5 minutes after three consecutive *yes* selections.

Steps to Solve the Problem: Did I . . . ?	Yes	No
Read the problem carefully?		
Restate the problem so that I know I understand it?		
Draw the problem out?		
Come up with a plan to solve the problem?		
Estimate what I thought the answer would be before completing it?		
Follow the plan and find the answer?		
Check the answer and review my steps?		

FIGURE 11.3. Self-report student response sheet for word problem strategy. Based on Montague (1992).

Monitoring Progress

Jim's progress was monitored by having him complete a story problem assessment each day that consisted of 10 items written to represent a standardized test of mathematics applications. All of the items applied single-digit multiplication within the story problem. He was not timed and was asked to show his work. One point was assigned for the correct answer. He also completed the assessment three times before beginning the intervention to establish a preintervention baseline. As shown in Figure 11.4, he completed 30% of the application problems correctly in baseline, but his performance immediately increased to 100% of the problems answered correctly during intervention, with an average of 97%. Therefore, the intervention seemed to help him more accurately complete story problems.

Conclusion

The strategies within cognitive therapy have potential to address the pandemic (Gutkin, 2012) in American schools because they follow an ecological approach to learning and consider both strategies and skills. Careful evaluation of skills to drive intervention, through an STI framework, allows

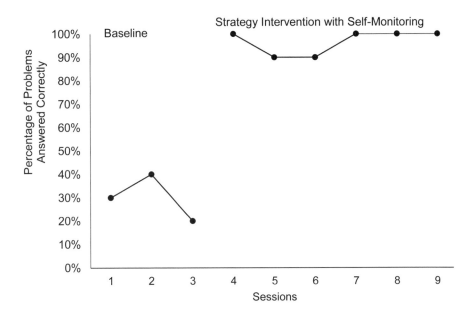

FIGURE 11.4. Jim's percentage of story problems correctly completed before and after intervention and self-monitoring.

interventionists to isolate the problem, provide an effective intervention that targets that specific problem, and monitor progress to quickly determine whether the intervention is having the desired effect. However, interventions for skills and strategies are more effective if they are implemented in partnership with families and if they consider multicultural issues.

The examples provided here illustrate how a skill-by-treatment model helped two students achieve more success with reading and completing mathematics story problems. The examples may help readers implement a similar approach with students with whom they work. Given the importance of reading and math to other behavioral and mental health needs and the growing pandemic in these important areas, we hope that readers will use this information to support the children and youth that they serve.

References

Afflerbach, P., Pearson, P. D., & Paris, S. G. (2008). Clarifying differences between reading skills and reading strategies. *Reading Teacher, 61,* 364–373.

August, D., McCardle, P., & Shanahan, T. (2014). Developing literacy in English language learners: Findings from a review of the experimental research. *School Psychology Review, 43,* 490–498.

Axelrod, M. I., Zhe, J. E., Haugen, K. A., & Klein, J. A. (2009). Self-management of on-task homework behavior: A promising strategy for adolescents with attention and behavior problems. *School Psychology Review, 38,* 325–333.

Baker, S., Gersten, R., & Lee, D. S. (2002). A synthesis of empirical research on teaching mathematics to low-achieving students. *Elementary School Journal, 103,* 51–73.

Barrouillet, P., Mignon, M., & Thevenot, C. (2008). Strategies in subtraction problem solving in children. *Journal of Experimental Child Psychology, 99,* 233–251.

Berkeley, S., Mastropieri, M. A., & Scruggs, T. E. (2011). Reading comprehension strategy instruction and attribution retraining for secondary students with learning and other mild disabilities. *Journal of Learning Disabilities, 44,* 18–32.

Bronfenbrenner, U. (1979). *The ecology of human development: Experiments by nature and design.* Cambridge, MA: Harvard University Press.

Brown, A. L., & Palincsar, A. S. (1989). Guided, cooperative learning and individual knowledge acquisition. In L. B. Resnick (Ed.), *Knowing, learning, and instruction: Essays in honor of Robert Glaser* (pp. 393–451). Hillsdale, NJ: Erlbaum.

Bub, K. L., McCartney, K., & Willett, J. B. (2007). Behavior problem trajectories and first-grade cognitive ability and achievement skills: A latent growth curve analysis. *Journal of Educational Psychology, 99,* 653–670.

Burns, M. K. (2002). Comprehensive system of assessment to intervention using curriculum-based assessments. *Intervention in School and Clinic, 38,* 8–13.

Burns, M. K. (2007). Reading at the instructional level with children identified as learning disabled: Potential implications for response-to-intervention. *School Psychology Quarterly, 22*, 297–313.

Burns, M. K. (2016). Effect of cognitive processing assessments and interventions on academic outcomes: Can 200 studies be wrong? *Communiqué, 44*(5), 1–6.

Burns, M. K., Codding, R. S., Boice, C. H., & Lukito, G. (2010). Meta-analysis of acquisition and fluency math interventions with instructional and frustration level skills: Evidence for a skill-by-treatment interaction. *School Psychology Review, 39*, 69–83.

Burns, M. K., & Mosack, J. L. (2005). Criterion-related validity of measuring sight-word acquisition with curriculum-based assessment. *Journal of Psychoeducational Assessment, 23*, 216–224.

Burns, M. K., & Parker, D. C. (2014). *Curriculum-based assessment for instructional design: Using data to individualize instruction.* New York: Guilford Press.

Burns, M. K., Petersen-Brown, S., Haegele, K., Rodriguez, M., Schmitt, B., Cooper, M., et al. (2016). Meta-analysis of academic interventions derived from neuropsychological data. *School Psychology Quarterly, 31*, 28–42.

Burns, M. K., Tucker, J. A., Frame, J., Foley, S., & Hauser, A. (2000). Interscorer, alternate-form, internal consistency, and test–retest reliability of Gickling's model of curriculum-based assessment for reading. *Journal of Psychoeducational Assessment, 18*, 353–360.

Burns, M. K., VanDerHeyden, A., & Boice, C. (2008). Best practices in delivery of intensive academic interventions. In A. Thomas & J. Grimes (Eds.), *Best practices in school psychology* (5th ed., pp. 1151–1162). Bethesda, MD: National Association of School Psychologists.

Burns, M. K., VanDerHeyden, A. M., & Jiban, C. L. (2006). Assessing the instructional level for mathematics: A comparison of methods. *School Psychology Review, 35*, 401–418.

Bryant, B., Wiederholt, J. L., & Bryant, D. P. (2004). *Gray Oral Reading Test.* Austin, TX: PRO-ED.

Christenson, S. L. (1995). Families and schools: What is the role of the school psychologist? *School Psychology Quarterly, 10*, 118–132.

Christenson, S. L. (2003). The family–school partnership: An opportunity to promote the learning competence of all students. *School Psychology Quarterly, 18*, 454–482.

Christenson, S. L. (2010). Engaging with parents: The power of information, responsiveness to parental need, and ongoing support for the enhanced competence of all students. *Communiqué, 29*, 20–24.

Christenson, S. L., & Carlson, C. (2005). Evidence-based parent and family interventions in school psychology: State of scientifically based practice. *School Psychology Quarterly, 20*, 525–528.

Christenson, S. L., Rounds, T., & Gorney, D. (1992). Family factors and student achievement: An avenue to increase students' success. *School Psychology Quarterly, 7*, 178–206.

Christenson, S. L., & Sheridan, S. M. (2001). *Schools and families: Creating essential partnerships for learning.* New York: Guilford Press.

Clark, F. B., & Kamii, C. (1996). Identification of multiplicative thinking in children in grades 1–5. *Journal for Research in Mathematics Education, 27,* 41–51.

Cox, D. D. (2005). Evidence-based interventions using home-school collaboration. *School Psychology Quarterly, 20,* 473–497.

Crabtree, T., Alber-Morgan, S. R., & Konrad, M. (2010). The effects of self-monitoring of story elements on the reading comprehension of high school seniors with learning disabilities. *Education and Treatment of Children, 33,* 187–203.

Cronbach, L. J. (1957). The two disciplines of scientific psychology. *American Psychologist, 12,* 671–684.

Cronbach, L. J., & Snow, R. E. (1977). *Aptitudes and instructional methods: A handbook for research on interactions.* Oxford, UK: Irvington.

Darney, D., Reinke, W. M., Herman, K. C., Stormont, M., & Ialongo, N. S. (2013). Children with co-occurring academic and behavior problems in first grade: Distal outcomes in twelfth grade. *Journal of School Psychology, 51,* 117–128.

Dettmers, S., Trautwein, U., Lüdtke, O., Kunter, M., & Baumert, J. (2010). Homework works if homework quality is high: Using multilevel modeling to predict the development of achievement in mathematics. *Journal of Educational Psychology, 102,* 467–482.

EnVisionMATH. (2011). Chicago: Scott Foresman-Addison Wesley.

Epstein, J. L. (1995). School/family/community partnership: Caring for the children we share. *Phi Delta Kappan, 76,* 701–712.

Esler, A. N., Godber, Y., & Christenson, S. L. (2008). Best practices in supporting school–family partnerships. In A. Thomas & J. Grimes (Eds.), *Best practices in school psychology* (5th ed., pp. 917–929). Bethesda, MD: National Association of School Psychologists.

Falkenberg, C. A., & Barbetta, P. M. (2013). The effects of a self-monitoring package on homework completion and accuracy of students with disabilities in an inclusive general education classroom. *Journal of Behavioral Education, 22,* 190–210.

Fan, X. T., & Chen, M. (2001). Parental involvement and students' academic achievement: A meta-analysis. *Educational Psychology Review, 13,* 1–22.

Fantuzzo, J., McWayne, C., Perry, M., & Childs, S. (2004). Multiple dimensions of family involvement and their relations to behavioral and learning competencies for urban, low-income children. *School Psychology Review, 33,* 467–480.

Fantuzzo, J., Tighe, E., & Childs, S. (2000). Family Involvement Questionnaire: A multivariate assessment of family participation in early childhood education. *Journal of Educational Psychology, 92,* 367–376.

Geary, D. C. (2004). Mathematics and learning disabilities. *Journal of Learning Disabilities, 37,* 4–15.

Geary, D. C., & Burlingham-Dupree, M. (1989). External validation of the strategy choice model for addition. *Journal of Experimental Child Psychology, 47,* 175–192.

Gersten, R., Fuchs, L., Williams, J., & Baker, S. (2001). Teaching reading comprehension strategies to students with learning disabilities: A review of research. *Review of Educational Research, 71,* 279–320.

Gersten, R., Jordan, N. C., & Flojo, J. R. (2005). Early identification and interventions for students with mathematics difficulties. *Journal of Learning Disabilities, 38,* 293–304.

Gickling, E. E., & Armstrong, D. L. (1978). Levels of instructional difficulty as related to on-task behavior, task completion, and comprehension. *Journal of Learning Disabilities, 11,* 559–566.

Gortmaker, V. J., Daly, E. J., III, McCurdy, M., Persampieri, M. J., & Hergenrader, M. (2007). Improving reading outcomes for children with learning disabilities: Using brief experimental analysis to develop parent-tutoring interventions. *Journal of Applied Behavior Analysis, 40,* 203–221.

Graue, M. E., Weinstein, T., & Walberg, H. J. (1983). School-based home instruction and learning: A quantitative synthesis. *Journal of Educational Research, 76,* 351–360.

Grolnik, W. S., Benjet, C., Kurowski, C. O., & Apostleria, N. H. (1997). Predictors of parent involvement in schooling. *Journal of Educational Psychology, 89,* 538–548.

Gustafsson, J. E. (2013). Causal inference in educational effectiveness research: A comparison of three methods to investigate effects of homework on student achievement: 1. *School Effectiveness and School Improvement, 24,* 275–295.

Gutkin, T. B. (2009). Ecological school psychology: A personal opinion and a plea for change. In C. B. Reynolds & T. B Gutkin (Eds.), *The handbook of school psychology* (4th ed., pp. 463–496). New York: Wiley.

Gutkin, T. B. (2012). Ecological psychology: Replacing the medical model paradigm for school-based psychological and psychoeducational services. *Journal of Educational and Psychological Consultation, 22,* 1–20.

Hagan-Burke, S., Gilmour, M. W., Gerow, S., & Crowder, W. C. (2015). Identifying academic demands that occasion problem behaviors for students with behavioral disorders: Illustrations at the elementary school level. *Behavior Modification, 39,* 215–241.

Heller, L. R., & Fantuzzo, J. W. (1993). Reciprocal peer tutoring and parent partnership: Does parent involvement make a difference? *School Psychology Review, 22,* 517–534.

Hook, C. L., & DuPaul, G. J. (1999). Parent tutoring for students with attention-deficit/hyperactivity disorder: Effects on reading performance at home and at school. *School Psychology Review, 28,* 60–75.

Jordan, N. C., Hanich, L. B., & Kaplan, D. (2003). A longitudinal study of mathematical competencies in children with specific mathematics difficulties versus children with comorbid mathematics and reading difficulties. *Child Development, 74,* 834–850.

Kane, H., & Boan, C. H. (2005). A review and critique of multicultural learning styles. In C. L. Frisby & C. R. Reynolds (Eds.), *Comprehensive handbook of multicultural school psychology* (pp. 425–456). Hoboken, NJ: Wiley.

Kazantzis, N., Whittington, C., & Dattilio, F. (2010). Meta-analysis of homework effects in cognitive and behavioral therapy: A replication and extension. *Clinical Psychology: Science and Practice, 17,* 144–156.

Kilpatrick, S., Swafford, J. F., & Findell, B. (2001). *Adding it up: Helping children learn mathematics.* Washington, DC: National Academies Press.

Langberg, J. M. (2011). *Homework, organization and planning skills (HOPS) interventions: A treatment manual.* Bethesda, MD: National Association of School Psychologists.

Langberg, J. M., Epstein, J. N., Becker, S. P., Girio-Herrera, E., & Vaughn, A. J. (2012). Evaluation of the Homework, Organization, and Planning Skills (HOPS) intervention for middle school students with ADHD as implemented by school mental health providers. *School Psychology Review, 41,* 342–364.

Lemaire, P., & Siegler, R. S. (1995). Four aspects of strategic change: Contributions to children's learning of multiplication. *Journal of Experimental Psychology: General, 124,* 83–97.

Lynch, A., Theodore, L. A., Bray, M. A., & Kehle, T. J. (2009). A comparison of group-oriented contingencies and randomized reinforcers to improve homework completion and accuracy for students with disabilities. *School Psychology Review, 38,* 307–324.

Lysynchuk, L. M., Pressley, M., & Vye, N. J. (1990). Reciprocal teaching improves standardized reading-comprehension performance in poor comprehenders. *Elementary School Journal, 90,* 469–484.

Mathematics computation administration and scoring guide. (2012). Bloomington, MN: Pearson.

McWayne, C., Hampton, V., Fantuzzo, J., Cohen, H., & Sekino, Y. (2004). A multivariate examination of parent involvement and the social and academic competencies of urban kindergarten children. *Psychology in the Schools, 4,* 364–377.

Merikangas, K. R., He, J. P., Burstein, M., Swanson, S. A., Avenevoli, S., Cui, L., et al. (2010). Lifetime prevalence of mental disorders in US adolescents: Results from the National Comorbidity Survey Replication—Adolescent Supplement (NCS-A). *Journal of the American Academy of Child and Adolescent Psychiatry, 49,* 980–989.

Montague, M. (1992). The effects of cognitive and metacognitive strategy instruction on the mathematical problem solving of middle school students with learning disabilities. *Journal of Learning Disabilities, 25,* 230–248.

Morgan, P. L., Farkas, G., Tufis, P. A., & Sperling, R. A. (2008). Are reading and behavior problems risk factors for each other? *Journal of Learning Disabilities, 41,* 417–436.

Murad, C. R., & Topping, K. J. (2000). Parents as reading tutors for first graders in Brazil. *School Psychology International, 21,* 152–171.

National Reading Panel. (2000). *Report of the National Reading Panel: Teaching children to read: An evidence-based assessment of the scientific research literature on reading and its implications for reading instruction: Reports of the subgroups.* Washington, DC: National Institutes of Health, National Institute of Child Health and Human Development.

Northwest Evaluation Association. (2004a). *Measures of academic progress for math.* Portland, OR: Author.

Northwest Evaluation Association. (2004b). *Measures of academic progress for reading.* Portland, OR: Author.

Parker, D. C., McMaster, K. L., & Burns, M. K. (2011). Determining an instructional level for early writing skills. *School Psychology Review, 40,* 158–167.

Perry, V., Albeg, L., & Tung, C. (2012). Meta-analysis of single-case design research on self-regulatory interventions for academic performance. *Journal of Behavioral Education, 21,* 217–229.

Powell-Smith, K. A., Shinn, M. R., Stoner, G., & Good, R. H. (2000). Parent tutoring in reading using literature and curriculum materials: Impact on student reading achievement. *School Psychology Review, 29,* 5–27.

Pressley, M., Borkowski, J. G., & O'Sullivan, J. T. (1985). Children's metamemory and the teaching of memory strategies. *Metacognition, Cognition, and Human Performance, 1,* 111–153.

Price, G. R., Mazzocco, M. M., & Ansari, D. (2013). Why mental arithmetic counts: Brain activation during single digit arithmetic predicts high school math scores. *Journal of Neuroscience, 33,* 156–163.

Raggi, V. L., Chronis-Tuscano, A., Fishbein, H., & Groomes, A. (2009). Development of a brief, behavioral homework intervention for middle school students with attention-deficit/hyperactivity disorder. *School Mental Health, 1,* 61–77.

Ramdass, D., & Zimmerman, B. J. (2011). Developing self-regulation skills: The important role of homework. *Journal of Advanced Academics, 22,* 194–218.

Reinecke, M. A., Dattilio, F. M., & Freeman, A. (2003). What makes for an effective treatment? In M. A. Reinecke, F. M. Dattilio, & A. Freeman (Eds.), *Cognitive therapy with children and adolescents: A casebook for clinical practice* (2nd ed., pp. 1–18). New York: Guilford Press.

Reinke, W. M., Lewis-Palmer, T., & Merrell, K. (2008). The classroom check-up: A classwide teacher consultation model for increasing praise and decreasing disruptive behavior. *School Psychology Review, 37,* 315–332.

Roberts, M. L., & Shapiro, E. S. (1996). Effects of instructional ratios on students' reading performance in a regular education program. *Journal of School Psychology, 34,* 73–91.

Rock, M. L. (2005). Use of strategic self-monitoring to enhance academic engagement, productivity, and accuracy of students with and without exceptionalities. *Journal of Positive Behavior Interventions, 7,* 3–17.

Scholin, S. E., & Burns, M. K. (2012). Relationship between pre-intervention data and post-intervention reading fluency and growth: A meta-analysis of assessment data for individual students. *Psychology in the Schools, 49,* 385–398.

Senechal, M. (2006). *The effect of family literacy interventions on children's acquisition of reading from kindergarten to grade 3: A meta-analytic review.* Portsmouth, NH: RMC Research.

Sheridan, S. M., & Gutkin, T. B. (2000). The ecology of school psychology: Examining and changing our paradigm for the 21st century. *School Psychology Review, 29,* 485–502.

Socie, D., & Vanderwood, M. (2016). Response to intervention for English learners. In S. Jimerson, M. K. Burns, & A. M. VanDerHeyden (Eds.), *Handbook of response to intervention: The science and practice of multitiered systems of support* (2nd ed., pp. 519–537). New York: Springer.

Spörer, N., Brunstein, J. C., & Kieschke, U. L. F. (2009). Improving students' reading comprehension skills: Effects of strategy instruction and reciprocal teaching. *Learning and Instruction, 19,* 272–286.

Star math. (2006a). Wisconsin Rapids, WI: Renaissance Learning.

Star reading. (2006b). Wisconsin Rapids, WI: Renaissance Learning.

Swanson, H. L., Trainin, G., Necoechea, D. M., & Hammill, D. D. (2003). Rapid naming, phonological awareness, and reading: A meta-analysis of the correlation evidence. *Review of Educational Research, 73,* 407–440.

Treptow, M. A., Burns, M. K., & McComas, J. J. (2007). Reading at the frustration, instructional, and independent levels: The effects on students' reading comprehension and time on task. *School Psychology Review, 36,* 159–166.

Tudge, J. R., Mokrova, I., Hatfield, B. E., & Karnik, R. B. (2009). Uses and misuses of Bronfenbrenner's bioecological theory of human development. *Journal of Family Theory and Review, 1,* 198–210.

U.S. Department of Education. (2015). *The nation's report card 2015.* Washington, DC: National Center for Education Statistics.

VanDerHeyden, A. M., & Burns, M. K. (2009). Performance indicators in math: Implications for brief experimental analysis of academic performance. *Journal of Behavioral Education, 18,* 71–91.

Vinoguard-Bausell, C. R., Bausell, R. B., Proctor, W., & Chandler, B. (1986). Impact of unsupervised parent tutors on word recognition skills. *Journal of Special Education, 20,* 83–90.

Williams, K. T. (2001). *Group reading assessment and diagnostic evaluation.* New York: Pearson.

Wood, S. J., Murdock, J. Y., Cronin, M. E., Dawson, N. M., & Kirby, P. C. (1998). Effects of self-monitoring on on-task behaviors of at-risk middle school students. *Journal of Behavioral Education, 8,* 263–279.

Zumbrunn, S., Tadlock, J., & Roberts, E. D. (2011). *Encouraging self-regulated learning in the classroom: A review of the literature.* Richmond, VA: Virginia Commonwealth University, Metropolitan Educational Research Consortium.

Cognitive-Behavioral Family Therapy

Norman B. Epstein
Stephen E. Schlesinger
HaeDong Kim

Theoretical Foundations

A hallmark of family therapy is its attention to interpersonal factors that influence the development of problems in family members' individual functioning. Child and adolescent problems can be influenced by intrapersonal characteristics such as innate temperament, and individually focused treatments described in this book have been demonstrated to be helpful. Nevertheless, there is substantial empirical evidence regarding effects of the family environment and specific parent–child interaction patterns on positive and problematic child functioning, pointing to the need for interventions that directly target those contextual factors. Parents commonly conceptualize child problems as primarily intrapsychic when they bring their offspring for psychological treatment, with such a view often reinforced by outsiders, such as school personnel, who make statements such as, "You need to get treatment for your child." The systemic theoretical foundation of family therapy models acknowledges influences of intrapersonal characteristics on both individual functioning (e.g., poor emotion regulation contributes to conduct problems) and family functioning (e.g., a child's emotion regulation problem is a stressor for other family members). The cognitive-behavioral family therapy (CBFT) approaches that we describe in this chapter capture both intrapersonal factors (family members' cognitions and emotional responses) and interpersonal factors (behavioral interaction patterns among family members) that influence a variety of child and adolescent presenting problems. The integration of those intrapersonal and interpersonal aspects of the family in assessment and treatment are a notable strength of CBFT. Although it can be tempting to focus on cognitions, emotional responses, and behaviors of one family member that appear to contribute to a child's presenting problem, it often is the combination of those factors in two or more members that results in a child's problem.

Thus the family is the unit of treatment in family therapy. There is substantial evidence that conflict between parents, as well as psychopathology in parents, has deleterious effects on child and adolescent emotional well-being and behavior, and the pathway from parental problems to child maladjustment is mediated by compromised parenting behavior (Foster et al., 2008; Kaczynski, Lindahl, Malik, & Laurenceau, 2006; Low & Stocker, 2005; Schulz, 2010). A parent who is distracted by psychological distress or couple relationship problems is less likely to guide and discipline a child in a warm, patient, consistent, and constructive manner. Consequently, family therapists assess parental functioning and intervene with it as appropriate. Even when a child is the "identified patient" due to his or her behavior, the focus on improving parents' skills leads to treating the whole family.

When parents who bring children to therapy are frustrated with them and blame them for problems such as oppositional behavior, the adults commonly experience some self-doubt regarding their competence as parents. Teachers, neighbors, and extended family members may have blamed them for their children's problems. Consequently, in family therapy it is crucial to identify contributions that parents make to family interactions that elicit or maintain child problems but to avoid blaming parents for those problems. Treatment builds on strengths and improves parents' skills and confidence. The framework that we describe emphasizes positive parental roles in addressing child and adolescent problems. Some problems involve a child exhibiting symptoms of a disorder (e.g., anxiety, attention-deficit/hyperactivity disorder [ADHD]) traditionally treated primarily with an individual focus, whereas others involve parent–child relations (e.g., parent–adolescent conflict).

A Cognitive-Behavioral Model of Family Functioning

In a cognitive-behavioral view of individual problems within a family context, family members' cognitions, emotional responses, and behaviors are seen as mutually influencing one another, both within each person and among family members (Dattilio, 1998, 2010; Dattilio & Epstein, 2016; Epstein & Falconier, 2014; Epstein & Schlesinger, 2003; Epstein, Schlesinger, & Dryden, 1988; Schwebel & Fine, 1994). For example, a thought (e.g., inferring that one's child is willfully disobeying orders) can produce emotions (e.g., anger) and behaviors (e.g., spanking). An emotion (e.g., anger) can influence cognitions (e.g., selectively noticing a child's unpleasant actions) and behaviors (e.g., yelling). Finally, a behavior (e.g., withdrawing from family members) can affect one's own emotions (e.g., decreased feelings of intimacy) or cognitions (e.g., concluding, "I must not care about them any longer, or else I would not be acting this way").

Family members mutually influence each other through interactive processes (e.g., the more a parent nags a child to comply with requests, the more the child withdraws, and the more the child withdraws, the more the parent nags). Members' behaviors constantly serve as events that are interpreted and evaluated by other members, eliciting emotional and behavioral responses. Once a cycle among family members has developed, a negative cognition, behavior, or emotion at any point in the pattern can lead to a negative spiral. For example, if one member misinterprets another's behavior as due to malicious intent and responds by disparaging the other, the other member may think, "I try my best, and all I get in return is criticism" and may leave the room in anger. Then the first individual might interpret the other's withdrawal negatively: "He doesn't care enough about me to listen to my feelings." Each person reacts to his or her cognitions about the other person as if they represent the absolute truth, and conflict can escalate quickly.

When more than two individuals are involved in an interaction, the events that family members observe become more complex than is the case with dyadic interactions (Epstein & Schlesinger, 1991). An individual is likely to observe the characteristics of the relationships among family members, such as noticing that two other members usually support each other's opinions during disagreements with the individual. Similarly, children commonly are aware of the degree to which their parents disagree about child-rearing practices and so forth. There is a vast array of events occurring during family interactions that are stimuli for the members' cognitive appraisals, emotional reactions, and behavioral responses, and these events can influence a child's presenting problems. Next we describe behaviors, cognitions, and emotional responses assessed and treated in CBFT.

Behavioral Patterns in Problematic Family Interactions

Behavioral interventions for family problems are based on an assumption that problematic behaviors are learned and can be reduced or replaced with more constructive behaviors through new learning processes. Operant learning principles regarding reinforcement, punishment, and extinction (Skinner, 1953) and social learning concepts regarding observational learning from models (Bandura, 1977; Rotter, 1954) are used to explain human learning, especially within interpersonal relationships. In the family of origin, a child learns skills and styles of communicating with others, both by observing parents and siblings and by being reinforced for certain actions and punished for others. Parents may model effective problem-solving skills or ineffective and even destructive approaches, such as aggressive behavior. In a CBFT framework, it is assumed that individuals develop both positive and negative behavioral responses through the same learning processes, and learning procedures can be used to modify problematic responses.

The major behaviors that are targeted in CBFT include (1) excesses of negative behaviors and deficits in pleasing behaviors among family members, (2) expressive and listening skills used in communication, (3) problem-solving skills, and (4) negotiation and behavior-change skills. The following are descriptions of these core behavioral foci.

Pleasing and Displeasing Behavior Exchanges

Social exchange theory (e.g., Thibaut & Kelley, 1959) conceptualizes an interpersonal relationship as an economic exchange in which each person's satisfaction is a function of the ratio of the benefits received to the costs incurred. It is assumed that in a satisfying relationship the parties exchange rewards in a reciprocal manner and restrain the escalation of negative exchanges. In contrast, relationship distress is associated with exchanges of aversive behavior. Consistent with a social learning perspective, research by Patterson and his colleagues (e.g., Patterson, 1982) demonstrated reciprocal coercion patterns in families, in which each member's behavior both elicits and reinforces aversive behavior in other members. Parents may reinforce their children's negative behavior by selectively paying attention to it and failing to notice and encourage positive behavior. In addition, parents may attempt to reduce children's negative behavior by means of aversive acts such as insults, threats, and physical punishment. Patterson (1982) stressed that, at best, those strategies suppress unwanted child behavior temporarily (while the punisher is present), and they teach children that aggression is an acceptable means of expressing dissatisfaction with other people. Thus parents can unwittingly teach a child to use aggression through modeling. Although a parent may be tempted to vent frustration by using aversive words and actions, doing so tends to contribute to more coercive exchanges between the child and parent. One of the tasks in CBFT is changing parents' beliefs that aggression is useful in developing more positive behavior in their children.

Communication Skills Deficits

Research on family communication commonly involves coding family interactions with a system that includes categories of specific positive and negative behavior (Eyberg, Nelson, Ginn, Bhuiyan, & Boggs, 2013; Hawes, Dadds, & Pasalich, 2013; Kerig & Lindahl, 2001; Patterson, 1982). Studies have indicated that distressed families exhibit higher rates of negative communication behaviors, less positive communication, and more escalating aversive exchanges than those that are not distressed.

Specific communication patterns have been identified as contributing to couple and family problems. For example, a demand–withdraw pattern involving one person pursuing while the other withdraws has been studied extensively in distressed couples (Christensen, Eldridge, Catta-Preta, Lim, & Santagata, 2006). It also can be observed in family interactions, with parents pursuing a child and the child withdrawing. Family members typically perceive linear causality in their interactions, with another person viewed as being at fault. A clinician's task is to help them understand the circular nature of their pattern and motivate each person to modify his or her contribution to it. Parents also often exhibit deficits in listening skills with children and adolescents and make requests that are vague or aggressive (Barkley, Robin & Benton, 2014; Eyberg, 1988; Forgatch & Patterson, 2010; Kazdin, 2008).

Thus some problems in communication among family members involve misinterpretations, in which messages that one person intends to send are received inaccurately. These discrepancies can result from faulty expression by the sender (e.g., vague messages, frequent topic shifts) or from ineffective listening by the recipient (e.g., formulating a rebuttal to the other person rather than attending carefully to what he or she is saying). At other times, family members complain that they cannot communicate when, in fact, they receive messages from each other clearly but find them unacceptable, either because the messages are sent in an aversive manner (e.g., a sarcastic tone) or because the recipient does not agree with the ideas expressed. It is crucial to distinguish among these different kinds of communication problems. When there are deficits in expressive and listening skills, communication skills training can be used. When family members send aversive messages, it also may be important to identify and modify emotions (e.g., strong anger) and cognitions (e.g., a parent's attribution that a child's misbehavior is caused by malicious intent) that can influence an individual's sending negative messages.

Problem-Solving Skills Deficits

Families inevitably are faced with a variety of problems that require them to work as a team to devise and implement solutions. Problem solving is a process that involves (1) clearly defining a problem in behavioral terms, (2) identifying possible solutions, (3) evaluating costs and benefits of each solution, (4) reaching family consensus on a solution, (5) implementing the solution (with each family member carrying out a specific role), and (6) evaluating the effectiveness of the solution, revising it if necessary (Barkley et al., 2014; Epstein & Baucom, 2002; Jacobson & Christensen, 1996; Mueser & Glynn, 1999). Many families have limited skills for this systematic, collaborative approach, so they become overwhelmed by problems and fail to generate solutions. Consequently, assessment of problem-solving skills and training in problem solving are important components of CBFT.

Behavior-Change Skills Deficits

As noted, members of many families tend to use coercive behavior (e.g., threats, punishment) to attempt to influence each other. Deficits in clear communication also interfere with change efforts. Behavioral family therapists emphasize advantages of family members making requests for increases in desired behavior rather than criticizing each other for negatives and of providing positive feedback for compliance (Barkley et al., 2014; Epstein & Falconier, 2014; Eyberg, 1988; Kazdin, 2008). As described in the section on treatment later in this chapter, CBFT clinicians often coach families in constructing behavioral contracts that specify the behavior changes that each member will make in order to implement a solution. Parents are aided in setting up contracts with children in which specific rewards and punishments are provided for specific types of positive and negative behavior, respectively (e.g., Barkley et al., 2014). Furthermore, many parents have heard about "time-outs" but implement them ineffectively (e.g., sending a child to his or her bedroom where toys are available), so clinicians assess skills in this area and may teach parents to use time-outs well as an alternative to punishment (Barkley et al., 2014; Kazdin, 2005, 2008).

Overall, even though many families seek assistance from CBFT clinicians based on concerns about the behavior of a child, the clinician assesses interaction patterns that involve many or all members of a family. The patterns identified in those assessments contribute to systemic interventions that alter the behaviors of parents as well as children.

Cognitions in Problematic Family Interaction

The forms of cognition that have become foci of CBFT were derived in part from cognitive models of individual psychopathology (e.g., Beck, 1976; Ellis, 1962) and partly from social psychological models of social cognition, such as attribution theory (cf. Arias & Beach, 1987). They include (1) *selective perceptions* about what events have occurred during family interactions, (2) *attributions* about why particular events occur, (3) *expectancies* (predictions) about the probabilities that particular events will occur in the future, (4) *assumptions* about the characteristics that family members and their relationships likely have, and (5) *standards* about the characteristics that family members and their relationships "should" have (Baucom & Epstein, 1990; Epstein & Baucom, 1993, 2002). An example of selective perception is a parent systematically noticing instances of a child's disobedient behavior and overlooking instances of compliance. A negative attribution may involve a parent inferring that a young child intentionally failed to clean up his or her room when instructed to do so without considering alternative causes of the noncompliance (e.g., the child's limited cognitive development for following through on a task, especially with vague instructions). A child may hold an inaccurate expectancy that her parents will punish her for earning less than an A grade on an exam and therefore hides the information from them. Having grown up being exposed to societal negative stereotypes about homosexual relationships, a gay man may hold an assumption that any close relationship he forms will be doomed to fail. Finally, an individual who holds a standard that partners who care about each other should always choose spending time together over independent activities is likely to be upset with her partner, who likes to spend periods of time alone reading. Robin and Foster (1989) described standards that contribute to parent–adolescent conflict, such as a parent's belief that "Young people have no right to challenge their parents' decisions" and an adolescent's belief that "My parents should be at least as lenient as my friends' parents."

A premise of CBFT is that these types of cognitions influence family members' satisfaction with their relationships and shape their behavior toward each other, and there is considerable empirical evidence that such influences occur. For example, partners who make negative attributions about each other's motives are more likely to communicate negatively with each other when discussing relationship problems (Bradbury & Fincham, 1992). In addition, extreme relationship standards are associated with relationship distress and negative couple communication (Baucom, Epstein, Rankin, & Burnett, 1996).

Emotional Responses Influencing Problematic Family Interactions

Emotions have very important roles in cognitive-behavioral approaches to family relationships. Because many individuals have difficulty differentiating among various emotions, it is crucial that therapists carefully inquire about the emotions that family members experience in specific situations. For example, individuals' negative emotions regarding events in their relationships can include anger, sadness, depression, anxiety, and so forth, or a combination of emotions, and each type of emotion may require a different form of therapeutic intervention. Thus it is important for CBFT clinicians to coach family members in identifying their emotional states and in using clear, direct communication skills to express those feelings constructively to each other (Dattilio & Epstein, 2016).

Difficulty regulating negative emotions contributes to family conflict and distress. In particular, intense anger commonly contributes to verbally and physically aggressive behavior, so interventions to improve anger management are a key component of CBFT for both partner aggression (Epstein, Werlinich, & LaTaillade, 2015) and parents' difficulty regulating anger toward children (Nicholson, Anderson, Fox, & Brenner, 2002; Sanders, Cann, & Markie-Dadds, 2003). Family members are taught a variety of strategies, including self-soothing methods (e.g., muscle relaxation), nonaggressive self-talk (e.g., "Even if my child's behavior is very frustrating, I can stay calm"), and use of "time-outs" in which individuals agree to distance themselves physically until they are calm.

In addition, shame responses, associated with a family member's condemnation by him- or herself or other family members for his or her behavior, commonly involve intense distress and dysfunctional coping, such as avoidance of other members (Epstein & Falconier, 2011). When parents use shaming as a discipline method, it is likely to backfire, as it tends to elicit depression and reduce the child's motivation. Consequently, family therapists need to identify ways in which family members attempt to elicit shame in other members and intervene to reduce that pattern.

Illustrative Review of CBFT

Based on social learning principles such as operant conditioning and a focus on circular interaction patterns among family members, Patterson (1971, 1982) developed behavioral interventions for families with children who exhibited aggressive and other problematic behavior. Patterson's approach, including its emphasis on behavioral observation and coding of discrete forms of family members' actions, served as a prototype for the behavioral family therapy programs that have followed. Those programs develop parents' skills at decreasing children's problematic behaviors and increasing their desirable behaviors, and they improve communication and problem-solving skills of the family as a group (Barkley et al., 2014; Blechman, 1985; Chronis, Chacko, Fabiano, Wymbs, & Pelham, 2004; Eyberg, 1988; Forgatch & Patterson, 2010; Kazdin, 1997, 2005; Webster-Stratton & Herbert, 1994). Although the child is commonly the "identified patient," parents' behaviors toward their children are modified significantly, making these systemic interventions. There is substantial evidence (e.g., Forgatch & Kjøbli, 2016; Kazdin, 1997) that parental skills training programs are effective, using outcome measures including parent and teacher ratings of child behavior in home and school settings, respectively, and institutional records such as school truancy and police contacts. Kazdin (1997) noted that, although many statistically significant improvements have been found, clinically significant change—that is, change that is sufficient to make a difference in daily life functioning and that has been examined in terms of statistical norms (Kendall, Marrs-Garcia, Nath, & Sheldrick, 1999)—has been less consistent, as has persistence of improvement over time.

Behavioral family therapy increasingly has been applied to a variety of child, adolescent, and adult problems. For example, parent–child interaction therapy (PCIT), created by Eyberg (1988), was developed to treat conduct (externalizing) problems of young children by training parents to use more effective commands combined with positive emotional connection with the child, and it has been demonstrated to be effective (Ward, Theule, & Cheung, 2016). PCIT applications have been expanded substantially; for example, in treating child internalizing problems (Carpenter, Puliafico, Kurtz, Pincus, & Comer, 2014), behavior problems associated with the autism spectrum (Masse, McNeil, Wagner, & Quetsch, 2016) and traumatic brain injury (Cohen, Heaton, Ginn, & Eyberg, 2012), and young children's anxiety disorders (Puliafico, Comer, & Pincus, 2012). Behavioral family therapy programs also have been developed and empirically supported for individuals with major mental disorders such as bipolar disorder and schizophrenia, providing conjoint interventions for all family members (McFarlane, 2016; Miklowitz & Chung, 2016). They include psychoeducation regarding the disorder and treatments, training in communication and problem-solving skills, and preparation for managing relapses (Morris, Miklowitz, & Waxmonsky, 2007; Mueser & Glynn, 1999).

Assessments and Measures of Outcomes

Assessments used with CBFT have been primarily self-report measures, some institutional data such as school records regarding truancy, and behavioral observation of parent–child interactions. We describe approaches for assessing family members' behaviors, cognitions, and emotional responses through clinical interviews, self-report questionnaires, and behavioral observation.

Assessment of Behavior

In cognitive-behavioral couple and family therapy (Dattilio & Epstein, 2016), the clinician initially interviews the family about the reasons for which they sought assistance and uses follow-up questions to specify presenting problems in behavioral terms. For example, when parents state that they are upset about a child's "constant arguing with us and disobedience," the therapist inquires about specific instances in which these problems occur and how each member of the family behaves. The goal is to conduct a functional analysis to identify antecedents and consequences for specific child behaviors.

Regarding self-report scales, it is common to ask parents and teachers to complete an inventory such as the Child Behavior Checklist (CBCL; Achenbach, 1991) to rate degrees to which a child exhibits various internalizing and externalizing symptoms. A variety of self-report measures of parenting behavior have been developed, although Hurley and colleagues (Hurley, Huscroft-D'Angelo, Trout, Griffith, & Epstein, 2014) reported that most lack evidence of sound psychometric properties. Among those with good psychometrics, the Parenting Scale (Arnold, O'Leary, Wolff, & Acker, 1993) has subscales assessing laxness (e.g., "When I say my child can't do something, I let my child do it anyway"), overreactivity (e.g., "Things build up and I do things I don't mean to"), and verbosity (e.g., "If saying no doesn't work right away, I keep talking and try to get through to my child"). Clinicians can use the Parenting Scale to identify forms of parenting that may benefit from skill development. The Alabama Parenting Questionnaire (APQ) also assesses aspects of parenting behavior (Shelton, Frick, & Wootton, 1996). Items were written for scales intended to measure involvement (e.g., "You play games or do other fun things with your child"), positive parenting (e.g., "You praise your child if he/she behaves well"), poor monitoring/supervision (e.g., "Your child goes out without a set time to be home"), inconsistent discipline (e.g., "You threatened to punish your child and then do not actually punish him/her"), and corporal punishment (e.g., "You slap your child when he/she has done something wrong"). The scale constructors administered the items separately to parents and children, using both interviews about the frequency of each behavior during the previous 3 days and global ratings of the frequency of each type of behavior on a scale ranging from 1 ("never") to 5 ("always"). Both types of reports from children had low reliability and failed to differentiate families with children with disruptive behavior diagnoses from normal control families. Both types of reports from parents performed well, with the exceptions of low reliability for interview responses regarding parental monitoring and supervision and those for corporal punishment with both formats. Thus the APQ has potential for screening parenting behavior.

Finally, behavior observation methods are a primary means of gathering objective data regarding parent–child behavior patterns, which can be used to assess initial family functioning and treatment outcome. A premise of CBFT is that constructive changes in parents' ways of trying to influence children's behavior will lead to improved child functioning. Consequently, Patterson's (1982) work with families of children with conduct problems that began in the 1960s involved observation of exchanges of aggressive behavior between parents and children during live family interactions.

Patterson and his colleagues developed a Family Interaction Coding System (FICS) that includes categories of coercive behavior (e.g., Command Negative, Humiliate, Noncompliance, Physical Negative, Whine). It is used to identify antecedents and consequences for aggressive acts during the ongoing sequence of behaviors among family members. The FICS also includes constructive behavior categories (e.g., Approval, Command, Compliance, Physical Positive). Researchers and clinicians can observe family interaction in the home as well as in the clinic or lab. Although observation methods are time-consuming, they are a hallmark of assessment in CBFT.

Eyberg et al.'s (2013) Dyadic Parent–Child Interaction Coding System (DPICS) is widely used for assessing interactions of parents and children participating in PCIT. DPICS coding involves instructing the parent and child to engage first in child-directed play (using a standard set of play materials in a clinic/lab room), then parent-directed play, and finally a clean-up period. The DPICS can be applied with live parent–child interactions or used later to code video-recorded interactions. The primary types of parent behavior that are coded focus on constructive versus negative forms of commands made to the child and child compliance versus noncompliance. Although mastering the DPICS can be time-consuming, it provides valuable data, and it provides a means of assessing outcomes of CBFT interventions. Even if a clinician chooses not to invest that degree of effort into full application of a coding system such as the DPICS, it is valuable to become familiar with the codes as a guide to observing family interactions.

Assessment of Cognitions

Several self-report measures of cognitions regarding couple relationships have been developed, such as Pretzer, Epstein, and Fleming's (1991) Marital Attitude Survey that assesses attributions about causes of problems in one's couple relationship (e.g., a partner's malicious intent or lack of love) and Baucom et al.'s (1996) Inventory of Specific Relationship Standards. However, there has been limited development of measures of cognition in parent–child relationships. The Parenting Sense of Competence (PSOC) scale (Gibaud-Wallston & Wandersman, 1978; Johnston & Mash, 1989) assesses generalized expectancies for effectiveness in parenting one's children, with items such as "I honestly believe I have all the skills necessary to be a good mother/father to my child." Johnston and Mash (1989) report good psychometric characteristics of the PSOC, so CBFT clinicians could use it for screening parents' self-efficacy expectancies. Roehling and Robin's (1986) Family Beliefs Inventory (FBI) was designed to assess unrealistic beliefs of parents and adolescents that exacerbate conflict and distress. It includes parental subscales assessing Ruination (that teenagers who are given too much freedom will ruin their futures), Obedience (that parents deserve their teenagers' absolute respect and obedience), Perfectionism (that teenagers should naturally behave perfectly), Malicious Intent (that teenagers misbehave with the intent to hurt parents), Self-Blame (that parents are at fault for their children's misbehavior), and Approval (that it is catastrophic if adolescents disapprove of their parents' child-rearing behavior). The adolescent subscales include Ruination (that parental restrictions will ruin the teenager's life), Unfairness (that it is catastrophic when the teenager's parents treat him or her unfairly), Autonomy (that parents should give teenagers complete freedom regarding rules and responsibilities), and Approval (that it is catastrophic if parents become angry with the teenager). Roehling and Robin (1986) found some associations between family members' levels of these beliefs and degrees of distress and conflict. The FBI has not been used often in publications, but clinicians could use it for screening regarding family members' beliefs about parent–adolescent relationships.

The primary method for assessing family members' cognitions in CBFT is live interaction with the individuals. Sometimes clients express cognitions spontaneously, as when a parent responds to a child's oppositional behavior by saying, "You have no respect for me" (an attribution) or says to the therapist, "He never does anything I ask him to do" (possible selective perception if the parent overlooks instances when the child complied). This assessment of cognitions occurs in conjunction with live observation of family behavioral interactions. At other times, the therapist needs to probe for cognitions, such as asking parents what standards they have for their adolescent's participation in family activities. During sessions, the therapist can look for nonverbal cues that a family member is reacting to another's behavior and ask what she or he was feeling and thinking at that moment. Sampling cognitions as they occur provides rich information about subjective experiences that cannot be assessed well with questionnaires.

Assessment of Emotions

It is important to identify family members' emotional states that either influence the occurrence of their cognitive and behavioral responses (e.g., a parent's persistent anger toward a child contributes to harsh parenting behavior) or are consequences of others' actions (a child shifts from a happy mood to anger when her parent turns off the television while she is watching a favorite show). Consequently, the most common means of collecting relevant information are clinical interviews about family interaction sequences (e.g., "What do you remember feeling just before you spanked your son?") and observation of family interaction with specific attention to cues of emotional responses and inquiries of family members about emotions that they experience at particular times. The richest data often come from simultaneously inquiring about behaviors, cognitions, and emotions as they play out during family sessions.

Treatment Strategies

The therapist can begin by giving the family a brief psychoeducational presentation regarding the interrelatedness of cognitions, behaviors, and emotions and how these three aspects of people's responses can influence family relationships. Examples can be given to illustrate how different thoughts (or emotions or behaviors) in the same situation can lead to different outcomes. This psychoeducational presentation is itself a cognitive intervention, as it is intended to broaden family members' thinking about their presenting problems.

It is imperative that the therapist emphasize that all family members need to experience sessions as a safe place for thinking about and solving family concerns. If parents brought a child to therapy with a goal of improving problematic behavior, the child is much more likely to learn positive things if the focus is on progress rather than past transgressions. It is also important to introduce the concept of circular causality and illustrate how family interactions are rarely linear ("Your ignoring me caused me to yell!") but are instead a cyclical process (yelling leads to ignoring, and ignoring leads to yelling). This perspective helps members each take responsibility for contributing to new positive patterns instead of treating one member as the cause of family problems.

The following interventions are for modifying behaviors, cognitions, and emotions. We separated them for clarity of presentation, but in practice the clinician commonly integrates the three types, due to mutual influences among them.

Interventions to Change Behaviors

Altering Behavioral Exchanges

As described earlier, families experiencing relational distress tend to exchange more negative behaviors and less positive behaviors than families that are not distressed. Based on social exchange theory, the goal is to increase positive behaviors and decrease negative ones. One pathway is to increase the family's engagement in enjoyable joint activities. The therapist guides the family in generating lists of activities that the members find pleasurable, focusing on those that are enjoyed by all members. The therapist can aid the process by providing a list of activities that other families enjoy (Baucom & Epstein, 1990). When parents select activities that they believe will be fun for the whole family without checking the child's or adolescent's preferences, they risk eliciting resistance from the youth. Clinicians encourage parents to explore youth's choices, stressing how allowing a child or adolescent to help select a family activity will produce good feelings between youth and parent.

The family can be coached in creating a list of negative behaviors that they exchange and that they will work toward decreasing while increasing the positives. These changes can be accomplished through behavioral contracts among family members. We emphasize "good faith" contracts in which members agree to enact particular positives or decrease particular negatives regardless of how other family members behave (avoiding a "standoff" of "I'll do my part when you do yours"). A number of books (e.g., Barkley et al., 2014; Eyberg & Funderburk, 2011; Patterson & Forgatch, 2005) are useful for teaching parents how to use contracts, as well as other parenting skills.

Therapists may need to identify and intervene with negative cognitions that some family members hold regarding others' actions in order to engage them in changing their behavior. For example, a parent who holds a standard that parents are "in charge" and children must follow their lead may resist allowing a child to voice preferences for family activities. The therapist can guide the parent in seeing how asking for the child's opinion boosts the child's self-esteem and does not mean that the parent has ceded power.

Communication Skills Training

Communication skills involve expressing one's thoughts and feelings to other family members and listening effectively, grasping the other's subjective experiences and conveying that empathy to the speaker by reflecting back the message that was received. CBFT texts (e.g., Epstein & Baucom, 2002; Mueser & Glynn, 1999) provide detailed instructions for conducting communication training. The therapist first teaches family members guidelines for effective expression and empathic listening, commonly using handouts that each person can refer to as needed. The therapist models constructive communication behavior to the family and then coaches the family members in practicing the skills with each other.

Problem-Solving Skills Training

As described earlier, the goals of problem-solving skills training are to guide a family toward a collaborative endeavor to define a problem in observable behavioral terms and then to create and implement a solution on which the family agrees, so everyone benefits. Initially, the therapist guides the family in describing the problem in terms of specific behaviors (e.g., the parents are ineffective in getting their two young children to go to bed by 8:30 P.M.), rather than globally (e.g., "The kids ignore what we want them to do."). The members who need to find a solution (in this case, the two parents) are then guided in brainstorming various possible solutions, without evaluating them at this point, to maximize creativity.

Subsequently, the members evaluate advantages and disadvantages of each proposed solution and then select a solution for which the advantages clearly outweigh the disadvantages. They then delineate each member's specific role in carrying out the solution. The family agrees to implement the solution during the upcoming week, evaluate its success in consultation with the therapist, and revise it if necessary (Epstein & Baucom, 2002; Mueser & Glynn, 1999).

Interventions to Modify Cognitions

A variety of interventions are used to modify family members' cognitions regarding interactions with other members. The cognitive restructuring process, based substantially on cognitive therapy procedures (Beck, Rush, Shaw, & Emery, 1979; Beck, 2011; Leahy, 1996), primarily consists of two components: (1) increasing self-awareness of one's cognitions and (2) evaluating the validity and utility of those cognitions and exploring alternative ways of thinking. The therapist can introduce the family to the concept of "automatic thoughts" (Beck et al., 1979) and emphasize that self-awareness of these thoughts is a skill that can be learned with practice. The therapist then guides family members in noticing their ongoing thoughts during family interactions (e.g., "What thoughts popped into your head as you were getting upset with her?"). The therapist also can educate family members about common errors or cognitive distortions (e.g., overgeneralizing, mind reading, dichotomous thinking, catastrophizing) and guide them in noticing when they have engaged in those information-processing errors.

The therapist then collaborates with the family to devise "homework" that they will conduct during the following week, such as logging their automatic thoughts and associated emotions and behaviors, either in writing or with one of the available phone cognitive therapy "apps." Homework logs are reviewed during the following session, helping family members increase self-awareness while providing feedback to each other about distressing cognitions and developing greater mutual empathy.

When implementing cognitive interventions with families, the therapist needs to consider the level of cognitive development of the children. Asking young children to elaborate their thoughts and evaluate them may be too abstract. Depending on the youth's cognitive development, it may be useful to ask, "What does your brain say to you when this happens?" When exploring alternative thoughts, the therapist can conduct a role play in which the therapist plays the role of one of the thoughts that the child expressed and the child is asked to tell the thought (the therapist) why it might not be true. Additionally, there are books and websites that provide age-appropriate cognitive-behavior therapy worksheets and metaphors for children (e.g., Huebner & Matthews, 2008).

Altering Selective Perceptions

Family members often recall the same event differently. The therapist can use this opportunity to demonstrate how people notice and remember different aspects of the same event and to emphasize that one should not assume that one has noticed everything about an event; other family members also noticed aspects of it. Review of homework logs can also sensitize the family regarding selective perceptions when members recorded different experiences of the same event.

As we have noted, parents who are globally upset with a child often have selective perceptions of the child's behavior, noticing instances of negative behavior and overlooking positive actions. The therapist can counteract that perceptual bias by pointing out the child's positive behavior during sessions and asking parents to keep daily logs of the child's behavior, especially of positive actions that the parents would like to increase.

Modifying Inaccurate Attributions

Modifying causal inferences about events is a widely used intervention in individual CBT (e.g., Beck, 2011; Beck et al., 1979; Leahy, 1996). In family therapy, other family members can provide data regarding factors that contribute to a member's behavior and examples of how multiple attributions can be made about an event. First, the therapist guides members in being aware that they make attributions about each other's (and their own) behavior. Then, the therapist guides them in performing a "logical analysis" of their attributions by questioning whether it makes sense that an individual's action was due to the particular cause that was inferred. Family members are encouraged to think of alternative explanations for the person's behavior. In order to minimize individuals' defensiveness in questioning their attributions, the therapist can emphasize that exploring alternative explanations does not necessarily mean that the prior one was wrong. Rather, thinking of alternative explanations can help one understand another person's behavior more thoroughly and reduce one's upset feelings toward him or her.

A powerful way of modifying negative attributions is to identify their occurrence immediately during a session. When a therapist notices a family member becoming upset with another member, the therapist can interrupt the interaction and ask the upset individual to explore his or her attributions. The therapist can use feedback from other members to help the individual test the accuracy of the inference. Initially, the upset member may be skeptical about alternative explanations, especially those provided by the member who "caused" them to be upset. However, as the therapist repeatedly encourages this process, members' ability to explore alternative explanations increases, resulting in less reactivity.

Modifying Inaccurate Expectancies

The process of modifying inaccurate expectancies or predictions that individuals make about others' future responses is similar to that used with attributions. While increasing an individual's awareness of his or her expectancies, the therapist also guides the family members to question whether the expectancies that they hold are logical outcomes. For example, after an adolescent fails to come home at a set curfew time and is punished for it, his parents may form an expectancy that he will be similarly unreliable if they allow him to go out with friends again. If the adolescent protests that he learned a lesson and will be home by the curfew time but the parents expect another violation, the therapist can coach them in examining how logical it is that they can predict the negative outcome with certainty. The family is then encouraged to explore other possible outcomes that could also happen, even if it feels like the possibility seems slim. Data from other family members and past events can be used to challenge the validity of rigid expectancies during sessions.

An effective way of modifying inaccurate expectancies is to have the family members conduct a real-life "behavioral experiment." Through these experiments, which are devised collaboratively with the therapist during a session, a family member's negative expectancy is tested during the week. For example, the parents allow the son to go out with friends, and the whole family has the opportunity to see whether the negative expectancy is confirmed or whether the son comes home on time.

Modifying Unrealistic or Inappropriate Assumptions and Standards

Family members are guided in becoming more aware of assumptions and standards that they hold, individually and collectively. They are encouraged to evaluate them through logical analysis (Does this assumption or standard make sense in the current situation?) and by examining the utility of living according to them. For example, a parent who believes that children should feel love consistently for their parents is guided in seeing that this belief inevitably leads to the parent feeling distressed, because children who are frustrated with parental rules sometimes express it by stating that they "hate" their parents.

Evaluating an assumption or standard can be conducted by creating lists of the advantages and disadvantages of holding a certain assumption or standard. The lists are reviewed, and a revised assumption or standard is created that maintains the individual's core value (e.g., that positive emotional bonds among family members are important) but is more flexible (e.g., allowing for the possibility of negative talk by upset children). The effects of the revised belief are then tested during the following week as an experiment.

It is imperative that a therapist is sensitive to discomfort in family members when they attempt to change long-standing beliefs. The therapist can explain beforehand that it is normal to feel discomfort and can encourage them to utilize sessions as a safe place to experiment with new assumptions and standards. Additionally, in a society such as the United States that is increasingly becoming culturally diverse, there may be intergenerational cultural tensions within some families. For example, tension may arise within a Vietnamese immigrant family from conflicting cultural standards regarding the role of a son according to Vietnamese standards versus American majority standards. The family members may hold a dichotomous view that they can only choose one cultural standard (either Vietnamese or American). However, a therapist can encourage the members to explore advantages and disadvantages of each cultural perspective and evaluate what could work for the family. The family can devise a revised standard that they can experiment with and fine-tune as needed. Thus they can experiment with a standard that values aspects of Vietnamese culture and American culture, and this process will gradually build toward a more bicultural approach to their family life in the United States.

Interventions to Modify Emotions

Increasing Awareness of Emotional States

When a family member is seemingly unaware of his or her emotions or claims to experience only a limited range of emotions, the therapist will work to increase emotional awareness. The therapist can guide the person in focusing on emotional states by cuing him or her to notice physical sensations and other cues, as well as the thoughts that accompany them (Epstein & Baucom, 2002; Epstein & Falconier, 2014). Coaching family members in expressive communication skills also contributes to enhanced awareness of emotional states.

Emotion Regulation Skills Training

When excessive experience and expression of emotions are adversely affecting the family, training in emotion regulation skills is needed. Emotion regulation can be increased by learning relaxation techniques, utilizing cool-down periods, or monitoring and challenging thoughts that cause the individual to become upset (Dattilio & Epstein, 2016). Also, the family can schedule times to discuss distressing issues, reducing members' dwelling on them at other times (Epstein & Baucom, 2002). For example, a therapist who was working with a single parent and her two children, ages 10 and 8, listened to them complaining about arguments that erupted among them on a daily basis when the mother noticed that the children had not completed chores that she had assigned to them. The therapist's questions about the typical sequence of events revealed that the mother quickly became angry when she noticed dirty dishes in the kitchen sink, for example, yelled at the children, and they became angry in return and yelled back at her. The family agreed with the therapist's feedback that their angry arguments only upset all of them and failed to resolve the conflict. The therapist proposed homework in which the family would have a meeting at the same time each week while seated in comfortable chairs and with no distractions such as television. The focus would be on discussing an ongoing contract regarding chores, including equitable distribution of chores between the two children, the mother's recording completed chores on a chart on the refrigerator, and her assigning points earned for each completed chore, which would accumulate to earn rewards such as computer time. The family agreed to discuss chores only during those meetings. Thus the mother would not bring up the topic if she noticed incomplete chores at other times; rather, she would relax her body and write herself a note to discuss the issue during the next family meeting. The children also agreed not to argue about each other's chore performance on individual days; rather, they could bring up concerns during family meetings.

CBFT therapists avoid singling out an individual family member for emotion regulation even if the assessment indicates that a particular member has more difficulty. The therapist may begin by describing an instance of an individual's emotion regulation difficulty but then tout the benefits of all family members moderating emotional responses so they can communicate clearly about their upsetting experiences and be heard well by the other members.

Applying Communication Skills to Expression of Emotions

Increasing awareness and learning to regulate emotions both lay the foundation for expressing emotions effectively to other family members. In CBFT, therapists guide family members in using good expressive and listening skills to express emotions in a nonblaming way and listen to each other's feelings empathetically.

Materials Used in Treatment

Because CBFT addresses child and adolescent problems by modifying the family system, it is important that the therapist have adequate office space to accommodate families of various sizes. It also is advantageous to have video recording equipment to capture family interactions. The therapist can stop a session and show the family the recording of an interaction that just occurred, so they can view their patterns, reexperience cognitions and emotions, and consider how the sequence among the members could have gone in a different direction if one or more members had responded differently. Between sessions, the therapist can review recordings to identify details about interactions that may be missed during the live session.

Given the importance of psychoeducation in CBFT, it is helpful to have a library of books and videos produced for a lay audience on relevant topics such as ADHD, child anxiety disorders, parenting skills, and so forth that the family can borrow. Handouts on communication and problem-solving skills, cognitive distortions, and other components of CBFT also are used during sessions and in homework. A supply of templates for constructing behavioral contracts is essential, as are forms for logging parents' observations of child behavior between sessions.

Factors Associated with Differential Outcomes

CBFT has been applied with diverse families, with evidence of wide applicability. Nevertheless, it is important to consider factors that may be associated with its effectiveness.

Severity of Individual and Relationship Problems

Kazdin (1997) reviewed literature on outcomes of parent management training and noted that severe child antisocial behavior and comorbid mental health problems predicted families' lower responsiveness to treatment. Marital discord, high stress in parents' lives, low socioeconomic status, single-parent status, a history of parental antisocial behavior, and harsh parenting also detracted from families' progress. A common thread among those parental factors is their interference with parents' abilities to devote time and attention to constructive parenting skills. Kazdin (1997) reported that supplemental sessions on improving parents' coping with stressors led to fewer dropouts, improved communication between parents, and improved child outcomes.

Culture

CBFT was developed primarily in Western cultures and was influenced by Western values, traditions, and forms of family functioning. Consequently, when implementing it with families from different cultures, it is crucial to assess and intervene in culturally sensitive ways. For example, in applying CBFT with families in China, Epstein et al. (2012) described how Chinese families commonly value its focus on problem solving and homework. However, their value of avoiding overt conflict and potential loss of face may result in their being uncomfortable with training in expressive communication skills and encouraging children to reveal their feelings to parents.

Case Example

Dave, a 45-year-old high school teacher, and Pamela, a 42-year-old administrative assistant, came to the first meeting with the family therapist because of their 17-year-old son Thomas's high-risk drug abuse and the impact it had on their family. Although the therapist used a portion of the session to gather assessment information, the immediate danger of Thomas's drug use required collaborating with the parents to devise a plan to ensure his safety. The therapist explored the parents' cognitions that had contributed to their hesitating to take more direct action; for example, their expectancy that putting pressure on Thomas would drive him away and precipitate a lethal overdose. As Dave and Pamela considered the substantial risks of avoiding confrontation, they decided to take steps toward implementing a treatment plan for Thomas and their whole family. It included a backup intensified safety plan of securing a bed for him in a detoxification center, evaluation for appropriate medications, and self-help group meetings, as well as individual therapy to address his propensity toward drug use after periods of abstinence.

During the assessment, the therapist gathered information about the marriage and family. Dave and Pamela had been married for 19 years. Thomas had been a robust infant and toddler. Angelina's birth was 2 years later, and she also was a healthy baby and toddler. The couple reported that adjusting to parenthood (especially Thomas's increasingly challenging conduct problems) and other stressors such as job workloads strained their marriage, with both partners increasingly feeling distant. Approximately a year before they sought therapy, Dave was worried enough about Pamela's emotional distancing that he asked her whether she was having an affair. Although she strongly denied an affair, she told him that she yearned for the closeness they used to have, with him or someone else. Each attributed the other's withdrawal to decreasing commitment. However, their concern about disengagement was insufficient to overcome their avoidance, and it took Thomas's second overdose to motivate them to seek help.

The therapist discussed factors that influenced the couple's feeling helpless regarding Thomas's substance use. Those included negative parent–child communication and the couple's own relationship issues that detracted from their ability to work as a team. The family therapy would include some couple sessions addressing their relationship and family sessions with both children to address family patterns, in addition to Thomas's individual substance abuse treatment. Dave and Pamela agreed to that approach.

During the subsequent family session, it was clear that Thomas was a bright student whose academic performance had deteriorated precipitously during ninth grade. Psychological and academic evaluations had revealed no learning difficulties but a marked decay in self-esteem in the transition from middle school to high school. During that transition, his circle of friends changed from academic strivers to adolescents with little interest in scholastic achievement and a propensity toward truancy and substance use. His parents' concern intensified when they became aware of his use of opiates. His overdoses became a constant source of dread and surveillance by Dave and Pamela.

Angelina was a gregarious and academically talented freshman in the same high school. Dave and Pamela agreed, with a guilty feeling, to Thomas's description of his sister as "the easier child." Angelina talked about the pride she felt in her accomplishments but also the strain the family endured as a result of her brother's drug use and her belief that "I need to lighten the load on the family by being good." Thomas stated that it was obvious his parents were disappointed in him and wished he was like his sister. When Pamela replied, "That's not so, Thomas; we think you are very smart, but you aren't using your ability," Thomas retorted, "That's bull!" When the therapist asked Thomas to elaborate, he said it was unlikely he could ever meet his parents' standards.

The therapist addressed the parents, suggesting that they cared a lot about Thomas and worried intensely about his well-being. The therapist also noted that they wanted to help Thomas but felt powerless. Because the family had scant knowledge about resources in the community that could address Thomas's substance use, the therapist provided information about local resources that Thomas could use individually to reduce his reliance on alcohol and drugs to cope with emotional distress. The therapist noted that conflicts among family members seemed to increase the stress in the home, which was not good for Thomas or anyone else in the family. If the family was willing to attend family therapy at the same time that Thomas focused on reducing his substance use, the improved atmosphere in the family could make it easier for him to make progress.

Because solely focusing on family dynamics risks the health and safety of the addicted individual through continued addictive behavior, the therapist referred Thomas to an individual therapist with experience treating addictions who could coordinate medical and self-help resources for him. However, the therapist emphasized that Thomas's substance use was not the sole source of stress in the family. Family therapy would focus on improving communication and problem solving among all family members.

One of the first goals of family therapy was to improve the communication process among all members. The therapist taught them about expressive and listening skills and had them practice in sessions, beginning with relatively benign topics before moving on to more conflictual issues. The therapist also focused on negative expectancies that members held about each other's behavior; for example, Pamela's expectancy that "Nothing I say to Dave will make a difference in the way he relates to me." This expectancy was addressed by asking both partners for examples they could think of in which Dave was influenced by a request from Pamela. In addition, the therapist coached the couple in setting up an "experiment" in which Pamela would make a request of Dave and he would agree to do so and then follow through. She requested that he take an hour away from his work one evening and take a walk around their neighborhood with her, talking but not about family problems. Dave agreed to do so, and at their next session both spouses reported that they took the walk and had a pleasant time.

The therapist also guided family members in examining assumptions that guided their thoughts about family life. For example, Thomas assumed that parents cannot understand their children's needs. This assumption was tested during a session by having Thomas use expressive skills to describe sources of stress in his life and experiences that led him to want to escape emotional distress through substance use. The therapist coached Pamela and Dave in using listening skills (and avoiding criticism of Thomas) to demonstrate that they could empathize with him, which they did fairly well. The therapist and family discussed how they had not been able to demonstrate the potential they had for understanding and supporting each other because their anxiety and frustration led the parents to pursue and lecture or to feel paralyzed and led Thomas to act out or withdraw.

Because unregulated emotions and poor communication resulted in misunderstandings and unresolved conflict, the therapist used portions of several sessions to teach the family emotion regulation skills (muscle relaxation, self-soothing strategies, calming self-talk), as well as skills for communication and problem solving. The therapist assigned homework for the family to practice the skills at home. With practice and feedback from the therapist, their skills improved, and they experienced increased confidence in their ability to change what previously seemed to be intractable patterns.

Because the assessment revealed that the family rarely demonstrated affection toward one another and made negative attributions about each other's intentions (a lack of caring), the therapist asked each member to explain to the others why she or he expressed so little affection. Some of the responses (e.g., "I'm afraid to show I care and then be rejected") helped modify attributions about negative intent. The therapist encouraged family members to "take risks by expressing some affection that may give you some encouraging results." This involved behavioral experiments at home. For example, Dave agreed to test his expectancy that Thomas would retreat if he expressed caring for him. The experiment involved Dave approaching Thomas, telling him that he means a lot to him, and giving him a hug. Dave stated, "I can't picture Thomas responding well to that!" but Thomas replied, "Well, I'll be surprised if you can get those words out!" At the next session the therapist inquired about the homework, and both Dave and Thomas reported that Dave did express caring verbally and through a hug and that Thomas was receptive. The therapist emphasized the importance of testing negative cognitions and replacing the pattern of distancing that developed among the family members over the years.

Given that distance in the couple relationship interfered with family cohesion, the therapist scheduled a few separate sessions with Pamela and Dave and coached them in using communication skills to discuss their visions for the future for themselves and their family. They developed a plan for balancing emotional intimacy in the marriage with maintenance of each partner's individuality, as well as steps to accept past hurts and to convey empathy for each other. The therapist helped them use problem-solving skills to resolve differences in their preferences. The therapist also maintained contact with Thomas's addictions therapist to ensure that the family therapy goals were consistent with those of his individual treatment.

References

Achenbach, T. M. (1991). *Manual for the Child Behavior Checklist/4–18 and 1991 profile*. Burlington: University of Vermont, Department of Psychiatry.

Arias, I., & Beach, S. R. H. (1987). Assessment of social cognition in the context of marriage. In K. D. O'Leary (Ed.), *Assessment of marital discord: An integration for research and clinical practice* (pp. 109–137). Hillsdale, NJ: Erlbaum.

Arnold, D. S., O'Leary, S. G., Wolff, L. S., & Acker, M. M. (1993). The Parenting Scale: A measure of dysfunctional parenting in discipline situations. *Psychological Assessment, 5*, 137–144.

Bandura, A. (1977). *Social learning theory*. Englewood Cliffs, NJ: Prentice-Hall.

Barkley, R. A., Robin, A. L., & Benton, C. M. (2014). *Your defiant teen: 10 steps to resolve conflict and rebuild your relationship*. New York: Guilford Press.

Baucom, D. H., & Epstein, N. (1990). *Cognitive-behavioral marital therapy*. New York: Brunner/Mazel.

Baucom, D. H., Epstein, N., Rankin, L. A., & Burnett, C. K. (1996). Assessing relationship standards: The Inventory of Specific Relationship Standards. *Journal of Family Psychology, 10*, 72–88.

Beck, A. T. (1976). *Cognitive therapy and the emotional disorders*. New York: International Universities Press.

Beck, A. T., Rush, A. J., Shaw, B. F., & Emery. G. (1979) *Cognitive therapy of depression*. New York: Guilford Press.

Beck, J. S. (2011). *Cognitive behavior therapy: Basics and beyond* (2nd ed.). New York: Guilford Press.

Blechman, E. A. (1985). *Solving child behavior problems at home and at school*. Champaign, IL: Research Press.

Bradbury, T. N., & Fincham, F. D. (1992). Attributions and behavior in marital interaction. *Journal of Personality and Social Psychology, 63*, 613–628.

Carpenter, A. L., Puliafico, A. C., Kurtz, S. S., Pincus, D. B., & Comer, J. S. (2014). Extending parent–child interaction therapy for early childhood internalizing problems: New advances for an overlooked population. *Clinical Child and Family Psychology Review, 17,* 340–356.

Christensen, A., Eldridge, K., Catta-Preta, A. B., Lim, V. R., & Santagata, R. (2006). Cross-cultural consistency of the demand/withdraw interaction pattern in couples. *Journal of Marriage and Family, 68,* 1029–1044.

Chronis, A. M., Chacko, A., Fabiano, G. A., Wymbs, B. T., & Pelham, W. E., Jr. (2004). Enhancements to the behavioral parent training paradigm for families of children with ADHD: Review and future directions. *Clinical Child and Family Psychology Review, 7,* 1–27.

Cohen, M. L., Heaton, S. C., Ginn, N., & Eyberg, S. M. (2012). Parent–child interaction therapy as a family-oriented approach to behavioral management following psychiatric traumatic brain injury: A case report. *Journal of Pediatric Psychology, 37,* 251–261.

Dattilio, F. M. (1998). Cognitive-behavioral family therapy. In F. M. Dattilio (Ed.), *Case studies in couple and family therapy: Systemic and cognitive perspectives* (pp. 62–84). New York: Guilford Press.

Dattilio, F. M. (2010). *Cognitive-behavioral therapy with couples and families: A comprehensive guide for clinicians.* New York: Guilford Press.

Dattilio, F. M., & Epstein, N. B. (2016). Cognitive-behavioral couple and family therapy. In T. L. Sexton & J. Lebow (Eds.), *Handbook of family therapy: The science and practice of working with families and couples* (4th ed., pp. 89–119). New York: Routledge.

Ellis, A. (1962). *Reason and emotion in psychotherapy.* New York: Lyle Stuart.

Epstein, N., & Baucom, D. H. (1993). Cognitive factors in marital disturbance. In K. S. Dobson & P. C. Kendall (Eds.), *Psychopathology and cognition* (pp. 351–385). San Diego, CA: Academic Press.

Epstein, N. B., & Baucom, D. H. (2002). *Enhanced cognitive-behavioral therapy for couples: A contextual approach.* Washington, DC: American Psychological Association.

Epstein, N. B., Berger, A. T., Fang, J. J., Messina, L., Smith, J. R., Lloyd, T. D., et al. (2012). Applying Western-developed family therapy models in China. *Journal of Family Psychotherapy, 23,* 217–237.

Epstein, N. B., & Falconier, M. K. (2011). Shame in couple therapy. In R. Dearing & J. P. Tangney (Eds.), *Shame in the therapy hour* (pp. 167–192). Washington, DC: American Psychological Association.

Epstein, N. B., & Falconier, M. K. (2014). Cognitive-behavioral therapies for couples and families. In J. L. Wetchler & L. L. Hecker (Eds.), *An introduction to marriage and family therapy* (2nd ed., pp. 259–318). New York: Brunner-Routledge.

Epstein, N., & Schlesinger, S. E. (1991). Marital and family problems. In W. Dryden & R. Rentoul (Eds.), *Adult clinical problems: A cognitive-behavioural approach* (pp. 288–317). London: Routledge.

Epstein, N. B., & Schlesinger, S. E. (2003). Treatment of family problems. In M. A. Reinecke, F. M. Dattilio, & A. Freeman (Eds.), *Cognitive therapy with children and adolescents: A casebook for clinical practice* (2nd ed., pp. 304–337). New York: Guilford Press.

Epstein, N., Schlesinger, S. E., & Dryden, W. (Eds.). (1988). *Cognitive-behavioral therapy with families.* New York: Brunner/Mazel.

Epstein, N. B., Werlinich, C. A., & LaTaillade, J. J. (2015). Couple therapy for partner aggression. In A. S. Gurman, J. L. Lebow, & D. K. Snyder (Eds.), *Clinical handbook of couple therapy* (5th ed., pp. 389–411). New York: Guilford Press.

Eyberg, S. (1988). Parent–child interaction therapy: Integration of traditional and behavioral concerns. *Child and Family Behavior Therapy, 10,* 33–46.

Eyberg, S., & Funderburk, B. (2011). *Parent–Child Interaction Therapy Protocol 2011.* Gainesville: University of Florida.

Eyberg, S. M., Nelson, M. M., Ginn, N. C., Bhuiyan, N., & Boggs, S. R. (2013). *Dyadic Parent–Child Interaction Coding System (DPICS) comprehensive manual for research and training.* Gainesville, FL: PCIT International.

Forgatch, M. S., & Kjøbli, J. (2016). Parent management training—Oregon model: Adapting intervention with rigorous research. *Family Process, 55,* 500–513.

Forgatch, M. S., & Patterson, G. R. (2010). Parent management training—Oregon model: An intervention for antisocial behavior in children and adolescents. In J. R. Weisz & A. E. Kazdin (Eds.), *Evidence-based psychotherapies for children and adolescents* (2nd ed., pp. 159–178). New York: Guilford Press.

Foster, C. E., Webster, M. C., Weissman, M. M., Pilowsky, D. J., Wickramaratne, P. J., Rush, A. J., et al. (2008). Course and severity of maternal depression: Associations with family functioning and child adjustment. *Journal of Youth and Adolescence, 37,* 906–916.

Gibaud-Wallston, J., & Wandersman, L. P. (1978, August). *Development and utility of the Parenting Sense of Competence Scale.* Paper presented at the meeting of the American Psychological Association, Toronto, Ontario, Canada.

Hawes, D. J., Dadds, M. R., & Pasalich, D. S. (2013). Observational coding strategies. In J. S. Comer & P. C. Kendall (Eds.), *Oxford handbook of research strategies for clinical psychology* (pp. 120–141). New York: Oxford University Press.

Huebner, D., & Matthews, B. (2008). *What to do when your temper flares: A kid's guide to overcoming problems with anger.* Washington, DC: Magination Press.

Hurley, K. D., Huscroft-D'Angelo, J., Trout, A., Griffith, A., & Epstein, M. (2014). Assessing parenting skills and attitudes: A review of the psychometrics of parenting measures. *Journal of Child and Family Studies, 23,* 812–823.

Jacobson, N. S., & Christensen, A. (1996). *Integrative couple therapy: Promoting acceptance and change.* New York: Norton.

Johnston, C., & Mash, E. J. (1989). A measure of parenting satisfaction and efficacy. *Journal of Clinical Child Psychology, 18,* 167–175.

Kaczynski, K. J., Lindahl, K. M., Malik, N. M., & Laurenceau, J. P. (2006). Marital conflict, maternal and paternal parenting, and child adjustment: A test of mediation and moderation. *Journal of Family Psychology, 20,* 199–208.

Kazdin, A. E. (1997). Parent management training: Evidence, outcomes, and issues. *Journal of the American Academy of Child and Adolescent Psychiatry, 36,* 1349–1356.

Kazdin, A. E. (2005). *Parent management training: Treatment for oppositional, aggressive, and antisocial behavior in children and adolescents.* New York: Oxford University Press.

Kazdin, A. E. (2008). *The Kazdin method for parenting the defiant child*. Boston: Houghton Mifflin Harcourt.

Kendall, P. C., Crawford, E., Kagan, E., Furr, J., & Podell, J. (2017). Child-focused treatment for anxiety. In J. R. Weisz & A. Kazdin (Eds.), *Evidence-based psychotherapies for children and adolescents* (3rd ed., pp. 17–34). New York: Guilford Press.

Kendall, P. C., Marrs-Garcia, A., Nath, S., & Sheldrick, R. C. (1999). Normative comparisons for the evaluation of clinical significance. *Journal of Consulting and Clinical Psychology, 67*, 285–299.

Kerig, P., & Lindahl, K. M. (2001). *Family observational coding systems: Resources for systemic research*. Mahwah, NJ: Erlbaum.

Leahy, R. (1996). *Cognitive therapy: Basic principles and applications*. Northvale, NJ: Aronson.

Low, S. M., & Stocker, C. (2005). Family functioning and children's adjustment: Associations among parents' depressed mood, marital hostility, parent–child hostility, and children's adjustment. *Journal of Family Psychology, 19*, 394–403.

Masse, J. J., McNeil, C. B., Wagner, S., & Quetsch, L. B. (2016). Examining the efficacy of parent–child interaction therapy with children on the autism spectrum. *Journal of Child and Family Studies, 25*, 2508–2525.

McFarlane, W. R. (2016). Family interventions for schizophrenia and the psychoses: A review. *Family Process, 55*, 460–482.

Miklowitz, D. J., & Chung, B. (2016). Family-focused therapy for bipolar disorder: Reflections on 30 years of research. *Family Process, 55*, 483–499.

Morris, C. D., Miklowitz, D. J., & Waxmonsky, J. A. (2007). Family-focused treatment for bipolar disorder in adults and youth. *Journal of Clinical Psychology: In Session, 63*, 433–445.

Mueser, K. T., & Glynn, S. M. (1999). *Behavioral family therapy for psychiatric disorders*. Oakland, CA: New Harbinger.

Nicholson, B., Anderson, M., Fox, R., & Brenner, V. (2002). One family at a time: A prevention program for at-risk parents. *Journal of Counseling and Development, 80*, 362–371.

Patterson, G. R. (1971). *Families*. Champaign, IL: Research Press.

Patterson, G. R. (1982). *Coercive family process*. Eugene, OR: Castalia.

Patterson, G. R., & Forgatch, M. S. (2005). *Parents and adolescents living together: Part 1. The basics* (2nd ed.). Champaign, IL: Research Press.

Pretzer, J., Epstein, N., & Fleming, B. (1991). Marital Attitude Survey: A measure of dysfunctional attributions and expectancies. *Journal of Cognitive Psychotherapy: An International Quarterly, 5*, 131–148.

Puliafico, A. C., Comer, J. S., & Pincus, D. B. (2012). Adapting parent–child interaction therapy to treat anxiety disorders in young children. *Child and Adolescent Psychiatric Clinics of North America, 21*, 607–619.

Robin, A. L., & Foster, S. L. (1989). *Negotiating parent–adolescent conflict: A behavioral family systems approach*. New York: Guilford Press.

Roehling, P. V., & Robin, A. L. (1986). Development and validation of the Family Beliefs Inventory: A measure of unrealistic beliefs among parents and adolescents. *Journal of Consulting and Clinical Psychology, 54*, 693–697.

Rotter, J. B. (1954). *Social learning and clinical psychology.* Englewood Cliffs, NJ: Prentice-Hall.

Sanders, M. R., Cann, W., & Markie-Dadds, C. (2003). The Triple P–Positive Parenting Programme: A universal population-level approach to the prevention of child abuse. *Child Abuse Review, 12,* 155–171.

Schulz, M. S. (Ed.). (2010). *Strengthening couple relationships for optimal child development: Lessons from research and intervention.* Washington, DC: American Psychological Association.

Schwebel, A. I., & Fine, M. A. (1994). *Understanding and helping families: A cognitive-behavioral approach.* Hillsdale, NJ: Erlbaum.

Shelton, K. K., Frick, P. J., & Wootton, J. (1996). Assessment of parenting practices in families of elementary school-age children. *Journal of Clinical Child Psychology, 25,* 317–329.

Skinner, B. F. (1953). *Science and human behavior.* New York: Macmillan.

Thibaut, J. W., & Kelley, H. H. (1959). *The social psychology of groups.* New York: Wiley.

Ward, M. A., Theule, J., & Cheung, K. (2016). Parent–child interaction therapy for child disruptive behaviour disorders: A meta-analysis. *Child and Youth Care Forum, 45*(5), 675–690.

Webster-Stratton, C., & Herbert, M. (1994). *Troubled families—Problem children: Working with parents: A collaborative process.* Chichester, UK: Wiley.

Index

The letter *f* following a page number indicates figure; the letter *t* indicates table.